Inhalation Toxicology

ILSI MONOGRAPHS

Sponsored by the International Life Sciences Institute

U. Mohr
Editor-in-Chief

Inhalation Toxicology

The Design and Interpretation of Inhalation Studies and Their Use in Risk Assessment

D. Dungworth G. Kimmerle J. Lewkowski
R. McClellan W. Stöber
Editors

Springer-Verlag
New York Berlin Heidelberg
London Paris Tokyo

Ulrich Mohr, Dr. med.
Professor of Experimental Pathology, Medizinische Hochschule Hannover, Institut für Experimentelle Pathologie, Konstanty-Gutschow-Straße 8, 3000 Hannover 61, FRG

Donald L. Dungworth, Ph.D., M.R.C.V.S
Department of Veterinary Pathology, University of California, Davis, CA 95616, USA

Georg Kimmerle, Dr. med.
Bayer AG, Institute for Toxicology, 5600 Wuppertal-Elberfeld, FRG

James Lewkowski, M.D.
Abbott Laboratories, Abbott Park, IL 60064, USA

Roger O. McClellan, D.V.M.
Inhalation Toxicology Research Institute, Lovelace Biomedical and Environmental Research Institute, P.O. Box 5890, Albuquerque, NM 87185, USA

Werner Stöber, Dr. rer.nat.
Fraunhofer Institute of Toxicology and Aerosol Research, Nikolai-Fuchs-Strasse 1, 3000 Hannover 61, FRG

Library of Congress Cataloging-in-Publication Data
Inhalation toxicology : the design and interpretation of inhalation studies and their use in risk assessment / D. Dungworth . . . [et al.] ; U. Mohr, editor-in-chief.
p. cm. – (ILSI monograph series)
Bibliography: p.
ISBN 0-387-17822-8 (U.S.)
1. Gases, Asphyxiating and poisonous–Toxicology. 2. Gases, Asphyxiating and poisonous–Physiological effect. 3. Toxicology–Animal models. 4. Toxicity testing. I. Dungworth, D. L. (Donald Lawrence) II. Mohr, U. (Ulrich) III. Series.
RA1245.I55 1988
615.9'1–dc 19

Typeset by Publishers Service, Bozeman, Montana.
Printed and bound by Arcata Graphics/Halliday, West Hanover, Massachusetts.
Printed in the United States of America.

9 8 7 6 5 4 3 2 1

ISBN 0-387-17822-8 Springer-Verlag New York Berlin Heidelberg
ISBN 3-540-17822-8 Springer-Verlag Berlin Heidelberg New York

Series Foreword

The International Life Sciences Institute (ILSI), a nonprofit, public foundation, was established in 1978 to advance the sciences of nutrition, toxicology, and food safety. ILSI promotes the resolution of health and safety issues in these areas by sponsoring research, conferences, publications, and educational programs. Through ILSI's programs, scientists from government, academia, and industry unite their efforts to resolve issues of critical importance to the public.

As part of its commitment to understanding and resolving health and safety issues, ILSI is pleased to sponsor this series of monographs that consolidates new scientific knowledge, defines research needs, and provides a background for the effective application of scientific advances in toxicology and food safety.

Alex Malaspina
President
International Life Sciences Institute

Contents

Part V. Risk Assessment of Airborne Toxicants

Contributors

The complete affiliations for all authors are given as footnotes to the opening pages of their chapters. These page numbers are given in the list below.

D.V. Bates, M.D., University of British Columbia 1

M.R. Becklake, M.D., McGill University 263

J.D. Brain, S.D. in Hyg., Harvard University 11

D. Cranz, B.S., School of Veterinary Medicine, University of California 25

R.G. Cuddihy, Ph.D., Lovelace Biomedical and Environmental Research Institute 167

A.R. Dahl, Ph.D., Lovelace Biomedical and Environmental Research Institute 41

D.L. Dungworth, Ph.D., M.T.C.V.S., School of Veterinary Medicine, University of California 209

J. St. George, Ph.D., School of Veterinary Medicine, University of California 25

T.R. Gerrity, Ph.D., US Environmental Protection Agency 139

R.C. Graham, M.A., Northrop Services Inc. 139

R.A. Griesemer, D.V.M., Ph.D., Oak Ridge National Laboratory 119

J. Heidsiek, M.S., School of Veterinary Medicine, University of California 25

D. Henschler, Dr. med., University of Würzburg 287

J. Heyder, Dr. phil. nat., Gesellschaft für Strahlen-und Umweltforschung m.b.H. 157

W. Holländer, Dr. rer. nat., Fraunhofer-Institut für Toxikologie und Aerosolforschung 67

D. Hyde, Ph.D., School of Veterinary Medicine, University of California 25

M.P.C. Ip, Ph.D., Case Western Reserve University 233

J. Kleinerman, M.D., Case Western Reserve University 233

T.R. Lewis, Ph.D., National Institute for Occupational Safety and Health 297

A. Mariassy, Ph.D., School of Veterinary Medicine, University of California 253

J.L. Mauderly, D.V.M., Lovelace Biomedical and Environmental Research Institute 243

R. Mermelstein, Ph.D., Xerox Corporation 103

F.J. Miller, Ph.D., US Environmental Protection Agency 139

U. Mohr, Dr. med., Medizinische Hochschule Hannover 209

P.E. Morrow, Ph.D., University of Rochester School of Medicine 103

S. Nishio, B.S. School of Veterinary Medicine, University of California 25

J.H. Overton, Ph.D., US Environmental Protection Agency 139

Dr. J. Pauluhn, Dr. rer. nat., Bayer AG-Institute für Toxikologie 87

C.G. Plopper, Ph.D., California Primate Research Center 25

N. Tyler, Ph.D., California Primate Research Center 25

M.J. Utell, M.D., University of Rochester Medical Center 273

A. Weir, M.A., School of Veterinary Medicine, University of California 25

D. Wilson, D.V.M., Ph.D., School of Veterinary Medicine, University of California 25

H.P. Witschi, M.D., University of California 195

H.C. Yeh, Ph.D., Lovelace Biomedical and Environmental Research Institute 169

Part I
Approaches to Assessing the Toxicity of Airborne Toxicants

CHAPTER 1

Standard-Setting as an Integrative Exercise: Alchemy, Juggling, or Science?

D.V. Bates[1]

Introduction

The setting of "standards" to protect the public health has a long history. General interest in the process, however, is recent, and has closely followed the economic implications of whatever standard has been set. At the present time it is reasonable to assume, first, that standards are required to protect the public health—particularly in instances where outright prohibition is impossible; second, that scientists will be involved in parts of that process; and, third, that attitudes to standard-setting will change as experience of the process is accumulated.

Not much attention has yet been given to the process of arriving at some single figure for such a standard. My purpose is to explore the questions of how different kinds of scientific data may be used in the process, and how relevant such data may be; of whether the exercise is scientific, or is better described as alchemy or juggling; and, finally, to draw some conclusions as to what the components are of any credible process of standard determination. In this discussion I shall mention, but not discuss, the economic and social factors that it is proper to consider before any standard is promulgated (1).

Observations on Different Kinds of Scientific Data

It is generally recognized that three types of data are required in standard-setting: all three are always reviewed when criteria documents are being prepared. Each of these requires individual discussion.

Animal Toxicology Data

This type of data has historically been the most important. Although the work is difficult and laborious, the proper use of controls and the care with which out-

[1]University of British Columbia, Vancouver BC, V6T 1W5, Canada.

comes must be measured are well understood. Such experiments are highly reproducible as a rule within a given species; the conclusions that may be drawn are usually statistically impeccable, and there is no ambiguity as to what has been shown. Problems arise when such data are discussed in relation to human data. Whittemore (2) has suggested ways in which such extrapolation might be formalized, but problems invariably remain—not least because there are always major differences between anatomical and physiological features between species and therefore, presumably, between animals and man. Thus, such questions as whether demonstrated interference in mucociliary clearance in the lungs of rabbits or donkeys can be assumed to apply to man, and if so at what dose levels, remain, and will remain, intractable. The fact that the (scientifically) most secure data are evidently the most difficult to relate to human exposure is at the core of the problem I am discussing. An exception may be the demonstration of carcinogenicity. It is properly considered as a rule that we must assume that materials shown to be carcinogenic in animals are carcinogenic to humans, though once again there are difficult problems in arriving at equivalent dose levels (3).

Acute Human Exposure

Episodes of accidental acute human exposure have in general indicated toxicity of high-level exposures, but as the dose level is rarely known with precision, such information is of little value in standard-setting. Over the last 20 years, clinical studies of acute human exposure to air pollutants have become an important component of the standard-setting process. The subjects exposed are usually carefully characterized, the dose level and level of physical activity are precisely known, and outcome variables such as increasing airflow limitation are well standardized. Useful information on the acute effects of gases such as ozone and SO_2 have been published, and it has been shown, for example, that asthmatic subjects (a not inconsiderable percentage of the "normal" population) react adversely to lower concentrations of SO_2 than do others. Hazucha (4) has shown that, in the case of ozone, data secured in different laboratories show very satisfactory consistency. He has also made the important observation that such studies show that although, for an individual subject, a "threshold" of no effect is a meaningful concept, there can be no equivalent threshold for a group or population. What takes its place in such instances is a statement of the kind: "On 2 h of exposure to x% of ozone with intermittent exercise, a statistically significant decrement in FEV_1 will occur in y% of a sample of normal individuals." The only way of defining a threshold for a group is by requiring that no decrement be observed in any individual, however large the sample.

There are two major difficulties with all these studies. The first is that they cannot reveal any possible long-term effects, and the second is that the importance of transient and reversible effects (on airflow, for example) remains to be defined. These problems are discussed later.

Epidemiological Data

Human population studies are necessarily central to any process of standard-setting. In relation to occupational exposures, the effect of a substance may be sufficiently "strong" for a dose-response relationship to be deducible even if the data on historical exposures are necessarily very approximate. This seems to be the case with the carcinogenicity of asbestos in conjunction with cigarettes. Enterline (5) has pointed out that a standard for exposure to asbestos may be set at such a low level that no future epidemiological studies could show whether there was or was not an adverse effect, as the population required to give such a study sufficient "power" would have to be impractically large. Epidemiological data on the effects of air pollutants usually suffer from inadequate exposure data and do not usually permit any kind of dose-response relationship to be deduced (6). What they do achieve, however, is an indication of whether or not existing levels of exposure are or are not associated with any consistent adverse effects, such as increased hospital admissions, or increased asthma attacks, over time. Such studies are therefore useful primarily in indicating whether or not existing levels of pollutants are likely to be having any adverse effects on the population.

Such data are invariably open to criticism, since the confounders in any such studies are multiple (6–9). The strength of the data depends on similar results from different populations and on the demonstration that the phenomenon was not a "one-shot" observation, but occurs over a long period of time. It is often objected that the scientific validity of any such associative studies is not comparable to the experimental data that can be secured from animal exposure data, and that therefore it should be accorded a lesser status in standard-setting.

From these brief comments, the problem confronting the evaluator of scientific data for the purposes of standard-setting becomes apparent. It may be summarized as follows:

1. Animal data are most secure scientifically, but their relevance to human data is difficult to establish.
2. Acute human laboratory exposure data are reproducible and well controlled, but the importance of transient reversible effects is questionable.
3. Human epidemiological data indicate the probability of the validity of a null hypothesis, but do not permit any precise dose-response relationship to be deduced, and the difficulty of their interpretation is compounded by the inevitable presence of many confounders.

Recognition that Data Are of Different Kinds

The problems I have described briefly in the previous paragraph are well known. Various aspects of them have been discussed is a variety of papers (10–12). What seems to be less well recognized, however, is that we are accustomed, in our daily lives, to using information of very different kinds. If I state, "I am wearing a brown pair of shoes," you know at once that you can look to see if this is true; it is a statement susceptible of immediate confirmation or refutation. If I say, "I enjoy listening to the violin," you are immediately aware that you will have to apply different criteria to determine if what I have said is likely to be true. You might conclude it was probably true if I showed you that I bought violin recordings or had concert tickets for a violin concerto in my pocket. What you are doing is using indirect methods to assess the probability that the statement is true. You would be hard put to give a numerical rating to the components of your judgment; such a rating would inevitably be strongly influenced by aspects of your experience and your knowledge of life in general.

From this simplistic example, I would draw two conclusions relevant to standard-setting:

1. In our daily decision-making, we more often use information of the second kind (that is, only indirectly susceptible of confirmation) than we use rigorous statistical data.
2. We take it for granted that we can make a decision based on inputs of varying "weights," since we do so all the time. We decide that it has become unsafe for us to use a chain saw up a tree, without knowing the statistics on accidents to people over the age of 50 who use chain saws up trees: we recognize that decisions have to be made without all the relevant data, and that the ability to do so correctly represents an advanced form of intelligence.

What is important is that we distinguish between these kinds of information in our thinking. It is not appropriate to characterize one type as scientific and the other as not, unless we are prepared to limit the perception of science to something much more confined than that recommended by Karl Popper, for example (13,14). If science deals with observations based on probability, then epidemiological data have as much claim to being scientific as experimental data, though, as I have suggested, they are different from them. However, I do not suppose that you can use any scientific criteria to form a judgment as to whether I am telling the truth when I say, "I have a headache."

Definition of the Problem of Setting a Standard

It is clear that a detailed review of the scientific data base is the first requirement in setting a standard (15,16). The United States Environmental Protection Agency (EPA), in its criteria documents, has set new standards for such work—probably because in the United States system (but not in the parliamentary tradition) standards may be appealed in courts, and it is necessary to prove to a court that all the relevant data have been reviewed. It is tempting to make prior judgments as to which studies are considered "key" to standard-setting, as Lippmann has suggested, in the interests of time-saving (16). However, such judgments are inherently suspect, as they may represent the inadvertent or concealed influence of values in that part of the process that is intended to be rigorously scientific;

they may also overemphasize the importance of animal toxicology (on the basis that this is "hard" data) compared to epidemiological studies (in which confounders are bound to be present). The importance of separating out value judgments in such matters, so that they can be seen for what they are, has been stressed by recent authors (17,18); indeed, the sensitization of all of us to the demarcation between factual criteria and value judgments (which often masquerade as science-based decisions) has been one of the positive results of discussion of these questions (18).

The review of the scientific data base should involve discussion round the table by those conversant with the data under review. It is a strength of the United States data that such discussions take place in the public domain.

The next part of the procedure of standard promulgation in the EPA involves the preparation of a staff paper. To quote from a recent example:

> This staff paper is intended to help bridge the gap between the scientific review of recent health effects information contained in the criteria document addendum and the judgments required of the Administrator in setting primary National Ambient Air Quality Standards for sulfur oxides (19).

Such a paper serves several purposes. It may calculate how many people would be exposed to a particular concentration of a pollutant; it may calculate the probability of an asthmatic citizen being exposed for a few minutes to a high SO_2 concentration from a single emission source under adverse meteorological conditions; it may comment on the possible significance of transient changes. In addition, it may approach the problem we are considering, namely, how to integrate disparate information. Another recent staff paper noted:

> When evaluating margins of safety for an annual standard, it is particularly important to examine the results of qualitative data from a number of epidemiological, animal, and air quality studies. These suggest concern for effects not directly evaluated in the studies used to develop the ranges. Such effects include damage to lung tissues contributing to chronic respiratory disease, cancer and premature mortality (20).

What is being considered here, among other things, is the possibility of long-term adverse effects existing but not yet being precisely measured. This quotation indicates the type of discussion that must precede a decision about a standard, but does not define it in detail. It is clear that different individuals will give different weight to such unquantifiable data. For example, in the case of ozone exposure, a cautious individual might give some weight to the following factors:

1. The acute adverse effect of ozone in humans lasts for several hours after exposure has ceased.
2. Ozone is a powerful oxidant, and oxidizing radicals are believed to be important in human lung disease.
3. Ozone is transported over long distances, and very large numbers of people are now exposed to it.
4. The components of what is assumed to be "normal aging," but which may be due to environmental factors, are poorly defined.

However, another individual might discount the first of these; dismiss the second as idle speculation; note, in relation to the third, that naturally occurring ozone exists anyway; and in relation to the fourth ask whether there are any data for humans indicating premature aging in oxidant atmospheres. After all, several men older than 50 do use chain saws up trees.

Such discussion must precede a decision about a standard. What must be considered is the congruence or lack of it between data from different fields, whether animal data and epidemiological studies indicate effects within the same general concentration range, and many other issues.

At this point, one might imagine that the whole exercise of standard-setting could be entirely subsumed by a formal risk analysis (21). As we all know, this process is now better understood than it used to be and can attain previously unimagined complexity. However, there is a danger that what are in fact value judgments get concealed in the process, rather than brought out for what they are (17). Nor is it easy to integrate the very different kinds of information that go into a standard-setting process. Thus, although recent papers have considered the role of risk analysis in environmental issues, they have not addressed its use in standard-setting (9,10,22).

In specific instances, when the epidemiological data are extensive enough for dose-response relationships to be deduced—as, for example, in assessing the risks of asbestos exposure (23)—formal risk assessment may well have a place, although even in that example the upper and lower limits of predictions are wide apart. There has also been useful discussion of the management of uncertainty, as, for example, in a recent NATO symposium volume (25), but the specific problems of standard-setting have not been addressed.

Integration of Disparate Information

The relevance of the title I chose should now be apparent. In alchemy, diverse data are thrown into a crucible, heat (political agitation) is applied, and we hope that "pure wisdom" (the standard) will flow out. We all know what juggling is, but we might note that a very high order of skill is needed when differently shaped objects are juggled—which is what we have to do, in the sense that animal, clinical, and epidemiological data have very different "shapes." Science starts the process by a rigorous consideration of the probable validity of the experimental approach, and the statistical criteria used in such studies; in the case of epidemiology, if science is the generation of refutable hypotheses, the scientific input consists in analyzing confounders, and deducing whether or not a given hypothesis has been refuted. The key to the problem of standard-setting, therefore, is to understand the process of integration of disparate information.

How do we normally perform this kind of integration? Those working in the growing field of artificial intelligence research have been edging up to this problem. Schank and Childers, in their book *The Cognitive Computer* (24) have written:

Any computer-understanding system must be able to understand new or unexpected situations. Real understanding requires the ability to establish connections between pieces of information for which no prescribed set of rules, or scripts, exist. We must be able to recognize general statements of connectivity between events when specifics are unavailable. We must have general principles for organizing seemingly disparate events in meaningful ways.

Such abilities are far beyond the capability of any contemporary computer. But we can recognize that the process requires the exercise of the most complex faculties of the human brain. What we are left with, therefore, is that standard-setting is indeed an integrative exercise, performed against a background of all the data, requiring judgment before decision. It is not reducible to a simple formula, nor is it likely to be made more simple in the future.

Defining a Credible Process of Standard-Setting

It is clear that the requirements for a credible standard-setting process are the following:

1. Total and critical literature review
2. Wide consultation and participation
3. Preparation of a staff paper to make explicit integrative aspects of a final standard
4. Clear separation of scientific considerations from economic or social reasons leading to modification of a standard

I said at the beginning that I was not going to discuss the way in which the political process is finally involved in a decision about a standard. This will, of course, be determined by political traditions. I would like to point out, however, that there seem to be three broad choices, as follows:

1. The "more or less democratic" process: this involves public disclosure of committee membership and minuted discussions; opportunity for interested groups or individuals to intervene, etc. It has been pioneered by the EPA in the United States; it is necessarily lengthy and expensive. Lippmann's valuable insider's review of the process is one of the most useful essays published on the procedure as a whole and the role of scientific advisory groups in particular (16).
2. The "more or less autocratic" process: this involves the selection of a small committee of experts and their meeting for a few days, followed by the issuing of a committee recommendation, bolstered by a small bibliography of papers that support whatever standard is proposed. This seems to be the procedure followed by the World Health Organization and some other bodies. It has the advantages of speed and economy.
3. The "more or less bureaucratic" process: this is followed by countries such as Canada with a parliamentary system in which court challenges of standards

are not possible. Small committees meet in private and advise the minister responsible on a confidential basis; the relevant government department then proposes a standard. In this process the scientific basis of a standard and its subsequent modification for political or economic reasons are inextricably mingled: the alchemy model. It is potentially the fastest and the cheapest process of all, but it is essentially closed.

Conclusion

I have considered the process of standard-setting as an integrative exercise because it seems to me that the public health is only adequately protected if there are standards, even if these are only goals. Such standard-setting is not an ephemeral pastime, but one likely to continue and expand in the future. I have concluded that the integration of disparate data is an extremely complex process; and in my opinion one that requires an open process if it is to be effective and credible. I think it is important that scientists in any of the relevant fields—and that must surely include all of us—give some thought to what is involved. They are of course entitled to take a cynical view of the whole process, as many do. But the quality of the exercise is only likely to be maintained if some scientists are prepared to devote time to it, and to the discussions which must be part of it. There is some danger that the process will be left only to lawyers if scientists vacate the field; and this, I know it will be agreed, would be a backward step.

It has been my purpose in this paper to stimulate interest in the process of standard-setting, so that readers will be encouraged to participate if called upon to do so.

References

1. Bates DV (1979) Air pollution: Political initiative, scientific reality and the process of decision-making. Lung 156:87–94
2. Whittemore AS (1982) Estimating human cancer risks from animal data. Electric Power Research Institute Conference Proceedings, Carmel. EA-4447, vol 1. (Research project 2378–7)
3. Whittemore AS, Grosser SC, Silvers A (1986) Pharmacokinetics in low dose extrapolation using animal cancer data. Fundam App Toxicol 7:183–90
4. Hazucha M (1987) Relationship between ozone exposure and pulmonary function changes. J Appl Physiol 62:1671–1680
5. Enterline PE (1983) Epidemiologic basis for the asbestos standard. Environ Health Persp 52:93–97
6. Epidemiology and air pollution (1985) Washington, National Academy Press
7. Lippmann M, Lioy PJ (1985) Critical issues in air pollution epidemiology. Environ Health Perspec 62:243–258
8. Whittemore AS (1986) Epidemiology in risk assessment for regulatory policy. J Chronic Dis (special issue in honor of Abraham M. Lilienfeld) 39:1157–1168

9. A national workshop on the role of epidemiology in the risk assessment process in Canada (1985) Science Council of Canada (publication number SS24–23)
10. Advances in health risk assessment for systemic toxicants and chemical mixtures (1985) Tox Indus Health 1(4)
11. Whittemore AS (1983) Combining pharmacokinetic and cancer bioassay data. EPRI Conference Proceedings, San Diego. EA-4447 vol. 2. (Research project 2378–7)
12. Alm AL (1985) Introductory remarks. Tox Indus Health 1(4):1–5
13. Magee B (1973) Popper. Fontana, London
14. MaClure M (1985) Popperian refutation in epidemiology. Am J Epidemiol 121:343–50
15. Bates DV (1983) Scientific components in standard setting. Environ Health Perspect 52:183–5
16. Lippmann M (1985) Role of science advisory groups in establishing standards for ambient air pollutants. Invited Plenary Lecture at 1985 Annual Meeting of the American Association for Aerosol Research, Albuquerque, New Mexico, 20th November 1985
17. Whittemore AS (1983) Facts and values in risk analysis for environmental toxicants. Risk Analysis 3:23–33
18. Regulating the regulators (1982) Science Council of Canada (report no. 35)
19. Draft addendum to 1982 OAQPS staff paper on air quality standards for sulfur oxides (1986) Office of Air Quality Planning and Standards, US Environmental Protection Agency, Washington, 12th Sept 1986
20. Draft addendum to 1982 OAQPS staff paper on air quality standards for particulate matter (1986) Office of Air Quality Planning and Standards, US Environmental Protection Agency, Washington, 12th Sept 1986
21. Cumming RB (1983) Risk assessment and the governmental policy-making process. Risk Analysis 3:1–3 (editorial)
22. Grima AP, Timmerman P, Fowle CD, Byer P (1986) Risk management and EIA: Research needs and opportunities. Background paper prepared for the Canadian Environmental Assessment Research Council. Ministry of Supply and Services, Canada (publication no. EN 107–3/5–1986E)
23. Nonoccupational health risks of asbestiform fibers. (1984) Washington, National Academy Press
24. Schank RC, Childers P (1984) The cognitive computer: On language, learning and artificial intelligence. Reading, Mass., Addison-Wesley
25. Wilkin L, Sutton A (eds) (1986) The management of uncertainty: Approaches, methods and applications. Nijhoff, Dordrecht. (NATO ASI series D: Behavioural and social sciences, no. 32)

CHAPTER 2

Species Differences in Inhalation Toxicology: Variations in Exposure–Dose Relationships and Macrophage Function

J.D. Brain[1]

Introduction

As emphasized throughout this symposium, human responses to toxic agents are often predicted from experiments done in other species such as rodents. In addition to obvious differences in body mass, anatomy, and life span, differences in metabolism among species are often substantial. For example, the oxygen consumption of rats per kilogram of body weight is 5.5 times greater than that of humans (2). Amino acid requirements, vitamin requirements, and xenobiotic metabolism also differ markedly (42). Differences in lifestyle such as nocturnal activity and coprophagy are also important when evaluating response to toxic agents. Despite these many differences, we are confronted with the necessity of extrapolating experimental results from animals to humans. Many different species have been used to assess the toxicity of chemicals and environmental pollutants; yet, although species differences are widely acknowledged, our understanding of the variability in response among commonly used laboratory animals is neither systematic nor complete.

Even within a single species, genetic differences are very apparent. All mice are not equal. Differences among strains may affect the susceptibility to disease, the nature of disease produced by a given pathogen, and immunologic competence (22,52,57). For example, Ranga and Kleinerman (47) reported that the blotchy mouse, a strain characterized by extensive connective tissue abnormalities in blood vessels and skin, had a different pattern of lung injury and repair after exposure to 20 ppm of NO_2 than did normal mice breathing the same atmosphere. Extrapolating results in laboratory animals to humans is valid only when the differences in response among species and strains are understood. At present, abstracting a comprehensive description of species differences from the literature is difficult because so many kinds of animals and types of exposures have been used in various combinations. Several theoretical and experimental contributions have been made, but the problem is far from solved.

[1]Harvard School of Public Health, 665 Huntington Avenue, Boston, MA 02115, USA.

In this chapter we first discuss two aspects of exposure to inhaled particles and gases in which species differences are known to exist. These aspects are deposition and clearance. Species may also vary in regard to the magnitude and type of biological response, but that essential topic will only be briefly discussed here. Finally, we examine the process of choosing suitable animal species as models of human disease or human physiologic responses, and the impact of species differences on establishing environmental quality standards.

Pulmonary Disease and Environmental Agents

Deposition

Palm and co-workers (43) studied retention of dust in the lungs of guinea pigs and small monkeys; the percentage of alveolar retention as a function of particle size was substantially the same as that found earlier in humans. Friedlander (19) used dimensional analysis to investigate deposition of particles in the lower lung. Kliment (32) identified several important physiologic variables involved in the deposition of aerosols that are independent of dimension (i.e., the dimensional units cancel each other out). He predicted the degree to which these "dimensionless groups" should vary among rats, guinea pigs, rabbits, and humans. Stauffer (53) has also used dimensional analysis to predict that sedimentation or turbulence-dominated deposition of inhaled aerosols should be constant, but that diffusion-dominated deposition should vary inversely with body weight. The predictions of McMahon and co-workers (34) differ from those of Stauffer (53) and suggest that diffusion-dominated deposition is also independent of body weight.

McMahon and co-workers (34) attempted to specify the physical mechanisms of particle deposition by identifying the controlling dimensionless variables. For example, the number of particles that deposit by impaction increases as the Stokes number increases. The Stokes number is the ratio of the stop distance of a moving particle to the characteristic dimension of the system. The Froude number, the ratio of the particle-sedimentation velocity to the flow-through velocity, is also a dimensionless variable, and controls the sedimentation of particles in the nose, pharynx, and large airways during normal breathing. Small particles diffuse more rapidly to the walls of pulmonary alveoli when the dimensionless diffusion time, expressed as DT/a^2, increases. In this variable, D is the diffusion coefficient (which depends directly on temperature and inversely on air viscosity and particle radius), T is the breath period, and a is the air-space diameter.

If all of the dimensionless groups varied with body weight, understanding the scaling rules for deposition of particles in the lungs would be complicated and difficult. Fortunately, although many important physiologic parameters such as breath period and ventilation change as body weight changes, competing effects generally cancel one another in the controlling dimensionless parameters. Thus, the fraction of a particular aerosol that is deposited is generally independent of body size.

McMahon and co-workers (34) used a "Noah's Ark" approach to test these ideas. They simultaneously exposed five different species (mice, hamsters, rats, rabbits, and dogs) to the same 0.78 μm aerosol of ^{198}Au and compared both total deposition and site of deposition. When the total amount of aerosol deposited was divided by the animal's body weight, it was found that the smaller animals received more particles per gram than the larger ones. However, as predicted by the theoretical analysis, the deposition fraction (collection efficiency) for both the lungs alone and the lung, nose, pharynx, and airways combined were substantially independent of body size.

Schum and Yeh (48) have developed a model for computing aerosol deposition in mammalian lungs that incorporates both breathing pattern and detailed anatomical models based on morphometric measurements. When they compared results predicted by their model to the experimental results obtained by Raabe and co-workers (46) in rats and hamsters, not only had the model correctly predicted total deposition, it had also correctly predicted that the highest relative deposition concentration was in the right apical lobe. Deposition models have also been developed for human lungs (13,65). The problem of species extrapolation is compounded by consistent, large, intersubject variations in humans; identifying the physiological or anatomical parameters responsible for this has been difficult (26).

In a recent article, Yu and Xu (66) developed theoretical models to predict the deposition of diesel exhaust particulates in humans and rats. Like McMahon and co-workers (34) they concluded that, despite their considerable differences in airway size and other variables, the percentage of inhaled particles depositing in the alveolar region was similar in rats and humans. However, the average dose per unit surface area was higher in rats.

In spite of some of these reassuring similarities for small particles, large particles, which are more likely to deposit in the nose and mouth, probably deposit in a more variable fashion among species. The nasopharynx is particularly variable. Patra (44) made silicone rubber casts of the nasopharyngeal region in human, baboon, rhesus monkey, dog, rabbit, guinea pig, rat, hamster, and mouse. Predictably, profound differences were apparent; while discussing the implications for aerosol deposition models, Patra (44) suggested that "simple scaling might not be sufficient to produce correct conclusions."

Clearance

Lung retention is determined not only by the amount of material deposited but also by the rates of clearance. The relative rates of deposition and clearance determine the retention—the amount of a substance present in the respiratory tract at any specified time. If exposure is continuous, then the equilibrium concentration (achieved when the clearance rate matches the deposition rate) equals the retention. It is the retention integrated over time as well as the metabolism and properties of the particles retained that is presumably related to the magnitude of the toxic response. Thus, the integrated dose to lung tissue is influenced by the speed and pathways of clearance. All aspects of clearance may show interspecies variation. We discuss below some mechanisms of clearance and what is known about how they differ among species.

Airway Clearance

Felicetti and co-workers (17) have shown that tracheal mucus velocity varies with species and is proportional to the 0.57th power of the tracheal surface area. They found that the linear velocity of intratracheally instilled ^{99m}Tc-macroaggregates of albumin in the trachea was higher in dogs than in smaller animals. If one includes nonmammalian species, the variability is even greater. Exposing boa constrictors to an inhaled, radiolabeled, submicrometric aerosol, Grant and co-workers (23) demonstrated that 41% of the aerosol that was still present 5 h after the end of exposure was retained in the trachea. In mammals, the percentage retained in the trachea is usually $<5\%$. This suggests that the mucociliary transport system is much slower in reptiles than in mammals. Grant and co-workers (23) also reported that less than 10% of the snake tracheal epithelium was ciliated, a small percentage compared to mammalian tracheal epithelium. While studying aerosol deposition and clearance in chickens, Mensah and Brain (36) showed that lung clearance of submicrometric particles was biphasic; during the fast phase, clearance rates exceeded what has been observed for hamsters or mice. Thomas (56) has developed a model describing the kinetics of clearance of inhaled particles in the respiratory tract of mice, rats, and dogs.

The fraction of material clearing via a given route varies among animal species, and, therefore, the pattern of pulmonary retention can differ markedly. Snipes and co-workers (50) studied retention of inhaled particles in dogs, rats, and mice for 850 days after a single exposure. Clearance to the blood, gastrointestinal tract, and lymph nodes was measured. Rats and mice cleared inhaled particles rapidly from the pulmonary region, and, except for a small proportion, transported most of the particles that appeared in lung-associated lymph nodes to the gastrointestinal tract. Dogs cleared particles at a slower rate, and more of the long-term clearance went to lung-associated lymph nodes. By comparing their data on retention patterns to human data from the literature, Snipes and co-workers (50) concluded that these patterns are similar in dogs and humans and that rodents are less suitable models for long-term retention of aerosols in humans.

The clearance of instilled microspheres of different diameters has also been measured both in rats (49) and dogs (50). In addition to demonstrating that microspheres >10 μm in diameter are tenaciously retained in the lung, these studies showed that microspheres with a diameter of 7–9 μm are retained differently in rats and dogs. Rats cleared these microspheres slowly (half-life = 580 days) via the mucociliary escalator, whereas dogs did not clear these particles at all except to translocate 0.2% to the tracheobronchial lymph nodes.

Lung Macrophages

Pulmonary macrophages are the primary protectors of the airway and alveolar surfaces. Their phagocytic behavior, migratory patterns, and lytic potential are often crucial in the prevention of pulmonary disease. Interspecies differences in the number of macrophages, their rates of phagocytosis, secretory function, and the rate of intracellular killing can lead to differences in susceptibility to pulmonary disease.

Phagocytosis is the classic function of the macrophage as described originally by Metchnikoff (37). Through this activity the lung surface is kept clean and sterile (6,24,28,29) and insoluble particles are prevented from penetrating on the alveolar epithelia. The latter function is essential; in humans, insoluble particles that remain on the surface have a biological half-life of days to weeks, whereas particles that penetrate alveolar epithelia remain for a half-life ranging from a few days to thousands of days (5). Thus, the rate of phagocytosis is critical to particle clearance from the nonciliated regions of the respiratory tract.

We have recently examined the rate at which insoluble gold particles are taken up by pulmonary macrophages in mice, hamsters, rats, and rabbits in situ. Gold particles were taken up most rapidly in hamsters, followed by rats, rabbits, and mice. Differences in macrophage size or number in the respiratory tract cannot completely account for the in vivo differences we observed. The numbers of macrophages recovered by lavage from hamsters, rats, and rabbits were approximately equal when expressed per gram of body weight (50,000 macrophages per gram of body weight) (33,59). Dogs, on the average, have about ten times more macrophages recoverable by lavage when expressed per gram of body weight (16,58).

Although in situ bioassays of macrophage function more accurately reflect the response of intact lungs to inhaled aerosols, in vitro bioassays may be preferable in several situations (3,31). In vitro assays permit various aspects of the clearance mechanism to be quantified under controlled conditions and also eliminate the difficulty of estimating actual dose, an inherent problem of in situ assays. Use of alveolar macrophages in vitro to predict inhalation hazards has been evaluated (1).

In vitro assays have been used to study the effects of many environmental agents on the phagocytic rate or viability of alveolar macrophages. Most of these studies have involved humans (12), mice (18), rats (10), or rabbits (7,14,21, 35,62). Despite the diversity of assays and environmental agents examined, none of these protocols has studied indices of phagocytosis and viability in alveolar macrophages simultaneously in different animal species.

To examine intrinsic macrophage ability across species, Valberg et al. (59) compared phagocytosis of colloidal gold target particles by lung macrophages from humans, hamsters, rabbits, rats, and mice. The macrophages were harvested from animal lungs and from nonsmoking human volunteers using bronchoscopic saline lavage. Cell concentrations were equalized and the rate of particle ingestion was measured at four concentrations of gold colloid, ranging from 10 μg/ml to 0.1 μg/ml.

The results, expressed as colloid uptake per cell, fell into three groups. Macrophages from hamsters and rabbits were very similar, as were those from rats and mice. At the lowest concentration of gold colloid, human macrophages took up twice as many particles as did macrophages from rabbits or hamsters; in turn, rabbit and hamster macrophages took up 1.7 times as many particles as those of rats or mice. When gold colloid concentrations were raised 100-fold, human macrophages took up 4.5 times as many as those from rats or mice, and seven times as many as hamster or rabbit macrophages. The rates of instilled colloidal gold uptake in situ in rabbits, hamsters, rats, and mice were not comparable to these data. Hamster colloid uptake exceeded rabbit uptake by a factor of three, and both rat and mouse by a factor of five. Note, however, that in situ uptake involves cell locomotion, whereas in a suspension assay contact between particles and macrophages is determined solely by collision frequency.

Inactivation of pathogens by macrophages has recently been of special concern (40). When the particles ingested by pulmonary macrophages are viable organisms, the efficiency with which the organisms are inactivated becomes a crucial factor in lung defense. The ability of the pathogen to cause lung damage and disease directly competes with the host's ability to mount an effective inactivation process. The efficiency of this defense mechanism varies from species to species. Huber and co-workers (30) have reviewed the literature on pulmonary antimicrobial defenses and have shown that the bactericidal activity of alveolar macrophages differs markedly among species. For example, rabbit alveolar macrophages avidly ingest and kill *Staphylococcus aureus*, whereas alveolar macrophages from rats ingest but have difficulty killing the same organisms. More recently, Nguyen and co-workers (41) reported that pulmonary macrophages from humans, rabbits, rats, and hamsters differed in their ability to phagocytize and kill pathogens. In the absence of serum opsonins, for example, human macrophages were able to phagocytize *S. aureus* Cowan I (protein A positive). In contrast, pulmonary macrophages lavaged from rabbit, rat, and hamster were unable to phagocytize *S. aureus* Cowan I and other nonopsonized bacteria in the test system studied.

Although pulmonary macrophages are the primary defenders of lung gas exchange surfaces, they do not always act alone. Polymorphonuclear leukocytes (neutrophils) appear in the lung in large numbers during inflammatory reactions (51). Differences among species in the phagocytic function, general behavior, enzymatic deficiencies, and metabolic pathways of these neutrophils may lead to differences in susceptibility to toxic agents. Higgins and co-workers (27), for example, have shown that the manner in which neutrophils dispose of H_2O_2 differs between species. They found that guinea pigs were more similar to humans than either rats or mice in this regard (27). Evidence also suggests that accumulation of neutrophils can cause tissue damage; thus chronic influx of these cells can actually lead to lung disease.

Less familiar species exhibit even greater variability in regard to the type and distribution of phagocytic cells in the respiratory tract. Warner and Brain (60) and Warner and co-workers (61) showed that calves have an extensive population of macrophages in the capillaries of their lungs. Large numbers of pulmonary intravascular macrophages have also been demonstrated in sheep (61). Morphometric methods applied to electron micrographs revealed that these macrophages occupied 15.3% of the intravascular volume and had 15.9 m^2 of free surface available for contact with blood. Intravascular macrophages were closely applied to 7.1% of the endothelial surface, including numerous short segments with 12–15 nm of membrane interspace, increased subplasmalemmal cytoplasmic density, and intercellular electron-dense material. We believe that pulmonary intravascular macrophages in sheep comprise an important component of their mononuclear phagocytc system. Furthermore, it is likely that these macrophages, through phagocytic uptake of pathogens, may contribute to pulmonary inflammation and injury.

The distribution of macrophages in bird lungs also represents a marked departure from our usual concept of the alveolar macrophage as the dominant pulmonary phagocytic cell. Stearns et al. (54) exposed ducks (*Anas platyrhynchos*) to a nontoxic iron oxide aerosol. The lungs were fixed with O_sO_4 vapor and examined by electron microscopy. We found that in birds different mechanisms handle particles deposited in the gas exchange region. In the mammalian lung, wandering alveolar macrophages are the primary defense against foreign particles, whereas in the bird lung we found no surface macrophages in the gas exchange region. Instead, a trilaminar substance unique to avian lungs which coats the atria and infundibula trapped inhaled particles. Unlike mammalian alveolar epithelial cells, which rarely ingest particles, epithelial cells in the atrial and infundibular regions of avian lungs exhibit extensive phagocytic activity. The cells then release particles into the subjacent connective tissue, where they are taken up by interstitial macrophages.

The differences in deposition and clearance mechanisms discussed above demonstrate that dose to the lungs at different times after exposure to a given agent is influenced by species. All species breathing the same aerosol or gas in the same atmosphere do not receive identical lung doses. Exposure concentration (e.g., mg/m^3 or ppm) is not an adequate description of lung dose. Ventilation, deposition fraction, lung anatomy, and clearance mechanisms vary systematically and irregularly among species and influence the local concentrations of retained aerosols and gases.

Biological Response

Even if different species received the same lung dose of a toxic particle or chemical, the extent of lung damage would not necessarily be identical. In addition to deposition and clearance, varying responses among species also reflect biochemical differences in the activation, degradation, excretion, or mechanism of action of a given agent. Different responses to toxic agents and environmental pollutants frequently reflect anatomical differences in site of uptake and cell distribution.

For example, ozone is recognized as a major component of oxidant smog and, in high concentrations, can impair the function of alveolar macrophages (11) and lead to severe lung damage (4). Changes in pulmonary function are detectable in humans at concentrations of ozone that are similar to those in smog. Although the mechanism by which ozone damages the tissues may be similar in different animal species (20), species differences in toxic response have been noted. Stokinger and co-workers (55) have shown that morbidity and mortality in animals exposed to chronic low levels (1 ppm) of ozone differ significantly with species. In particular, mortality of rats and guinea pigs was 33% and 30% respectively, whereas the mortality of dogs was zero. These differences in mortality and lung pathology after exposure to ozone appear to be related to efficiency of nasopharyngeal removal of ozone: nasopharyngeal ozone removal has been found to be more efficient in the dog than in either the rabbit or guinea pig (38), and this results in significant differences in the dose of ozone that reaches the cells of the lung parenchyma in the exposed animals.

Interspecies differences in the fine structure of the respiratory tract can affect the degree and distribution of damage after exposure to harmful aerosols or gases. Several studies have shown that rats develop lesions in the terminal bronchioles and alveoli of proximal alveolar ducts after exposure to ozone (8), whereas monkeys are primarily affected in the respiratory bronchiole (15). The distribution of damage is determined in part by the structure of the respiratory tract epithelia. Respiratory bronchioles are well developed in Macaque monkeys and are lined by nonciliated epithelium comprised of cuboidal cells interspersed among squamous cells (9). Nonrespiratory bronchioles are very short or nonexistent. Rats, on the other hand, do not have well-developed respiratory bronchioles; the pulmonary acinus is simpler, and terminal bronchioles open into alveolar ducts.

In addition to these anatomic differences (e.g., the importance of respiratory bronchioles), differences at the cellular and enzymatic level may also influence the response of the lungs to inhaled agents. Plopper and co-workers (45) examined six species of mammals and examined the ultrastructure of cells in the trachea. They concluded that: "(1) mucous and serous cells are not common to the tracheal epithelial lining of all mammalian species; (2) there is significant interspecies heterogeneity in the abundance, distribution and ultrastructure of tracheal secretory cells; (3) potential differences in the roles of nonciliated cells in tracheal function exist within tracheal epithelial populations and between species." Hadly and Dahl (25) examined the concentration of cytochrome P_{450}-dependent monooxygenases in the nasal membranes of six different species. The existence of extensive differences in the concentrations of various enzymes in the nasal epithelium suggests that possible variations in nasal metabolism must be considered when evaluating hazards associated with inhaled toxins.

Implications for Research

The goal of inhalation toxicology is to provide enough information to protect the public from the harmful effects of environmental agents. This usually requires determining the particulate and gas concentrations of environmental agents beyond which adverse effects are manifest in a defined percentage of the population. More importantly, environmental quality standards should protect subsets of the population with preexisting disease or with an increased susceptibility to specific agents. For obvious ethical reasons, human subjects have not been used to investigate the full spectrum of toxic effects evoked by environmental agents. Thus, extrapolating results from animal experiments to humans remains a major challenge for toxicology. The species differences we have discussed directly relate to the determination of environmental quality standards and the measurement of potential toxicity of environmental agents to humans. For these determinations, the choice of suitable animal species for the study of toxicity and the selection of appropriate models for human disease is essential.

Weil (63,64) has published guidelines for predicting through experimental studies how safe a material is for humans. He recommends the use of "species that biologically handle the material as similarly as possible to man" (64). Mohr (39) also gives a very useful discussion of factors influencing the choice of species and strain. It is clear that the metabolism, absorption, excretion, storage, and other physiological aspects of any animal model studied must be considered. Because all of these factors are usually not well understood in a single species of laboratory animal, several animal species should be used, at least initially. Neither taxonomic closeness to human beings, per se, nor logistic convenience is sufficient justification for the choice of a particular animal species.

Conclusion

Many differences in dose and response to toxic agents have been identified among animal species and between humans and animals. However, the catalog is far from complete, and many more systematic experiments need to be done. Extrapolating results from animal studies to humans would be greatly aided by better understanding of the underlying mechanisms that govern reactions to toxic agents. Experiments that compare animal cells to human cells in vitro can provide insight in this regard. Better models of human disease need to be developed, and to this end, closer cooperation between epidemiologists, pathologists, and toxicologists should be encouraged.

References

1. Aranyi C, Gardner DE, Huisingh JL (1981) Evaluation of potential inhalation hazard of particulate silicious compounds by in vitro rabbit alveolar macrophage test: application to industrial particulates containing hazardous impurities. In: Dunnom DD

(ed) Health effects of synthetic silica particulates. Document No. ASTM-STP-732. American Society for Testing Materials, Philadelphia, pp 48–61
2. Badeer HS (1974) Effect of hypothermia on circulation: vertebrates. I. Physiological variables. In: Altman PL, Dittmer DS (eds) Biological data book, vol. 3, 2nd edn. Federation of American Societies for Experimental Biology, Bethesda, pp 1740–1742
3. Beck BD, Brain JD (1983) Predicting the pulmonary toxicity of particulates using damage indicators in lung lavage fluid. In: Wagner WL, Rom WN, Merchant JA (eds) Health issues related to metal and nonmetallic mining. Butterworth, Boston, pp 83–104
4. Bouhuys A, Gee JBL (1980) Environmental lung disease. In: Isselbacher KJ, Adams RD, Braunwald E, Petersdorf RG, Wilson JD (eds) Principles of internal medicine. McGraw-Hill, New York, pp 1213–1233
5. Brain JD (1980) Macrophage damage in relation to the pathogenesis of lung disease. Environ Health Perspect 35:21–28
6. Brain JD (1985) Macrophages in the respiratory tract. In: Fishman AP, Fisher AB (eds) Handbook of physiology, sect 3: The respiratory system, vol 1: Circulation and nonrespiratory functions. American Physiological Society, Bethesda, MD, pp 447–441
7. Camner P, Lundborg M (1977) Alveolar macrophages and teflon particles coated with carbon and metals. In: Pulmonary macrophage and epithelial cells. US Energy Research and Development Administration Technical Information Center, Springfield Va, pp 405–413 (ERDA symposium series no. 43)
8. Castelman WL, Dungworth DL, Tyler WS (1973) Cytochemically detected alterations of lung acid phosphatase reactivity following ozone exposure. Lab Invest 29:310–319
9. Castleman WL, Gillespie J, Kosch P, Schwartz L, Tyler WS (1979) The role of non-human primates in environmental pollution research. In: Lee SD, Mudd JB (eds) Assessing toxic effects of environmental pollutants. Ann Arbor Science Publishers, Ann Arbor, pp 15–29
10. Castranova V, Bowman L, Reasor MJ, Miles PR (1980) Effects of metallic ions on cellular and subcellular properties of rat alveolar macrophages. Toxicol Appl Pharmacol 53:14–23
11. Coffin DL, Gardner DE, Holzman RS, Wolock FJ (1968) Influence of ozone on pulmonary cells. Arch Environ Health 16:633–636
12. Cohen AB, Cline MJ (1971) The human alveolar macrophage: isolation, cultivation in vitro, and studies of morphologic and functional characteristics. J Clin Invest 50:1390–1398
13. Davies CN (1982) Deposition of particles in human lungs as a function of particle size and breathing pattern: an empirical model. In: Walton WH (ed) Inhaled particles V. Pergamon, Oxford, pp 119–135
14. Dubreuil A, Bouley G, Boudene C (1979) In vitro cytotoxicity of cadmium microparticles for rabbit pulmonary alveolar macrophages. Scand J Work Environ Health 5:211–216
15. Dungworth DL, Castleman WL, Chow CK, Mellick PW, Mustafa MG, Tarkington B, Tyler WS (1975) Effect of ambient levels of ozone on monkeys. Fed Proc 34:1670–1674
16. Felicetti SA, Silbaugh SA, Muggenburg BA (1975) Effect of time post-exposure on the effectiveness of bronchopulmonary lavage in removing inhaled ^{145}Ce in fused clay from beagle dogs. Health Phys 29:89–96

17. Felicetti SA, Wolff RK, Muggenburg BA (1981) Comparison of tracheal mucous transport in rats, guinea pigs, rabbits, and dogs. J Appl Physiol 51:1612–1617
18. Fisher GL, McNeil KL, Whaley CB, Fong J (1978) Attachment and phagocytosis studies with murine pulmonary alveolar macrophages. J Reticuloendothel Soc 24:243–252
19. Friedlander SK (1964) Particle deposition by diffusion in the lower lung: application of dimensional analysis. Am Ind Hyg Assoc J 25:37–42
20. Goldstein BD (1977) Cellular effects of ozone. Rev Environ Health 2:117–202
21. Graham JA, Gardner DE, Waters MD, Coffin DL (1975) Effect of trace metals on phagocytosis by alveolar macrophages. Infect Immun 11:1278–1283
22. Grahn D (1958) Acute radiation response of mice from a cross between radiosensitive and radioresistant strains. Genetics 43:835–843
23. Grant MM, Brain JD, Vinegar A (1981) Pulmonary defense mechanisms of *Boa constrictor*. J Appl Physiol 50:979–983
24. Green GM, Kass EH (1964) The role of the alveolar macrophage in the clearance of bacteria from the lung. J Exp Med 119:167–176
25. Hadley WM, Dahl AR (1983) Cytochrome P-450-dependent monooxygenase activity in nasal membranes of six species. Drug Metab Dispos 11:275–276
26. Heyder J, Gebhart J, Stahlhofen W, Stuck B (1982) Biological variability of particle deposition in the human respiratory tract during controlled and spontaneous mouth-breathing. In: Walton WH (ed) Inhaled particles V. Pergamon, Oxford, pp 137–147
27. Higgins CP, Baehner RL, McCallister J, Boxer LA (1978) Polymorphonuclear leukocyte species differences in the disposal of hydrogen peroxide (H_2O_2). Proc Soc Exp Biol Med 158:478–481
28. Hocking WG, Golde DW (1979) The pulmonary-alveolar macrophage I. N Engl J Med 301:580–587
29. Hocking WG, Golde DW (1979) The pulmonary-alveolar macrophage II. N Engl J Med 301:639–645
30. Huber GL, Johanson WG Jr, LaForce FM (1977) Experimental models and pulmonary antimicrobial defenses. In: Brain JD, Proctor DF, Reid LM (eds) Respiratory defense mechanisms, part 2. Dekker, New York, pp 983–1022
31. Kavet RI, Brain JD (1980) Methods to quantify endocytosis: a review. J Reticuloendothel Soc 27:201–221
32. Kliment V (1973) Similarity and dimensional analysis: evaluation of aerosol deposition in the lungs of laboratory animals and man. Folia Morphol (Praha) 21:59–64
33. Mauderly JL (1977) Bronchopulmonary lavage of small laboratory animals. Lab Anim Sci 27:255–261
34. McMahon TA, Brain JD, LeMott SR (1977) Species differences in aerosol deposition. In: Walton WH (ed) Inhaled particles IV. Pergamon, Oxford, pp 23–33
35. Medinsky MA, Cuddihy RG, Hill JO, McClellan RO (1981) Toxicity of selenium compounds to alveolar macrophages. Toxicol Lett 8:289–293
36. Mensah GA, Brain JD (1982) Deposition and clearance of inhaled aerosol in the respiratory tract of chickens. J Appl Physiol 53:1423–1428
37. Metchnikoff E (1905) Immunity in infective diseases. Cambridge University Press, Cambridge
38. Miller FJ (1979) Biomathematical modeling applications in the evaluation of ozone toxicity. In: Lee SD (ed) Assessing toxic effects of environmental pollutants. Ann Arbor Science Publishers, Ann Arbor, pp 263–286

39. Mohr U (1982) Methods of testing carcinogens: principles and limitations. Expl Biol Med 7:186–194
40. Nathan CF, Murray HW, Cohn ZA (1980) The macrophage as an effector cell. N Engl J Med 303:622–626
41. Nguyen B-YT, Peterson PK, Verbrugh HA, Quie PG, Hoidal JR (1982) Differences in phagocytosis and killing by alveolar macrophages from humans, rabbits, rats, and hamsters. Infect Immun 36:504–509
42. Oser BL (1981) The rat as a model for human toxicological evaluation. J Toxicol Environ Health 8:521–542
43. Palm PE, McNerney JM, Hatch T (1956) Respiratory dust retention in small animals: a comparison with man. AMA Arch Ind Health 13:355–365
44. Patra AL (1986) Comparative anatomy of mammalian respiratory tracts: the nasopharyngeal region and the tracheobronchial region. J Toxicol Environ Health 17: 163–174
45. Plopper CG, Mariassy AT, Wilson DW, Alley JW, Nishio SJ, Nettesheim P (1983) Comparison of nonciliated tracheal epithelial cells in six mammalian species: ultrastructure and population densities. Exp Lung Res 5:281–294
46. Raabe OG, Yeh HC, Newton GJ, Phalen RF, Velasquez DJ (1977) Deposition of inhaled monodisperse aerosols in small rodents. In: Walton WH (ed) Inhaled particles IV. Pergamon, Oxford, pp 3–21
47. Ranga V, Kleinerman J (1981) Lung injury and repair in the blotchy mouse. Am Rev Respir Dis 123:90–97
48. Schum M, Yeh HC (1980) Theoretical evaluation of aerosol deposition in anatomical models of mammalian airways. Bull Math Biol 42:1–15
49. Snipes MB, Clem MF (1981) Retention of microspheres in the rat lung after intratracheal instillation. Environ Res 24:33–41
50. Snipes MB, Boecker BB, McClellan RO (1983) Retention of monodisperse or polydisperse aluminosilicate particles inhaled by dogs, rats, and mice. Toxicol Appl Pharmacol 69:345–362
51. Sorokin SP (1977) Phagocytes in the lungs: incidence, general behavior, and phylogeny. In: Brain JD, Proctor DF, Reid LM (eds) Respiratory defense mechanisms, part 2. Dekker, New York, pp 711–848
52. Staats J (1966) The laboratory mouse. In: Green EL (ed) Biology of the laboratory mouse. McGraw-Hill, New York, pp 1–9
53. Stauffer D (1975) Scaling theory for aerosol deposition in the lungs of different mammals. J Aerosol Sci 6:223–225
54. Stearns RC, Barnas GM, Walski M, Brain JD (1987) Deposition and phagocytosis of inhaled particles in the gas exchange region of the duck *Anas platyrhynchos*. Resp Phys 67:23–36
55. Stokinger HE, Wagner WD, Dobrogorski OJ (1957) Ozone toxicity studies: III. Chronic injury to lungs of animals following exposure at a low level. AMA Arch Ind Health 16:514–522
56. Thomas RG (1972) An interspecies model for retention of inhaled particles. In: Mercer TT, Morrow PE, Stober W (eds) Assessment of airborne particles. Thomas, Springfield, Ill, pp 405–455
57. Upton AC (1970) Comparative observations on radiation-induced myeloproliferative disorders in animals and man. In: Clarke WJ, Howard EB, Hackett PL (eds) Myeloproliferative disorders of animals and man. US Atomic Energy Commission,

Division of Technical Information Extension, Oak Ridge, Tenn, pp 149–170 (AEC symposium series no. 19)
58. Valberg PA, Wolff RK, Mauderly JL (1985) Redistribution of retained particles: effect of hyperapnea. Am Rev Respir Dis 131:273–280
59. Valberg PA, Brain JD, Pikus AA, Stearns R (1988) Phagocytic rates for pulmonary macrophages lavaged from rabbit, rat, hamster, and mouse. Exp Lung Res (submitted)
60. Warner AE, Brain JD (1984) The ruminant reticuloendothelial system includes phagocytic intravascular pulmonary macrophages. J Leukocyte Biol 36:388a
61. Warner AE, Barry BE, Brain JD (1986) Pulmonary intravascular macrophages in sheep: morphology and function of a novel constituent of the mononuclear phagocyte system. Lab Invest 55:276–288
62. Waters MD, Gardner DE, Aranyi C, Coffin DL (1975) Metal toxicity for rabbit alveolar macrophages. Environ Res 9:32–47
63. Weil CS (1970) Editorial. Toxicol Appl Pharmacol 17(2):i-ii
64. Weil CS (1972) Guidelines for experiments to predict the degree of safety of a material for man. Toxicol Appl Pharmacol 21:194–199
65. Yeh HC, Schum GM (1980) Model of human lung airways and their application to inhaled particle deposition. Bull Math Biol 42:461–480
66. Yu CP, Xu GB (1986) Predictive models for deposition of diesel exhaust particulates in human and rat lungs. Aerosol Sci Technol 5:337–347

CHAPTER 3

Cell Populations of the Respiratory System: Interspecies Diversity in Composition, Distribution, and Morphology

C.G. Plopper,[1,2] A. Weir,[1,2] J. St. George,[1,2] N. Tyler,[1] A. Mariassy,[3] D. Wilson,[1,3] S. Nishio,[2] D. Cranz,[2] J. Heidsiek,[2] and D. Hyde[1,2]

Introduction

A major site for pulmonary injury resulting from exposure to environmental toxicants is the epithelial lining of respiratory airways. This appears to be the case for a wide range of compounds that have been tested for their toxicity to the respiratory system, whether these compounds are administered by inhalation or other systemic means. The extrapolation to humans of inhalation toxicology studies using animal models assumes comparability in the structure and function of the respiratory system of these model species and humans. The underlying assumption is that data obtained in model species can be extrapolated to humans. The primary consideration of this study is that the tracheobronchial epithelium of most mammalian species commonly used as models may not adequately reflect the condition in human conducting airways. This study focuses on the epithelial population lining the tracheobronchial airways (trachea, bronchi, and bronchioles) of the mammalian respiratory system. We will consider the following questions concerning the epithelial populations of conducting airways:

1. Is the composition of the epithelial populations similar in the same portion of the airway in different species?
2. Does the relative abundance of epithelial cell types vary in the same airway level in different species?
3. Is the composition of epithelial populations the same in all airway levels of the tracheobronchial tree in one species?
4. Are the secretory products contained in these epithelial cell types similar in the same airway level of different species?

---

[1]California Primate Research Center, University of California, Davis CA 95616, USA.

[2]Department of Anatomy, School of Veterinary Medicine, University of California, Davis CA 95616, USA.

[3]Department of Veterinary Pathology, School of Veterinary Medicine, University of California, Davis CA 95616, USA.

5. Does the cytochemical composition of the secretory product vary in cells in different portions of the tracheobronchial tree in the same species?
6. Is the organization the same in the centriacinar region of different species?

Types of Airway Epithelial Cells

Ultrastructure

At least eight types of epithelial cells have been identified lining the conducting respiratory airways (1–4). Not only do they differ in ultrastructure but they are considered to differ in both function and sensitivity to inhaled toxicants. These cell types include ciliated cells, basal cells, mucous goblet cells, Clara cells, serous cells, small mucous granule cells, neuroendocrine cells, brush cells, and a variety of intermediate forms. The ultrastructure of some of these cell types is illustrated in Figs. 3.1–3.3. Basal cells (Fig. 3.1a) are characterized as very small, flattened cells tightly attached to the basal lamina and not extending to the airway lumen (5). They have a small cytoplasm-to-nucleus ratio, and the cytoplasm is filled primarily with intermediate filaments. There are large numbers of desmosomes attaching the basal cell to the surrounding epithelial cells. The ciliated cell (Fig. 3.1a) is attached to the basal lamina and extends to the luminal surface. Its apical surface contains large numbers of cilia interspersed with long microvilli. The majority of the cytoplasm is more electron-lucent than other epithelial cell types, and the apical region of the cytoplasm is filled with mitochondria. Several secretory cell types have been identified in various portions of the conducting airway tree. These include the mucous goblet cell (Fig. 3.1a), Clara cell (Fig. 3.1b), and serous cell (Fig. 3.1c). These three cell types are considered to be secretory because their cytoplasm contains relatively large numbers of spherical, membrane-bound inclusion bodies which have been identified as secretory granules. The mucous goblet cell (Fig. 3.1a) is described as being filled with large granules of varying electron density (6,7). The nucleus is compressed at the basal side of the cell and there are few organelles interspersed in the cytoplasm between individual granules. The Clara cell (Fig. 3.1b) is characterized by smaller, electron-dense granules in its apical cytoplasm (3,4,8). The majority of the cytoplasm is filled with large numbers of organelles. These include abundant agranular endoplasmic reticulum on the apical side of the nucleus and a significant amount of granular endoplasmic reticulum in the perinuclear cytoplasm. The serous cell (Fig. 3.1c) is characterized primarily by large numbers of electron-dense secretory granules, and the cytoplasm is filled with granular endoplasmic reticulum and Golgi apparatus (6).

Morphometry of Secretory Cells

One of the major questions that arises in characterizing different types of secretory cells within the conducting airway tree is the degree of difference between

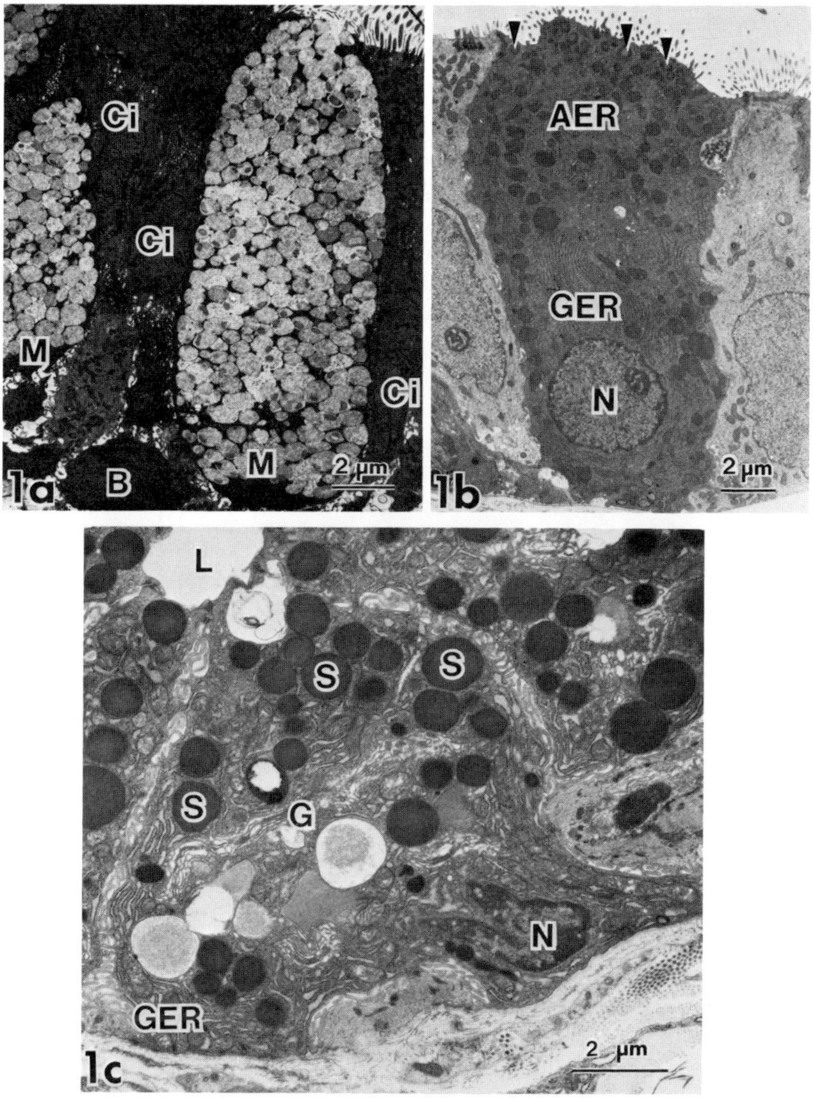

Fig. 3.1a-c. Ultrastructural features of tracheobronchial epithelium. **a**. Epithelium of the trachea of the adult sheep with basal cells (B), ciliated cells (Ci) and mucous goblet cells (M). **b**. Clara cell in trachea of the rabbit. The nucleus (N) is in the basal portion of the cell surrounded by granular endoplasmic reticulum (GER). Agranular endoplasmic reticulum (AER) fills the majority of the apical portion of the cell. Mitochondria and small electron-dense granules (*arrowheads*) are intermixed with AER in the apex of the cell. **c**. Serous cell in the submucosal glands of the rhesus monkey. The nucleus (N) is basal. The majority of the cell is filled with GER, a prominent Golgi apparatus (G) and electron-dense secretory granules (S). These cells face onto the lumen of the submucosal acinus (L). For details, see refs. 6, 8, 37.

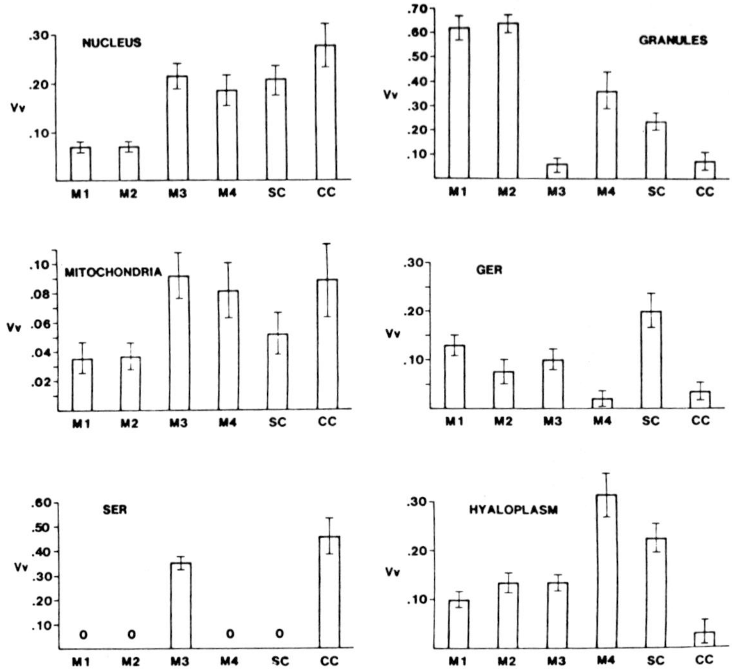

Fig. 3.2. Morphometric comparison of the proportions of cellular components in different epithelial cell types lining tracheobronchial airways of the sheep. Vv, volume fraction; M1, M2, M3, M4, mucous cells; SC, serous cells; CC, Clara cells.

these cell types. One method to determine the degree of difference would be morphometric comparison of the relative amount of cellular space occupied by different cellular organelles. Such a study has been done in sheep airways (Fig. 3.2) (6). By ultrastructural morphological characteristics, four types of mucous cells, serous cells of submucosal glands, and Clara cells are described. As Fig. 3.2 illustrates, there is considerable variation in the proportion of cell volume that is occupied by different cellular components between different airway epithelial cell types of the sheep. The proportion of the cell volume occupied by the nucleus can vary from below 10% to almost 30%. The secretory granule content ranges from approximately 5% in Clara cells and small mucous granule (M3) cells to well over 60% in some types of mucous cells.

Mitochondrial abundance varies from as little as 3.5% to almost 10%. Only two of these cell types, the Clara cell and small mucous granule cell, have significant amounts of smooth endoplasmic reticulum. There are also differences in abundance of granular endoplasmic reticulum and in organelle-free cytoplasm.

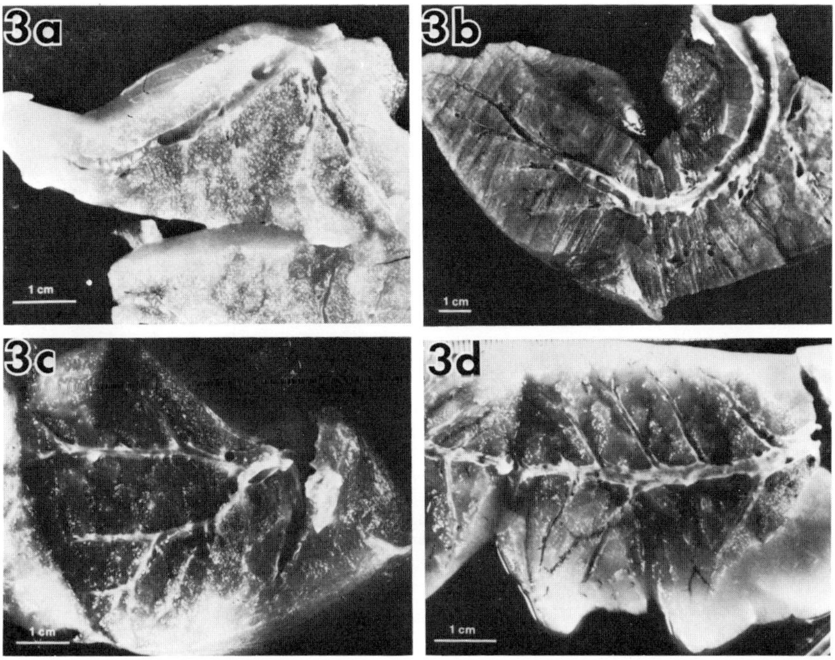

Fig. 3.3a-d. A comparison of the airway branching patterns in the cranial lobe of four species following airway microdissection: **a** rabbit, **b** sheep, **c** bonnet monkey, **d** cat. For details, see ref. 12.

Abundance of Epithelial Cells

Trachea

The composition of the epithelial population of the trachea has been shown to differ from species to species (1,2,5,9–11). Table 3.1 compares the epithelial populations of the distal third of the trachea of six different mammalian species (5). There is wide variability not only in the total abundance of the entire cell population, as measured by number of cells per millimeter of basal lamina, but also in the relative percentage of specific cell types within the population. The number of cells per unit length of basal lamina varies by a factor of almost four. The relative proportion of basal cells varies by a factor of almost ten. Only the proportion of ciliated cells seems to be relatively constant. The predominant secretory cell type varies in different species. Even when the same cell type is present, its relative abundance is not the same in different species [compare Table 3.1 to (11)].

Table 3.1. Comparison of abundance and percentage (%) of cell types in tracheas of six mammalian species

			Percentage						
Species	N	Total nuclei	Basal cells	Ciliated cells	Clara cells	Mucous goblet cells	Serous cells	Other cells	Uniden-tified
Sheep	5	414.3[a] (+33.2)	28.5	30.6	-0-	5.1	-0-	35.9	-0-
Bonnet monkey	3	266.0 (±12.0)	31	41	-0-	8	-0-	16	4
Cat	3	273.0 (±15.0)	37.3	36.1	-0-	20.2	-0-	5.4	1.1
Rabbit	3	210.9 (±29.7)	28.2	43.0	17.6	1.3	-0-	-0-	9.4
Rat	3	147.9 (±3.1)	13.4	40.6	-0-	0.5	39.2	-0-	6.2
Hamster	3	151.4 (±11.2)	5.6	47.5	41.4	-0-	-0-	-0-	5.3

Source: Reprinted with permission from ref. 5. Copyright 1983, Hemisphere Publishing Corporation.
[a]Mean ± 1 S.D., number of nuclei per millimeter.

Bronchi and Bronchioles

Microdissection Approaches

The intrapulmonary airways progress to the parenchymal gas exchange area by an extensive branching pattern. To characterize the epithelial populations in the airway tree, it is necessary to define the location of airways to be sampled in terms of branching pattern from the trachea and the region within a particular lung lobe. The most effective way that we have found to perform such a localization is to microdissect the airway trees from the lobar bronchus down to the centriacinar region (12). As Fig. 3.3 illustrates, microdissection of intrapulmonary airways not only allows high selectivity but also demonstrates the variability in the branching pattern in different species. This approach allows comparisons of the toxic response in the same airway level in different species, in different airway levels of the same species, and in different airway levels and regions of a single lobe of one individual.

Abundance of Epithelial Cells

Comparing the epithelial populations of intrapulmonary airways in different species demonstrates that variation occurs both in the relative proportions of specific cell types by airway generation and within the same species. Figure 3.4 compares the relative abundance of the major cell types in the airway trees of the three species that we have evaluated (8,13,14). There are distinct distributional differences in the abundance of basal cells, mucous cells, Clara cells, and ciliated cells. Additionally, there is considerable variation in the numbers of generations between the trachea and the most distal terminal bronchiole in these three species. The percentage of basal cells in these species generally decreases in more distal airways; however, the number of airway generations in which they are found, as well as their proportion of the population, varies from species to species. The most standard feature appears to be the presence of ciliated cells. Secretory cells vary in abundance and type of cell present. The proportion of brush cells in the rat lung also varies between the trachea (3%), lobar bronchus (0%), terminal bronchiole (1.4%), and first alveolar duct bifurcation (10.1%) (15).

Centriacinar Region

Architecture

The centriacinar region is the area of junction between the conducting airways and the gas exchange area, or parenchyma. There are two different arrangements for this junctional region (16). In most of the smaller species, and some of the larger, there are several generations of nonalveolarized bronchioles and a single very short, or absent, alveolarized bronchiole that directly joins alveolar ducts (Fig. 3.5). Species that have this arrangement include the horse, ox, sheep, pig, rabbit, guinea pig, hamster, gerbil, rat, and mouse. In all of these species the epithelial population is simple cuboidal, with approximately equal numbers of ciliated and nonciliated, or Clara, cells (3,4). A number of other species have an extensive transition zone between nonalveolarized bronchioles and alveolar duct in the form of long, alveolarized bronchioles, or respiratory bronchioles (Fig. 3.5c,d). Species that have few nonalveolarized, noncartilaginous bronchioles and several generations of alveolarized bronchioles include the macaque monkey (17,18), dog (19,20), and cat (21,22). Species in which there are several generations of nonalveolarized, noncartilaginous bronchioles and several generations of alveolarized bronchioles include the human (23,24) and ferret (25). Respiratory bronchioles are characterized as having the luminal surface lined by epithelial populations characteristic of more proximal conducting airways, i.e., simple cuboidal epithelium, interrupted by alveolar outpocketings lined by epithelial populations characteristic of alveoli in the gas exchange areas. In the three species in which this region has been studied—dog (26), cat (21,22,26), and macaque monkey (17,18)—the bronchiolar epithelial population consists almost entirely of nonciliated cells completely encircling respiratory bronchiole in the cat and the dog and on the side opposite the pulmonary artery of the macaque monkey.

Clara Cell Ultrastructure

Interspecific variation exists in the ultrastructural characteristics of the nonciliated (Clara) cells lining the respiratory and terminal bronchioles (4,26–28). A quantitative comparison of the ultrastructural features of the nonciliated

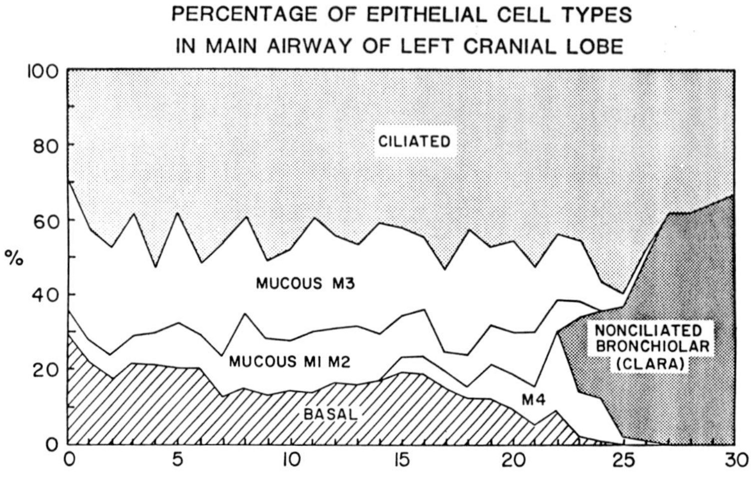

a

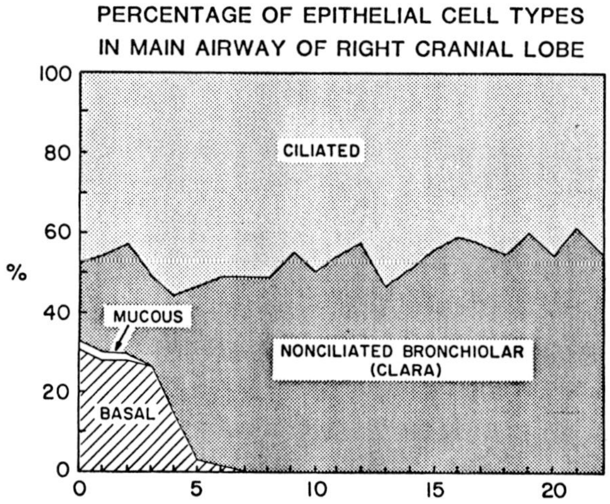

b

Fig. 3.4a-c. A comparison of the relative abundance of the identifiable cell types throughout the tracheobronchial tree in three species: **a** sheep, **b** rabbit, **c** rhesus monkey. The airway generation number equals the number of generations of branching from the trachea (no. 0) to the most distal bronchiole. For details, see refs. 8, 13, 14.

bronchiolar cells in three species (29) is presented in Fig. 3.6. In a large number of species (horse, sheep, rabbit, guinea pig, rat, hamster, and mouse), more than 40% of the cytoplasm is occupied by agranular endoplasmic reticulum (Fig. 3.6). The nucleus is the second most predominant component, followed by mitochondria. Glycogen comprises approximately 10% or less of the cell

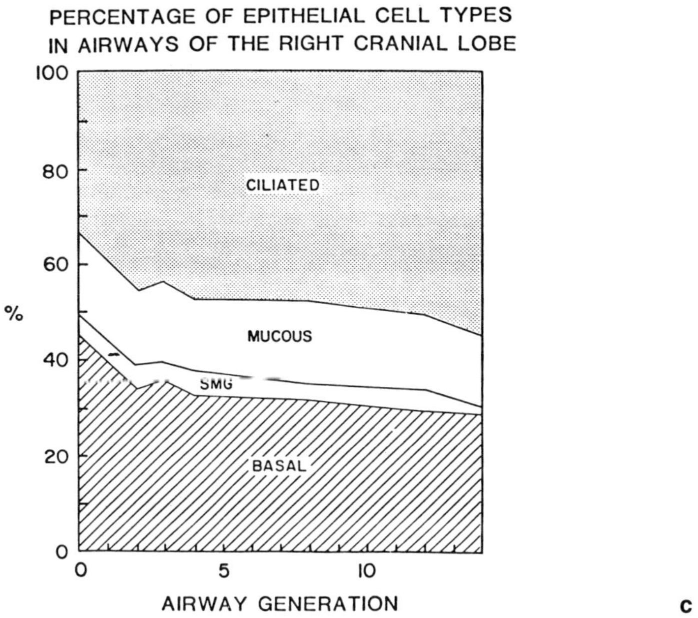

Fig. 3.4. (*Continued*)

volume in these species (Fig. 3.6a). In other species the Clara cell contains primarily glycogen (Fig. 3.5b). In the ox, cat, and dog, more than 60% of the cytoplasmic volume is glycogen. Other extranuclear components, including agranular endoplasmic reticulum and mitochondria, make up a relatively small proportion of the cell volume. Primate species (Fig. 3.6c) do not have an abundance of either endoplasmic reticulum or glycogen in the nonciliated cells lining respiratory bronchioles. These cells have a smaller volume than in the other species (Fig. 3.6c), and the largest component is the nucleus. While a large percentage of the cell is organelle-free hyaloplasm (Fig. 3.6c), other organelles comprise <10% of the cell volume.

Secretory Granule Carbohydrate Content

Carbohydrate Histochemistry

Conventional carbohydrate cytochemical methods have demonstrated a wide variation in the carbohydrate content of secretory cells between species (30–35). The periodic acid Schiff reaction in combination with Alcian blue (AB/PAS) is used to distinguish between neutral (PAS+) and acidic (AB+) glycoconjugates. High iron diamine in sequence with Alcian blue (HID/AB) is used to distinguish

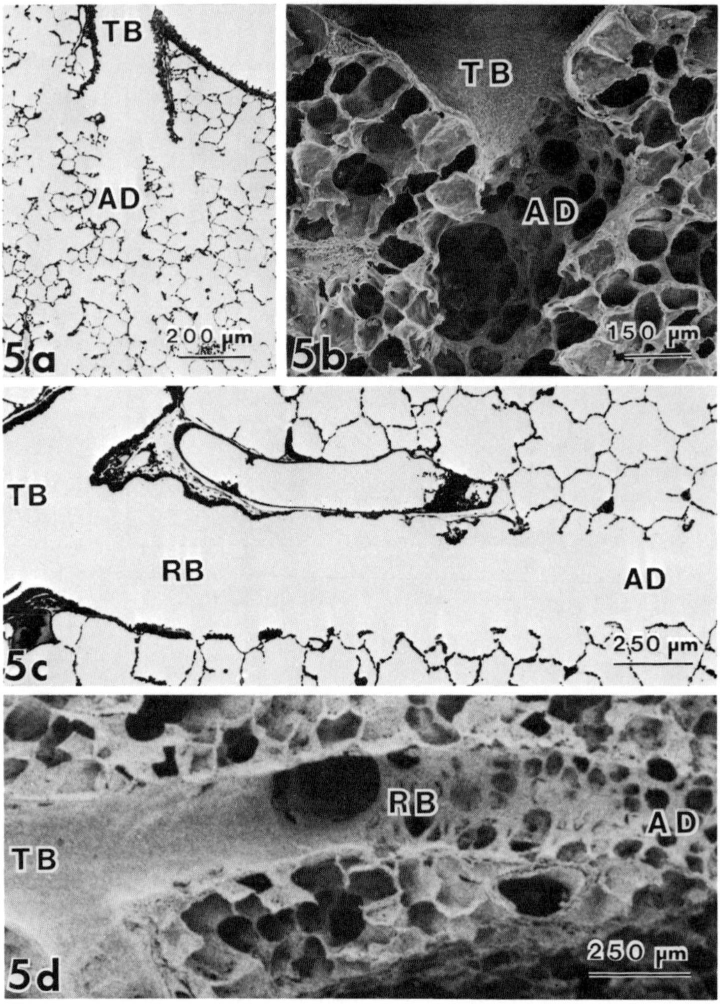

Fig. 3.5a-d. A light microscopic and scanning electron microscopic comparison of the centriacinar region with two different types of architectural organization, the short, or poorly developed, respiratory bronchiole (**a** mouse, **b** rat) and the well-alveolarized respiratory bronchiole (**c** and **d** cat). TB, terminal bronchiole; RB, respiratory bronchiole; AD, alveolar duct. For details, see ref. 16.

between sulfated (AB+, HID+) and nonsulfated (AB+, HID−) acidic glycoconjugates. While the mucous cell is usually the predominant secretory cell in the trachea, for some species this is not the case (Table 3.2). In species in which the Clara or serous cell is the predominant secretory cell, the majority of the secretory product is a neutral glycoconjugate. In species in which mucous goblet cells are the predominant secretory cell type, the majority of the secretory product is

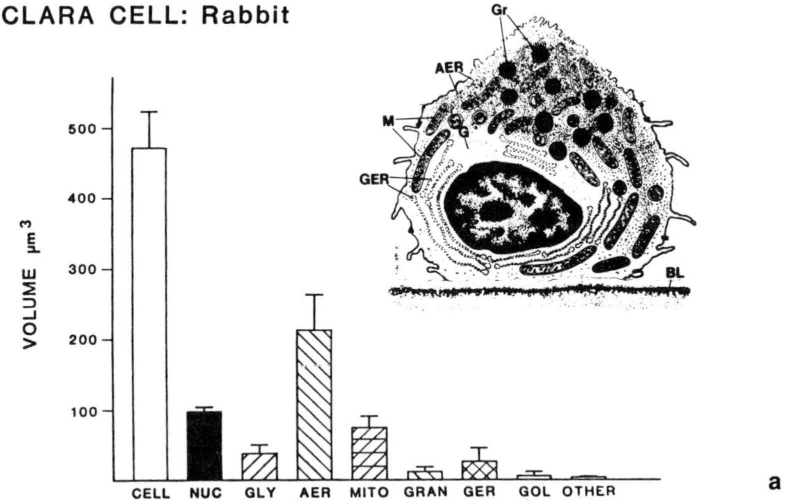

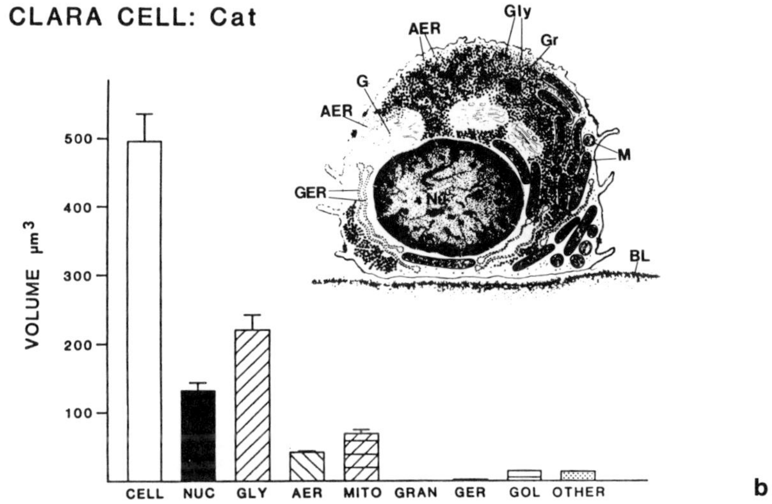

Fig. 3.6a-c. Morphometric comparison of the volumes of cellular components in the Clara cells of three species: **a** rabbit, **b** cat, **c** bonnet monkey, NUC, nucleus; GLY, glycogen; AER, agranular endoplasmic reticulum; MITO, mitochondria; GRAN, secretory granules; GER, granular endoplasmic reticulum; GOL, Golgi apparatus; OTHER, other components and hyaloplasm. For details, see ref. 29.

an acidic glycoconjugate. In some species, such as the rhesus monkey, all the secretory cells contain an acidic sulfated glycoconjugate. In other species, such as the sheep, some mucous goblet cells contain sulfated glycoconjugates and others contain sialoglycoconjugates. As Table 3.3 demonstrates, there is considerable variability in glycoconjugate composition in the submucosal glands. In serous cells the secretory product is neutral, and in mucous cells it is either a sialo- or a sulfomucin.

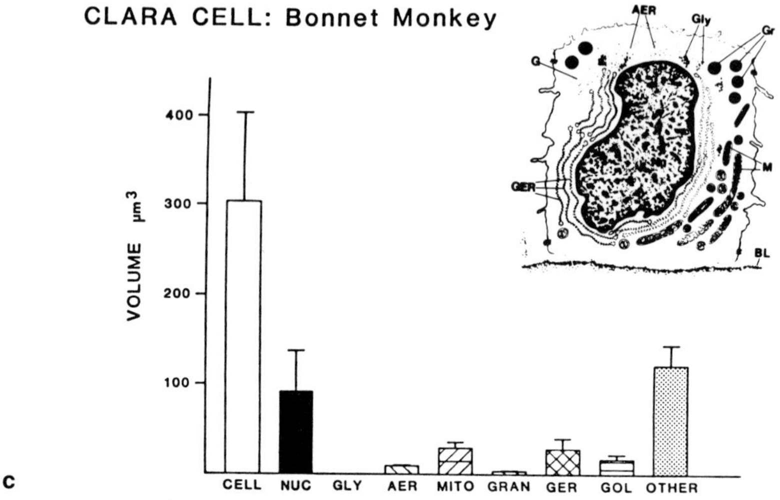

Fig. 3.6. (*Continued*)

Table 3.2. Comparison of carbohydrate content of tracheal epithelium

Species	Cell type	Abundance	Carbohydrate content		
			PAS	AB	HID
Hamster (36)	Clara	+++	+	−	−
Rat (38)	Serous	+++	+	−	−
	Mucous	+	+	+	−
Rabbit (35)	Mucous	+	+	+	+
	Clara	+++	+/−	−	−
Sheep	Mucous	++	+	+	+ and −
Rhesus (34)	Mucous	++	+	+	+
Human (33)	Mucous	+++	+	+	+ and −

Table 3.3. Comparison of carbohydrate content of tracheal submucosal glands

Species	Abundance	Secretory cell	Carbohydrate content		
			PAS	AB	HID
Hamster[a]	?	?	?	?	?
Rat (35)	+	Serous	+	−	−
		Mucous	+	+	+
Rabbit	+/−	Mucous	+	+	+
Sheep	++	Serous	+	−	−
		Mucous	+	+	+
Rhesus (37)	++	Serous	+	−	−
		Mucous	+	+	+
Human (33)	+++	Serous	+	−	−
		Mucous	+	+	+ and −

[a] No submucosal glands described for hamsters.

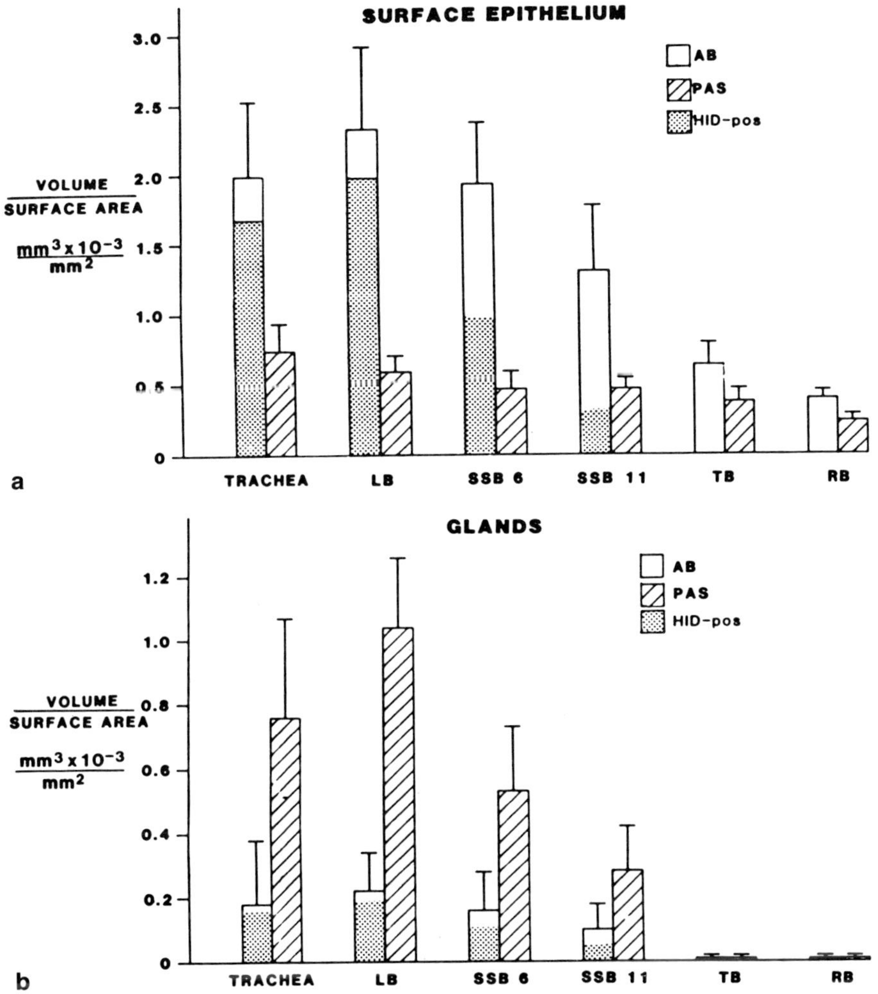

Fig. 3.7a,b. Morphometric comparison of the volume of stored secretory product per unit basal lamina in the tracheobronchial tree of the rhesus monkey: **a** surface lining epithelium, **b** submucosal glands. LB, lobar bronchus; SSB6, 6th generation intrapulmonary bronchus; SSB11, 11th generation intrapulmonary bronchus; TB, terminal bronchial; RB, respiratory bronchial. For details, see ref. 14.

Quantitation

Not only may the glycoconjugate composition of the secretory cells of one airway, such as the trachea, vary between species, but the type and relative abundance of glycoconjugates can vary between airway levels in the same species. Computerized morphometric assessment of the volume of the secretory product per unit surface area demonstrates that there is considerable variation in the amount of glycoconjugate stored in airway epithelium of the rhesus monkey (Fig. 3.7). Not only is there a more than twofold difference in the amount of secretory material stored when comparing the trachea with terminal and respiratory bronchioles, but there is a difference in the type of product being stored (Fig. 3.7a). The product is predominantly sulfated in proximal airways and acidic nonsulfated in more distal airways. The amount of product stored in submucosal glands of the rhesus conducting airways shows the same degree of variability (Fig. 3.7b). However, our observations indicate the secretory product in the glands is predominantly a neutral glycoconjugate (Fig. 3.7b).

Conclusion

This comparative overview of tracheobronchial epithelial composition emphasizes the high degree of diversity found in different species of mammals. Epithelial populations of the tracheobronchial tree vary (a) in the same airway level in different species, (b) in different airway levels in the same species, (c) in types of cells present in all airways, (d) in the overall abundance of secretory product and number of cells, (e) in carbohydrate content of the secretory granule, (f) in the amount of stored secretory product, and (g) in the ultrastructural composition of the same cell type in different species.

It is unclear what impact this wide diversity in the tracheobronchial tree of different species will have on our ability to extrapolate findings from animal models to humans. Care must be taken when extrapolating information from experiments employing animal models to humans. This study emphasizes the need for careful selection of animal species for specific types of exposure and precise selection of the site for assessment of the reactivity within the lung. It should be emphasized that comparative inhalation toxicologic studies are still needed in order to assess how this diversity will affect the reaction of the respiratory system to the same environmental toxicant.

Acknowledgment. This work was supported in part by NIH Grants HL28978, ESO0628, and DRR00169.

References

1. Breeze RG, Wheeldon EB (1977) The cells of the pulmonary airways. Am Rev Respir Dis 161:705–777
2. Jeffery PK (1983) Morphologic features of airway surface epithelial cells and glands. Am Rev Respir Dis 128:S14–S20
3. Plopper CG (1983) Comparative morphologic features of bronchiolar epithelial cells: The Clara cell. Am Rev Respir Dis 128:S37–S41

4. Widdicombe JG, Pack RJ (1982) The Clara cell. Eur J Respir Dis 63:202–220
5. Plopper CG, Mariassy AT, Wilson DW, Alley JL, Nishio SJ, Nettesheim P (1983) Comparison of nonciliated tracheal epithelial cells in six mammalian species: Ultrastructural and population densities. Exp Lung Res 5:281–294
6. Mariassy AT, Plopper CG (1984) Tracheobronchial epithelium of the sheep: II. Ultrastructural and morphometric analysis of the epithelial secretory cell types. Anat Rec 209:523–534
7. Jeffery PK (1977) Structure and function of mucus-secreting cells of cat and goose airway epithelium. Ciba Found Symp 5–19
8. Plopper CG, Halsebo JE, Berger WJ, Sonstegard KS, Nettesheim PK (1983) Distribution of nonciliated bronchiolar epithelial (Clara) cells in intra- and extrapulmonary airways of the rabbit. Exp Lung Res 5:79–98
9. Reid L, Jones R (1979) Bronchial mucosal cells. Fed Proc 38:191–196
10. Wilson DW, Plopper CG, Hyde DM (1984) The tracheobronchial epithelium of the bonnet monkey: A quantitative ultrastructural study. Am J Anat 171:25–40
11. Pack RJ, Al-Ugaily LH, Morris G (1981) The cells of the tracheobronchial epithelium of the mouse: A quantitative light and electron microscopic study. J Anat 132: 71–84
12. Plopper CG, Mariassy AT, Lollini LO (1983) Structure as revealed by airway dissection: A comparison of mammalian lungs. Am Rev Respir Dis 128:S4–S7
13. Mariassy AT, Plopper CG (1983) Tracheobronchial epithelium of the sheep. I. Quantitative light microscopic study of epithelial cell abundance and distribution. Anat Rec 205:263–275
14. Heidsiek JG, Hyde DM, Plopper CG, St George JA (1985) Computerized quantitation of mucosubstances in pulmonary airways of rhesus monkeys. Am Rev Respir Dis 131:A386
15. Chang L-Y, Mercer R, Crapo JD (1986) Differential distribution of brush cells in rat lung. Anat Rec 216:49–54
16. Tyler WS (1983) Comparative subgross anatomy of lungs. Am Rev Respir Dis 128:S32–S36
17. Castleman WL, Dungworth DL, Tyler WS (1975) Intrapulmonary airway morphology in three species of monkeys: A correlated scanning and transmission electron microscopic study. Am J Anat 152:107–122
18. Tyler NK, Plopper CG (1985) Morphology of the distal conducting airways in rhesus monkey lungs. Anat Rec 211:295–303
19. Freeman G, Stephens R, Coffin D, Stara J (1973) Changes in dog's lungs after long-term exposure to ozone. Arch Environ Health 26:209–216
20. Hyde D, Orthoefer J, Lum H, Tyler WS, Dungworth DL (1978) Morphometric and morphologic evaluation of pulmonary lesions in beagle dogs chronically exposed to high ambient levels of air pollutants. Lab Invest 38:455–469
21. Hyde DM, Plopper CG, Weir AJ, Murnane RD, Warren DL, Last JA (1985) Peribronchiolar fibrosis in lungs of cats chronically exposed to diesel exhaust. Lab Invest 52:195–206
22. Plopper CG, Hyde DM, Weir AJ (1983) Centriacinar alterations in lungs of cats chronically exposed to diesel exhaust. Lab Invest 49:391–399
23. Clara M (1937) Zur histobiologie des bronchial Epithels. Z Mikrosk Anat Forsch 41:321–347
24. Hayak H. von (1960) *The human lung*. Hafner, New York

25. Hyde DM, Samuelson DA, Blakeney WH, Kosch PC (1979) A correlative light microscopy, transmission and scanning electron microscopy study of the ferret lung. Scan Electron Microsc 3:891–898
26. Plopper CG, Mariassy AT, Hill LH (1980) Ultrastructure of the nonciliated bronchiolar epithelial (Clara) cell of mammalian lung. II. A comparison of horse, steer, sheep, dog, cat. Exp Lung Res 1:155–169
27. Plopper CG, Mariassy AT, Hill LH (1980) Ultrastructure of the nonciliated bronchiolar epithelial (Clara) cell of mammalian lung. I. A comparison of rabbit, guinea pig, rat, hamster, mouse. Exp Lung Res 1:139–154
28. Plopper CG, Hill LH, Mariassy AT (1980) Comparative ultrastructure of the nonciliated bronchiolar epithelial (Clara) cell of mammalian lung. III. A study of man with comparison of 15 mammalian species. Exp Lung Res 1:171–180
29. Hyde DM, CG Plopper: Cell and organellar volumes of nonciliated bronchiolar cells of rabbits, cats and monkeys. Anat Rec 208:77A
30. Spicer SS, Schulte BA, Thomopoulos GN (1983) Histochemical properties of the respiratory tract epithelium in different species. Am Rev Respir Dis 128:S20–S25
31. Spicer SS, Mochizuki I, Setser ME, Martinez JR (1980) Complex carbohydrates of rat tracheobronchial surface epithelium visualized ultrastructurally. Am J Anat 158:93–109
32. Marsan C, Cava E, Lougnon J, Roujeau J (1978) Cytochemical and histochemical characterization of epithelial mucins in human bronchi. Acta Cytol (Baltimore) 22:562–565
33. Spicer S, Chakrin L, Wardell J Jr, Kendrick W (1971) Histochemistry of mucosubstances in the canine and human respiratory tract. Lab Invest 25:483–490
34. St. George JA, Nishio SJ, Plopper CG (1984) Carbohydrate cytochemistry of rhesus monkey tracheal epithelium. Anat Rec 210:293–302
35. Plopper CG, St. George JA, Nishio SJ, Etchison JR, Nettesheim P (1984) Carbohydrate cytochemistry of tracheobronchial airway epithelium of the rabbit. J Histochem Cytochem 32:209–218
36. Emura M, Mohr U (1975) Morphological studies on the development of tracheal epithelium in the Syrian golden hamster. I. Light microscopy. Versuchstierk 17:14
37. St. George JA, Nishio SJ, Cranz DL, Plopper CG (1986) Carbohydrate cytochemistry of rhesus monkey submucosal glands. Anat Rec 216:60–67
38. McCarthy C, Reid L (1964) Acid mucopolysaccharide in the bronchial tree in mouse and rat (sialomucin and sulphate). Q J Exp Physiol 49:81–84

CHAPTER 4

Comparative Metabolic Basis for the Disposition and Toxic Effects of Inhaled Materials

A.R. Dahl[1]

The purpose of this report is to review the metabolism of inhaled xenobiotic materials in the respiratory tract, to indicate when interspecies differences occur, and to suggest how these species differences in metabolism may affect the toxicity of inhaled materials.

Introduction

The fate of a portion of material that is inhaled may parallel the fate of material administered either intravenously or orally. Thus, a portion of the material deposited in the pulmonary region may diffuse into the blood and be transported via the blood first to the heart and from there throughout the body. This portion of the inhaled material shares the fate of intravenously administered material. On the other hand, inhaled material, especially particles, deposited in the nose or the upper airways of the lung may be transported by mucociliary clearance to the alimentary tract. From there its fate is identical to that of an orally administered dose of the same material. Both intravenous and oral routes of administration, therefore, to some degree represent valid models for inhalation exposure. In their simplest expression, however, both models overlook the contribution of xenobiotic metabolism within the respiratory tract to the fate of inhaled materials. This is an important oversight: inhaled material that is metabolized in the respiratory tract may have toxicity different from material cleared as the parent molecule. The unique toxic consequences of the inhalation route of exposure are derived, in large part, from the contribution of respiratory tract metabolism to the fate of inhaled materials.

Reactive metabolites may exert toxic effects not only on respiratory tract tissue, but on tissues to which they are transported. For instance, reactive metabolites formed in the lung may be transported to the heart via the circulation and may affect the cardiovascular system, or reactive metabolites that are formed in the airways of the lungs or in the nose may be transported via mucociliary clearance

[1]Inhalation Toxicology Research Institute, Lovelace Biomedical and Environmental Research Institute, P.O. Box 5890, Albuquerque, NM 87185-5890, USA.

to the alimentary tract, where they may exert toxic effects on the esophagus, forestomach, or other tissues of the alimentary tract. Thus, the tissues at risk to the effects of potentially toxic metabolites formed in the respiratory tract are different from those at risk from metabolites formed in the liver or other organs.

The importance of respiratory tract metabolism is evident when there are conflicting data from studies involving the toxicity of an inhaled vapor in two or more animal species. In many cases, the spectrum of tumors or other toxic effects will differ from species to species, or they may be present in one and totally absent in another. It is important to understand why these different toxic effects occur so that data obtained in animal studies can be interpreted and extrapolated with confidence to expected effects in humans. Often, the differences in toxic effects may be rooted in differences in the metabolic fate of the inhalant in the respiratory tract.

Deposition of Inhalants in the Respiratory Tract

Inhaled particles deposit to a substantial extent in both the nose and the lung (Fig. 4.1). The factors affecting particle deposition in various animal species have

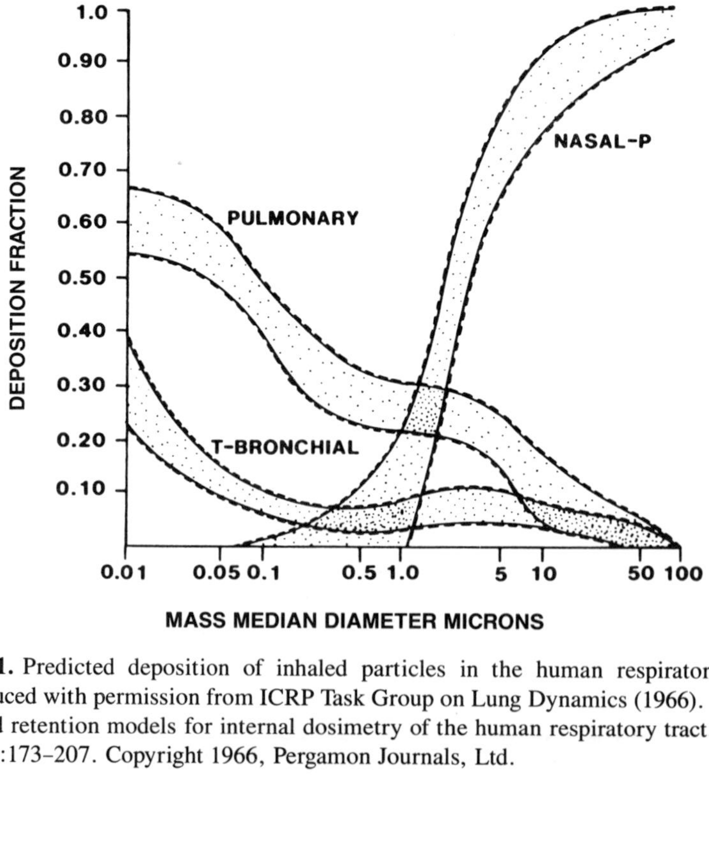

Fig. 4.1. Predicted deposition of inhaled particles in the human respiratory tract. Reproduced with permission from ICRP Task Group on Lung Dynamics (1966). Deposition and retention models for internal dosimetry of the human respiratory tract. Health Phys 12:173–207. Copyright 1966, Pergamon Journals, Ltd.

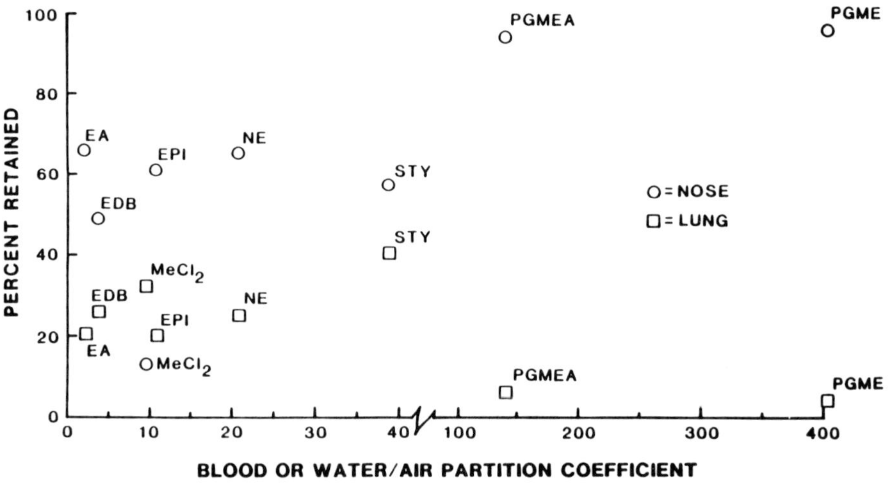

Fig. 4.2. Nasal and lung contributions to uptake of inhaled vapors as a function of blood or water/air partition coefficients. (Adapted from ref. 3.)

been the subject of considerable research (1,2) and will not be discussed here; this section will be concerned with the factors affecting uptake of vapors in the respiratory tract.

Inhaled vapors, even those with relatively high volatility and low water solubility, may be largely absorbed in the nasal cavity rather than in the lungs, although lung uptake may also be substantial (3) (Fig. 4.2). The deposition of vapors in the respiratory tract may differ among animal species (4). The initial deposition of vapors is greater in the anterior part of the nose than in the posterior area where the olfactory mucosa occurs (5). Unless they are highly reactive with tissue, however, most vapors reentrain in the air stream after initial deposition. Unless deposited molecules are removed by uncatalyzed reaction, metabolism, or absorption into the blood, successive reentrainments of deposited vapor molecules result in movement toward the gas exchange regions of the lung. For inhalation of many irritant vapors, however, it is the nose, particularly the anterior part, that is most prone to toxic effects (6). Thus, toxic effects are more often related to the deposition of vapors than to the intrinsic sensitivity of the target tissue, since the olfactory tissue at the back of the nasal cavity is more sensitive than tissue in the anterior part of the nose (7–10).

Metabolic activating capacity presents a third aspect governing toxicity, in addition to deposition and intrinsic tissue sensitivity. For example, inhalation of the water-soluble procarcinogen dimethylnitrosamine causes tumors from cells originating in the olfactory tissue (11), where, as discussed later, the preponderance of the activating enzymes occur.

Inhaled vapors provide substantial amounts of substrate to activating enzymes in all tissues of the respiratory tract. Similar results are obtained for inhaled particles (1,2). Thus, inhalation of both vapors and particles provides substantial substrate for xenobiotic metabolizing enzymes in both nasal and lung tissues. As

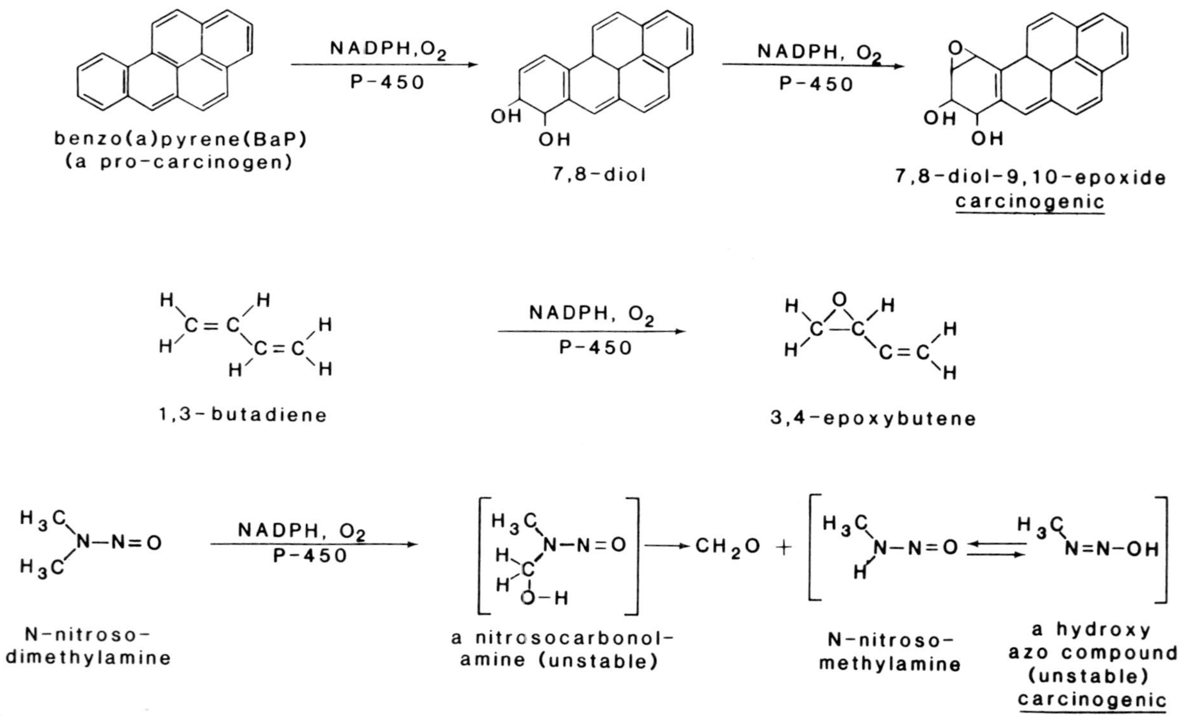

Fig. 4.3. Some cytochrome P_{450}-catalyzed reactions that occur in the respiratory tract: BaP (50), butadiene (51), nitrosamines (19).

alluded to in the case of dimethylnitrosamine, metabolism in these tissues may have important effects on the toxicity of inhalants.

Respiratory Tract Xenobiotic Metabolism

Phase I Enzymes

Monooxygenases

The monooxygenases include the cytochromes P_{450} and the flavin-containing monooxygenases. A wide variety of chemical reactions are catalyzed by these enzymes (Figs. 4.3,4.4). The cytochrome P_{450}-catalyzed oxidation of benzo(*a*)-pyrene (BaP) leads to , among other products, benzo(*a*)pyrene-7,8-epoxide. This is hydrolyzed to the 7,8-diol which, in turn, is recycled through the cytochrome P_{450} system to yield the 7,8-diol-9,10-epoxide, an ultimate carcinogen. The metabolism of BaP illustrates an important principle: often it is not the inhaled compound which is the toxicant, but a metabolite. BaP is metabolized to toxic products in the nasal cavity of the Syrian hamster (12), in the isolated perfused lung of rats (13), and by tracheal and bronchial tissue of a number of species (14).

Butadiene is a common industrial chemical used in the rubber industry. In chronic toxicity tests it has been shown to cause cancer in rats and mice (15,16). Oxidation of butadiene by cytochrome P_{450} results in the genotoxic monoepoxide

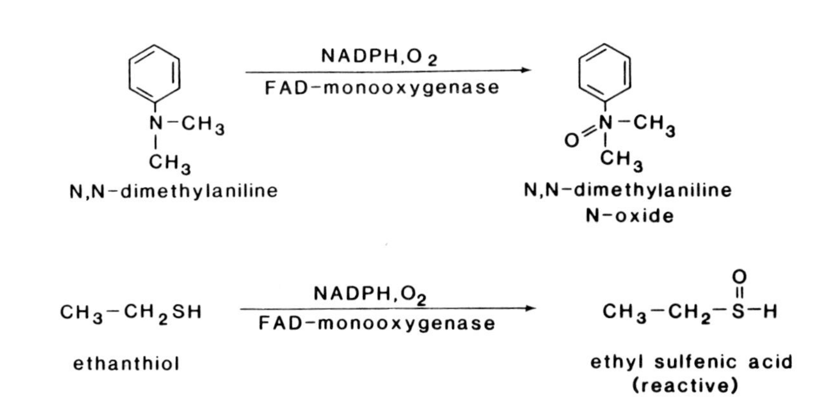

Fig. 4.4. Some reactions catalyzed by cytochrome P_{450} and FAD-monooxygenase (42).

(Fig. 4.3). It is further metabolized to the diepoxide which is also genotoxic (17). Metabolism of butadiene occurs in lung tissue (18).

Nitrosamines are common environmental carcinogens that require metabolic activation (19). The metabolism of nitrosamines is illustrated by dimethylnitrosamine which, through the intermediacy of a nitrosocarbonolamine, is metabolized to *N*-nitrosomethylamine in equilibrium with a diazo compound, the putative genotoxin (Fig. 4.3). The nitrosamines are interesting because they are often respiratory tract carcinogens (19). The tissues of the nasal cavity are particularly susceptible to nitrosamine-caused tumors (20). This susceptibility corresponds well with the high metabolic activity of nasal tissue towards nitrosamines (21–24).

Flavin-containing monooxygenase (FAD-MO) is the second major monooxygenase responsible for xenobiotic metabolism. It occurs in both nasal and lung tissues (25–27). Flavin-containing monooxygenase typically oxidizes at a heteroatom rather than at a carbon atom. This is illustrated for *N,N*-dimethylaniline and further illustrated for ethanthiol (Fig. 4.4). *N,N*-Dimethylaniline is metabolized by cytochrome P_{450} to an unstable carbonolamine which spontaneously decomposes to *N*-methylaniline and formaldehyde (Fig. 4.4). The same substrate may be metabolized by the FAD-MO. In this case, however, the product is *N,N*-dimethylaniline *N*-oxide (Fig. 4.4). These equations illustrate an important point: a compound may be a substrate for more than one enzyme.

Not only can a given compound be a substrate for more than one enzyme, but often a given substrate may be metabolized by respiratory tract enzymes to a

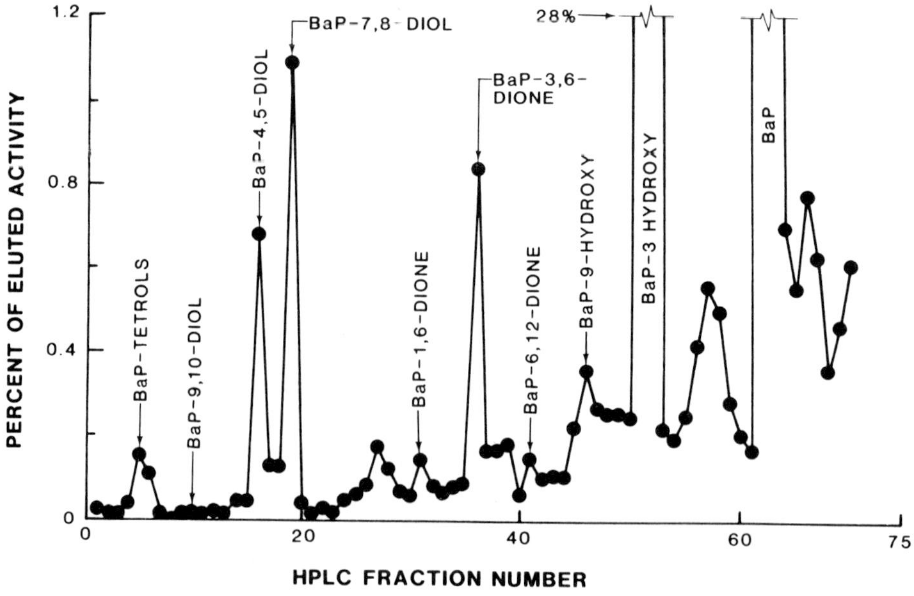

Fig. 4.5. HPLC profile of BaP metabolites from hamster nasal metabolism (12).

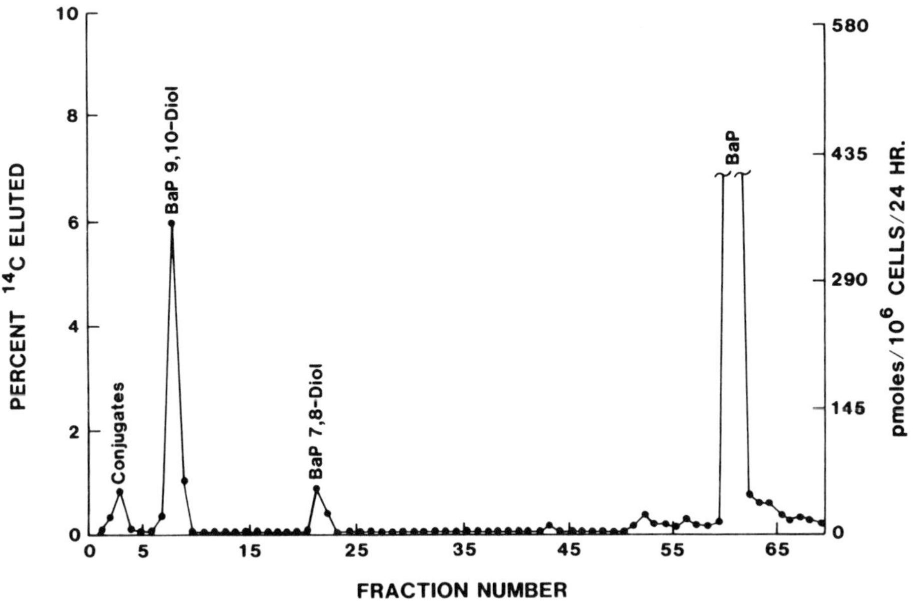

Fig. 4.6. HPLC profile of BaP metabolites from hamster nasal metabolism (52).

variety of products. For example, many metabolites result from metabolism of BaP placed on the nasal mucosa of the Syrian hamster (Fig. 4.5). Among the metabolites are BaP-7,8-diol, a precursor of the BaP-7,8-diol-9,10-epoxide, an ultimate carcinogen (Fig. 4.3). Although metabolism of BaP in the Syrian hamster nasal cavity leads to a complex spectrum of metabolites, rat lung epithelial cells metabolize BaP to relatively few products (Fig. 4.6). Still included among the metabolites, however, is the BaP-7,8-diol which may be further metabolized to a carcinogenic product (see Fig. 4.3).

The concentrations of cytochrome P_{450} present in the various portions of the respiratory tract vary among animal species (Fig. 4.7). Of particular interest is the finding that human lung has relatively little cytochrome P_{450} compared to human liver. (Nasal enzymes in man have not been measured.) In humans there is, however, considerable individual variability in the amount and types of cytochromes P_{450} present (28). Both the hamster and the rabbit have high concentrations of nasal cytochromes P_{450} relative to the liver. Except in the mouse, the lungs in all species tested have less cytochrome P_{450} per milligram microsomal protein than do the nasal cavity or the liver (Fig. 4.7).

The capacity of respiratory tract tissues to metabolize xenobiotics varies among animal species (29). The metabolism of aniline to parahydroxyaniline, for example, proceeds much more rapidly in the nasal tissue of the Syrian hamster than in nasal, lung, or liver tissue of other species (Fig. 4.8). Aniline hydroxylation is especially well catalyzed in rabbits by an isozyme of cytochrome P_{450}

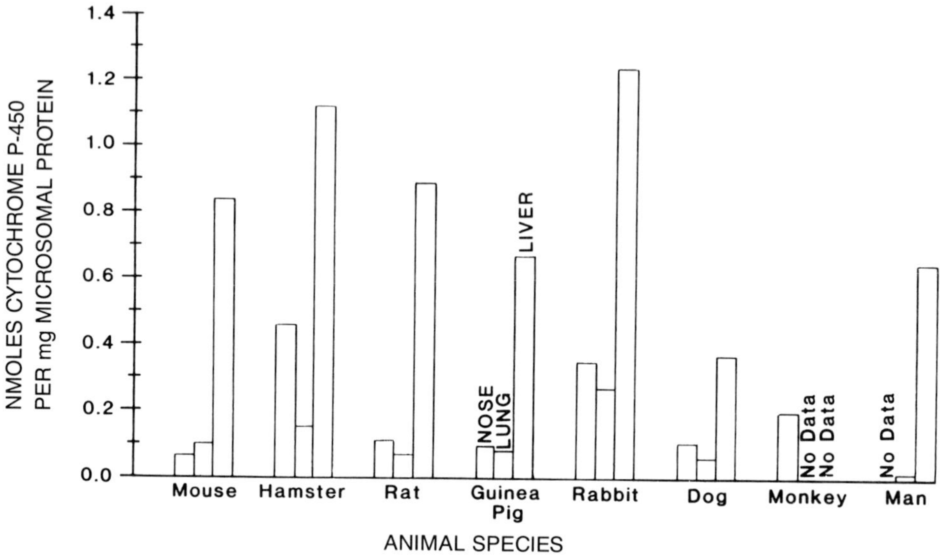

Fig. 4.7. Comparative microsomal concentrations of cytochrome P_{450} in liver, nose, and lung of eight species (20,28,29).

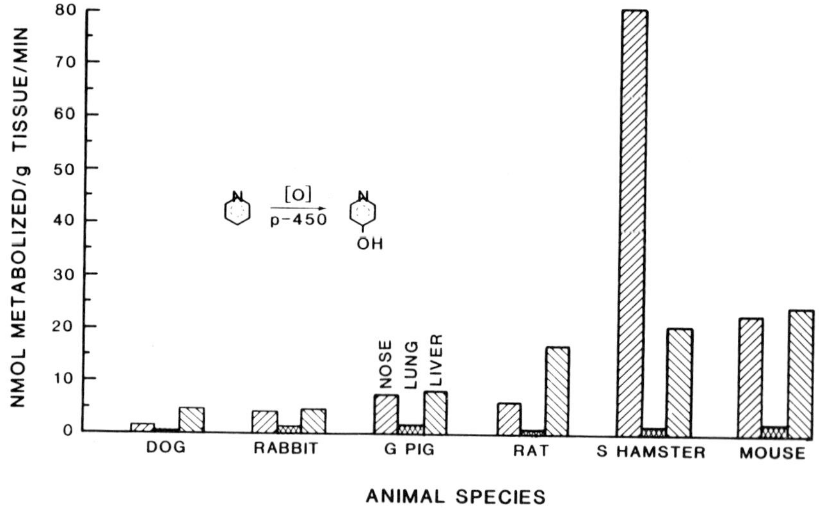

Fig. 4.8. Aniline hydroxylase in noses, lungs, and livers of six species (29).

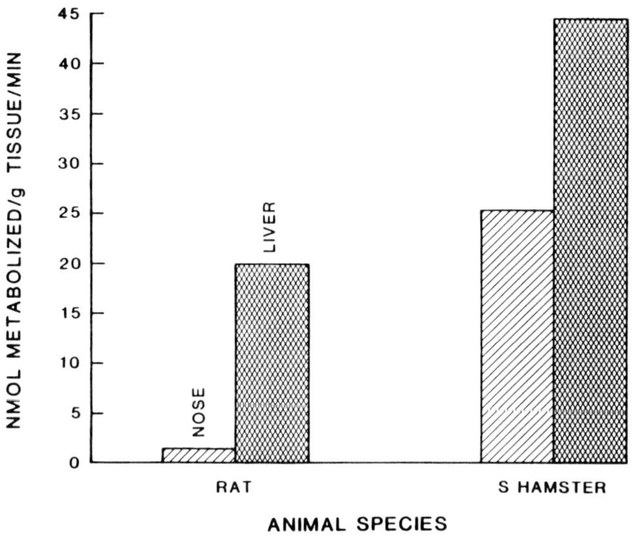

Fig. 4.9. Diethylinitrosamine *N*-deethylase in rat and hamster nasal tissue and liver (24).

termed P_{450} LM3a (30). This isozyme is inducible by ethanol and is associated not only with the metabolism of aniline but also with the metabolism of alcohols to aldehydes (30) and with the metabolism of nitrosamines (22). Cytochrome P_{450} LM3a is an important constitutive enzyme in rabbit nasal mucosa (31).

Isozymes with substrate specificities similar to those of P_{450} LM3a are, apparently, present in the nasal cavities of many species. The aniline hydroxylase activity is relatively high in most species examined (Fig. 4.8). The relative ratios of activities between rat and hamster tissues found for aniline hydroxylase activity are also found for diethylnitrosamine *N*-deethylase activity (Fig. 4.9). The nasal tissue capacity to metabolize diethylnitrosamine correlates directly with the susceptibility of rats and hamsters to diethylnitrosamine-induced nasal tumors (24).

One cannot generalize on the rate of production of potentially toxic metabolites in a tissue based solely upon cytochrome P_{450} content. Predictions of metabolism rates for different substrates should be viewed with caution because the rate of formation of potentially toxic metabolites varies among tissues and also depends on the substrate examined. For instance, the rates of metabolism for BaP and nitropyrene by rat lung, liver, and nasal microsomes are highly variable. BaP is poorly metabolized in both respiratory tract tissues but well metabolized by the liver. Nitropyrene, in contrast, is metabolized best by nasal tissue, liver tissue metabolism is nearly the same as that of nasal tissue, and lung tissue metabolism comes in a distant third to the other two (Fig. 4.10).

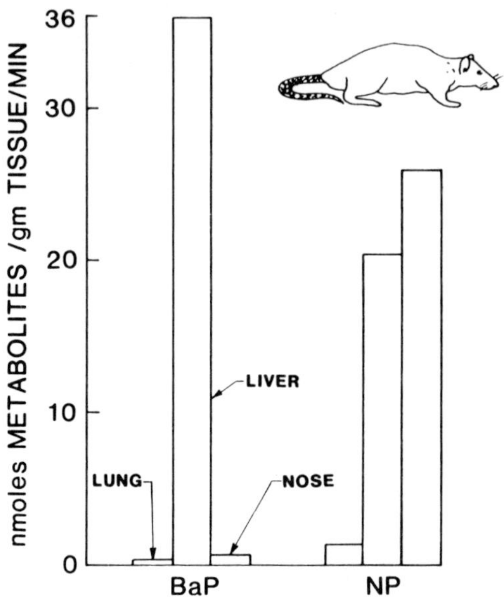

Fig. 4.10. The rates of metabolism of BaP and nitropyrene (*NP*) in lung, liver, and nose of rats (37,53).

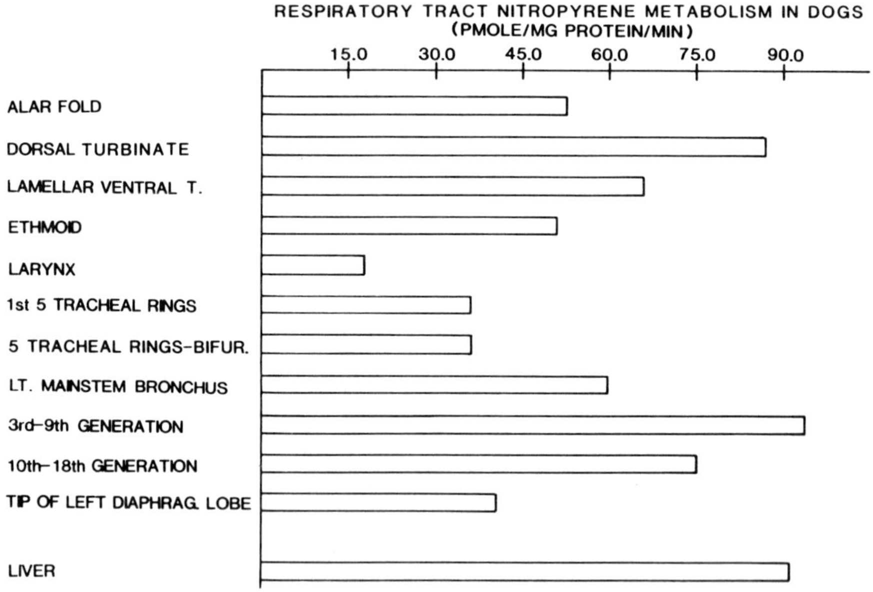

Fig. 4.11. Metabolism of nitropyrene in discrete parts of the dog respiratory tract (J.A. Bond, personal communication.)

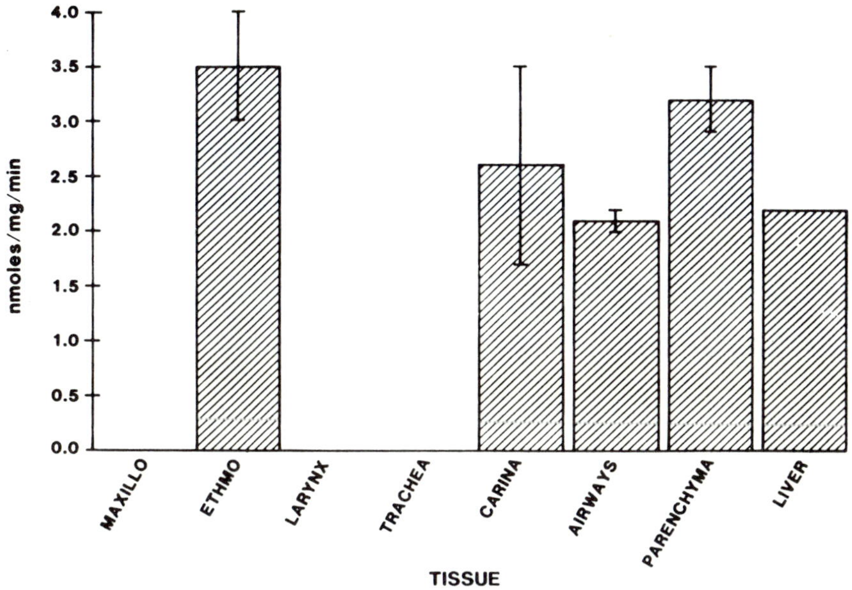

Fig. 4.12. Distribution of FAD-containing monooxygenase in discrete parts of the respiratory tract (25).

Discrete regions of the nasal cavity and the lungs have been examined for enzyme activity (Fig. 4.11). All regions of the nasal cavity have considerable metabolic activity towards nitropyrene. The activity is high in the dorsal turbinate and then decreases as one proceeds to the larynx. Proceeding from the larynx to the bronchi, where P_{450}-containing Clara cells occur (32,33), there is increased metabolic capacity. FAD-MO distribution in the respiratory tract is similar to the distribution of cytochrome P_{450} (Fig. 4.12).

Dehydrogenases and Hydrolases

The dehydrogenases and hydrolases include alcohol and aldehyde dehydrogenases, carboxylesterases, and epoxide hydrolases. Each of these enzymes is found in the respiratory tract (34–38). Comparison of reactions catalyzed by some of these enzymes shows how different compounds can be metabolized to the same products and, hence, may exhibit the same toxicities (Fig. 4.13). Thus, ethanol is metabolized by alcohol dehydrogenase to acetaldehyde. Acetaldehyde, in turn, is metabolized by aldehyde dehydrogenase to acetic acid. On the other hand, vinyl acetate can be metabolized by completely different enzymes, carboxyl esterases, to acetic acid and the unstable intermediate, vinyl alcohol, which rearranges to acetaldehyde (39). This acetaldehyde can be further metabolized by aldehyde dehydrogenase to acetic acid. Thus, acetaldehyde and acetic

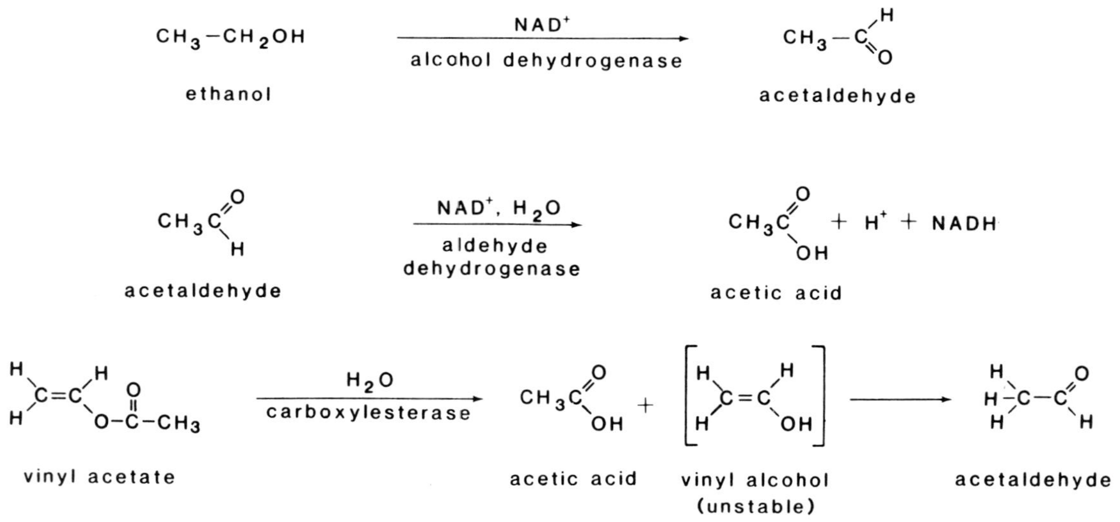

Fig. 4.13. Comparison of products of metabolism of ethanol and vinyl acetate (39,42).

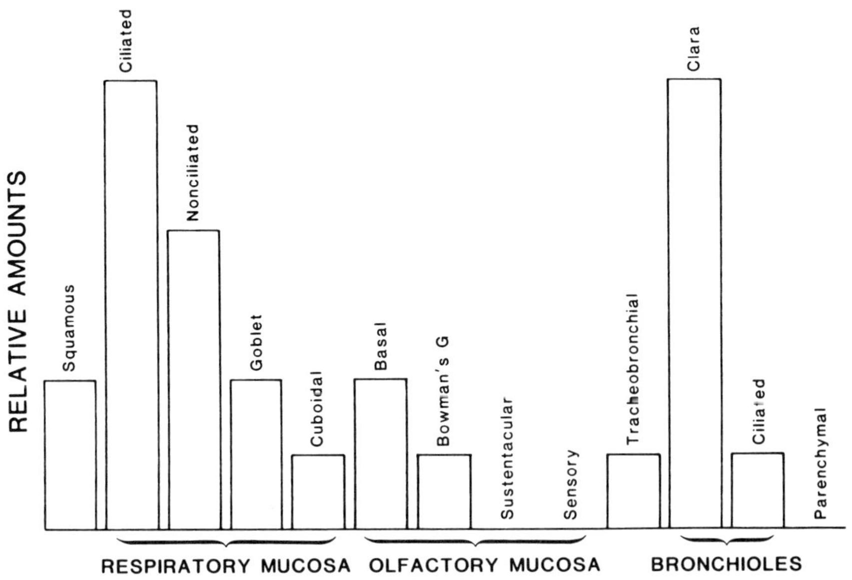

Fig. 4.14. Cellular distribution of aldehyde dehydrogenase in rat respiratory tract cells (34).

acid arising as metabolites from entirely different molecules, could lead to similar toxic responses.

Aldehyde dehydrogenase is not uniformly distributed among the cells of the rat respiratory tract (Fig. 4.14). The ciliated cells of the nasal respiratory mucosa have high levels of aldehyde dehydrogenase activity, whereas the cells of the olfactory mucosa, including Bowman's gland cells and basal cells, have less activity. This is a reversal of the usual order for enzyme distribution in the nasal cavity: for most enzymes, the olfactory mucosa has higher activity than does the respiratory mucosa (40). Descending towards the lungs, a familiar pattern recurs: low concentrations of the xenobiotic metabolizing enzyme in the anterior tracheobronchial tree, and high concentrations in the lower airways, especially in the Clara cells. Interestingly, the nonciliated Clara cells in the lungs have high levels of aldehyde dehydrogenase activity, whereas high levels are associated with ciliated cells in the nasal respiratory epithelium.

The capacity of the tissues of the respiratory tract to metabolize esters to carboxylic acids and alcohols or phenols varies with the ester to be hydrolyzed. In rabbit maxillo-or ethmoturbinate tissue, β-butyrolactone is more readily metabolized than is amyl acetate. Phenyl acetate under the same conditions, however, is more than twice as good a substrate for the nasal tissues than is the potential carcinogen β-butyrolactone (Fig. 4.15).

In the rabbit, the ethmoturbinates have higher capacity to metabolize β-butyrolactone than do the tissues from the liver or the maxilloturbinates. These

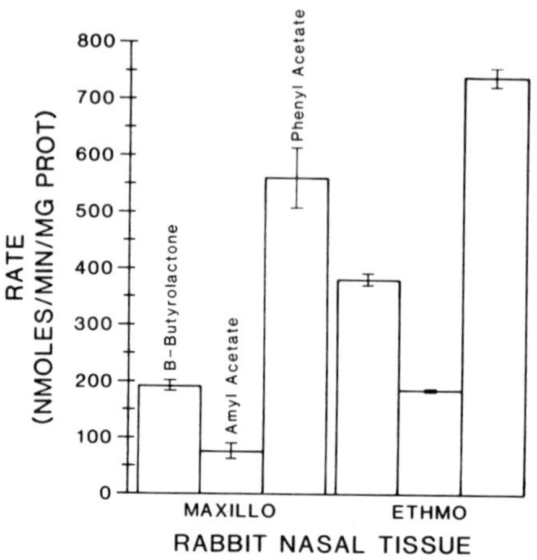

Fig. 4.15. Rates of hydrolysis of β-butyrolactone, amyl acetate, and phenyl acetate by rabbit nasal carboxylesterase (36).

tissues, in turn, have considerably higher activities than do trachea and lung tissues (Fig. 4.16). In rats, on the other hand, activities for maxillo- and ethmoturbinates are about equal to each other and both have higher activities than trachea and lung tissue but lower activities than liver tissue (see Fig. 4.16). The Syrian hamster tissues exhibit a distribution pattern for β-butyrolactonase activity similar to that of rabbit tissues. For the carboxylesterase activities, therefore, there seems to be high variability among tissues, among substrates, and among animal species, so that generalizations cannot be made.

Phase II Enzymes (Transferases) and Epoxide Hydrolase

The phase I enzyme, epoxide hydrolase, is included in this section along with the phase II transferases to illustrate competition for substrate between phase I and phase II enzymes. Styrene oxide is a substrate both for epoxide hydrolase and glutathione transferase (Fig. 4.17). Reaction catalyzed by either of these enzymes probably results in detoxification of the substrate. Metabolites of epoxide hydrolases, which occur in both lung (38) and nasal tissue (37), are virtually always less toxic than epoxides, all of which are reactive compounds. In some cases, however, as illustrated for BaP metabolism (see Fig. 4.3), the resulting diol may be a precursor for an ultimate carcinogen. Thus, epoxide hydrolase may figure obliquely in the chain of events that produces the ultimate toxicant. Glutathione transferase metabolism, on the other hand, can lead directly to toxic products. Thus, the nasal carcinogen, dibromoethane, is metabolized by glutathione transferase to a conjugate that spontaneously loses a bromide ion to form a carcinogenic episulfonium ion (41) (see Fig. 4.17).

Glutathione transferase occurs in the nasal cavity (37), as well as in the lung (38). A second transferase that has been demonstrated in both the nasal cavity (37) and the lung (38) is UDP-glucuronyl transferase (see Fig. 4.17). Products of

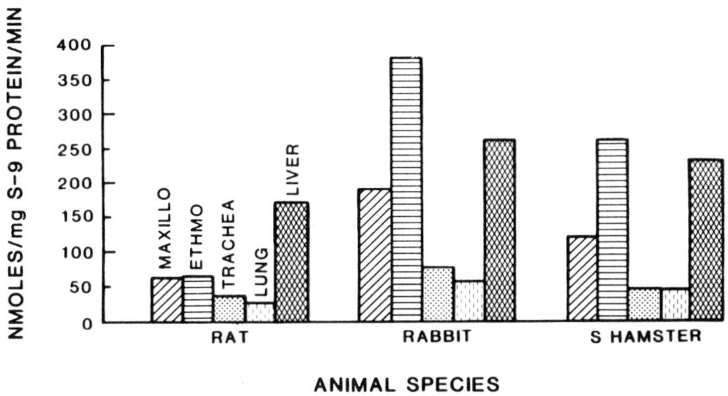

Fig. 4.16. Comparison of hydrolysis rates of β-butyrolactone in rat, rabbit, and hamster respiratory tract tissues and liver (36).

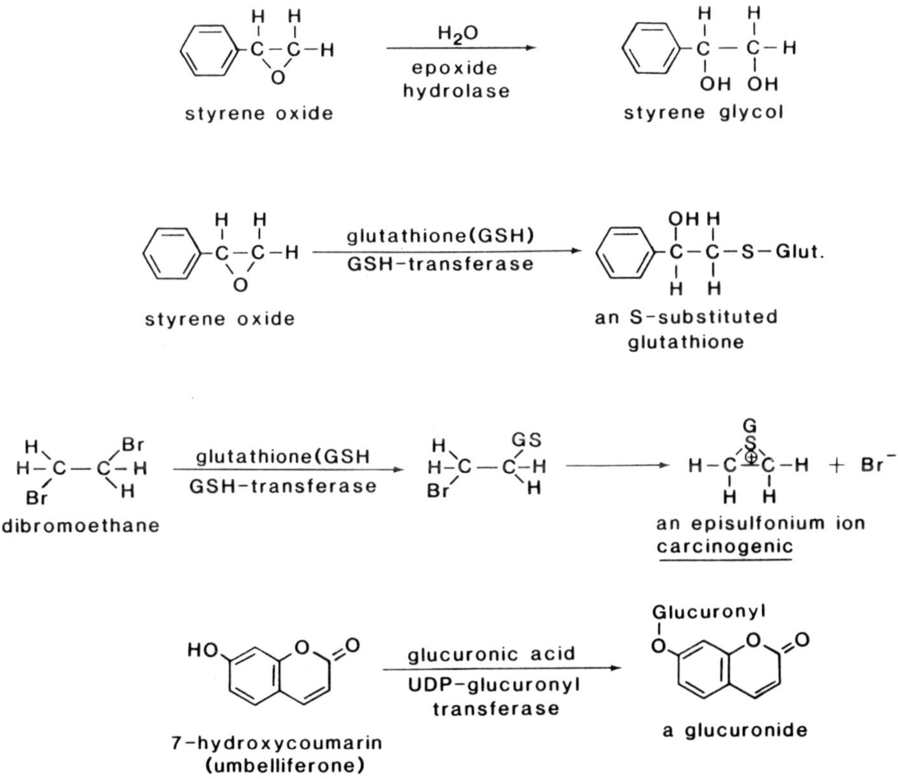

Fig. 4.17. Some reactions catalyzed by epoxide hydrolase, glutathione transferase and UDP-glucuronyl transferase (42).

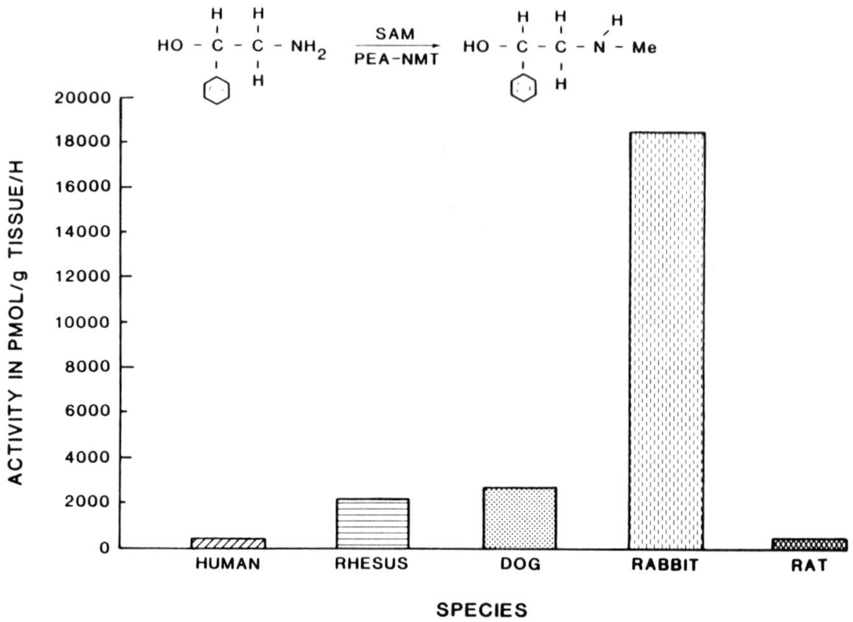

Fig. 4.18. Phenylethanolamine *N*-methyl transferase in lungs of five species (43).

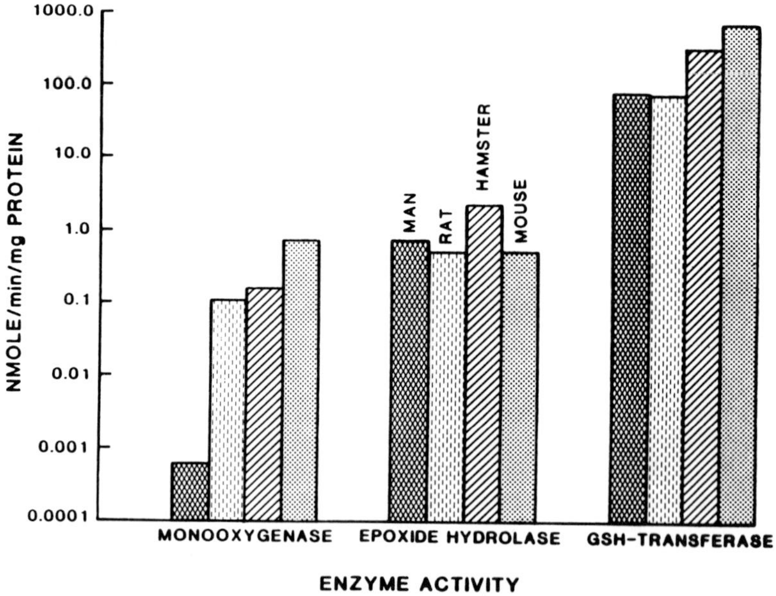

Fig. 4.19. Comparison of 7-ethoxycoumarin monooxygenase, benzo[*a*]pyrene epoxide hydrolase, and 2,4-dinitrochlorobenzene glutathione *S*-transferase activities in lung tissues of man, rat, hamster and mouse.

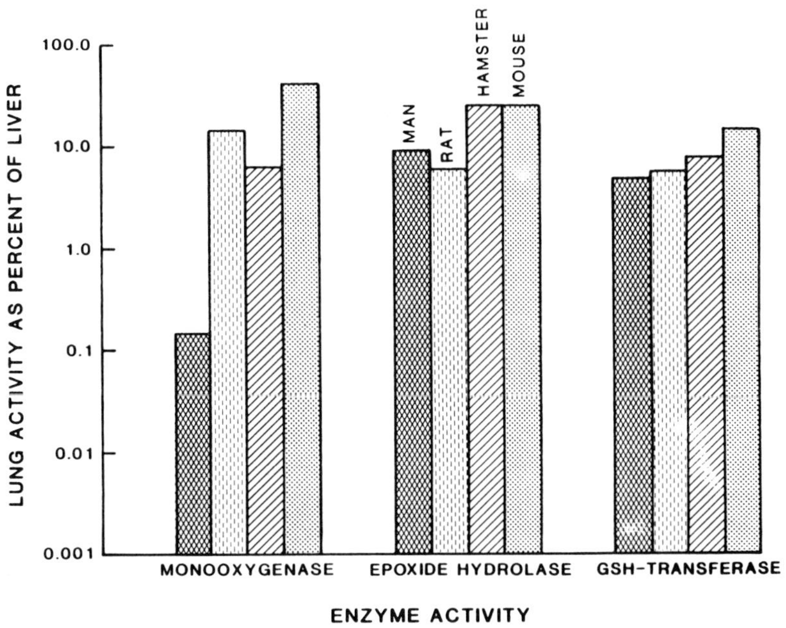

Fig. 4.20. Comparison of lung and liver activities of 7-ethoxycoumarin monooxygenase, benzo[*a*]pyrene epoxide hydrolase, and 2,4-dinitrochlorobenzene glutathione *S*-transferases in four species (54).

metabolism catalyzed by this enzyme are almost always less toxic than the substrate molecule.

N-Methyltransferase is an enzyme that catalyzes the transfer of a methyl group from *S*-adenosyl-L-methionine to carbon-bonded nitrogen atoms (42). Its role in the metabolism of xenobiotics is rarely considered with regard to the fate of inhalants. It may, however, play a significant role, along with similar enzymes that catalyze methylation of oxygen and sulfur heteroatoms. The enzyme is found, in highly variable concentrations, in the lungs of a variety of species, including humans (Fig. 4.18) (43).

It is instructive to compare a typical activating enzyme to enzymes that usually detoxify their substrates. In human lung tissue, the detoxifying enzymes—epoxide hydrolase and glutathione transferase—are both present in higher amounts than the activating enzyme activity cytochrome P_{450}-dependent 7-ethoxycoumarin deethylase (Fig. 4.19). Similar favorable ratios occur for glutathione transferase in rats, hamsters, and mice (Fig. 4.19). The favorable ratios do not, however, guarantee that all toxic products are harmlessly detoxified. A fraction of them may encounter and react with critical cell proteins or DNA before encountering a detoxifying enzyme, no matter how high the concentration of detoxifying enzyme may be.

The ratio of the capacity of the lung to metabolize xenobiotics to the capacity of the liver may vary greatly among animal species (Fig. 4.20). Humans, in particular, have relatively little monooxygenase activity towards 7-ethoxycoumarin in the lung contrasted to the liver. It is important to bear in mind, however, that some lung cell types (for instance, the Clara cells) may have enhanced metabolic capacity (32,33). Moreover, different substrates may present a substantially different picture.

The tissue levels of activating and deactivating xenobiotic metabolizing enzymes towards a specific substrate may vary among different animal species. The metabolism of the rodent carcinogen, butadiene, by cytochrome P_{450} has been discussed (see Fig. 4.3). Its metabolism to the monoepoxide is catalyzed by rat and mouse lung tissue. This activity was not detected, however, in monkey or human lung tissue (Fig. 4.21). Epoxide hydrolase hydrolyzes butadiene oxide to the diol, which is presumably less toxic. This enzyme activity occurs in fairly similar concentrations in mouse, rat, monkey, and human lung tissue (see Fig. 4.21). Both mice and rats are susceptible to cancers from inhaled butadiene (15,16), but the information shown in Fig. 4.21 indicates that monkeys and people may be less susceptible to the toxic effects of butadiene than are the laboratory rodents.

Induction and Inhibition of Respiratory Tract Xenobiotic Metabolizing Enzymes

Lung cytochromes P_{450} are inducible (44). For example, the capacity of lung microsomes to metabolize nitropyrene (NP) is significantly enhanced by pretreatment with 3-methylcholanthrene (Fig. 4.22). In contrast, phenobarbitol, an inducer of some liver cytochromes P_{450}, is not an effective inducer of lung cytochrome P_{450}-dependent NP-hydroxylase (45).

Nasal P_{450} is more difficult to induce than is lung P_{450}, although induction has been observed (37,46). Nasal cytochromes P_{450}, however, are inhibited by low concentrations of methylenedioxyphenyl (MDP) compounds such as isosafrole (Fig. 4.23). Thus, nasal cytochrome P_{450}-dependent hexamethylphosphoramide (HMPA) *N*-demethylase is over 50% inhibited by 5 micromolar isosafrole. This concentration of isosafrole barely affected the liver enzyme activity (see Fig. 4.23). MDP compounds are common in the environment, occurring in insecticide aerosols and in a large number of natural products (47).

Respiratory Tract Enzymes in the Ames Mutagenicity Test

The use of liver-derived S-9 homogenate as the activating enzyme source in the Ames test may not be entirely appropriate when one is examining the genotoxicity of inhalants. For example, the tobacco constituent *N*-nitrosopiperidine (NPIP) is activated to a genotoxin in the Ames test by rat nasal enzymes but not by rat

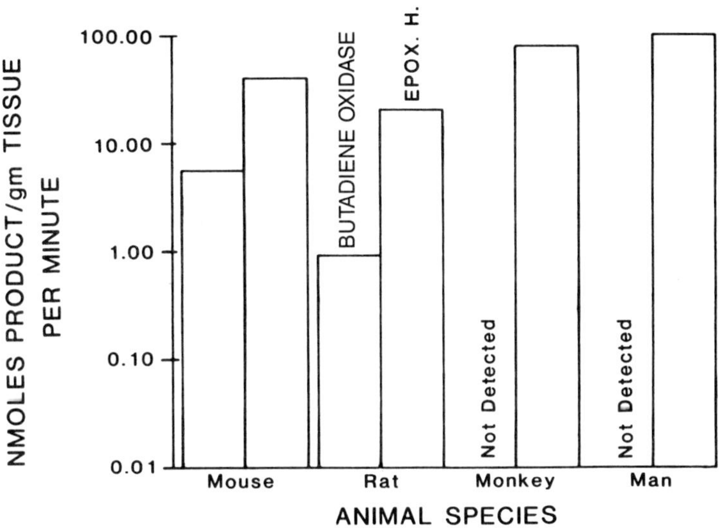

Fig. 4.21. Comparison of butadiene oxidase and epoxide hydrolase activities in the lungs of mice, rats, monkeys, and man (18).

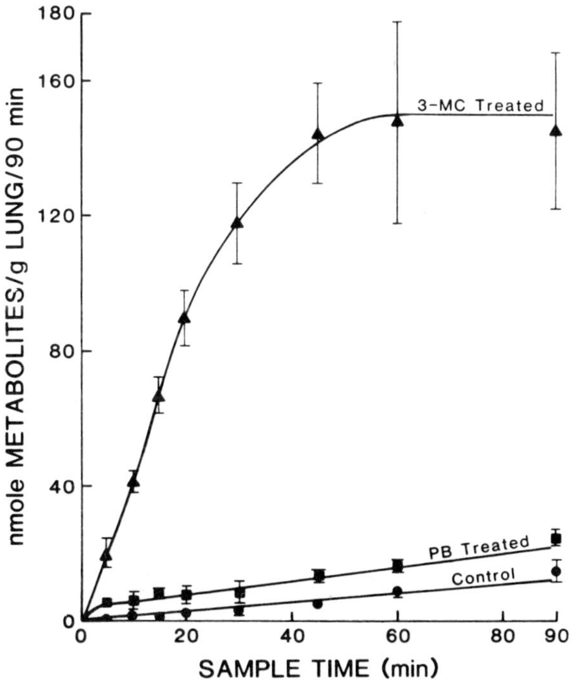

Fig. 4.22. Effect of pretreatment with cytochrome P_{450} inducers on the metabolism of 1-nitropyrene in the rat isolated perfused lung (45). 3-MC, 3-methylcholanthrene; PB, phenobarbitol.

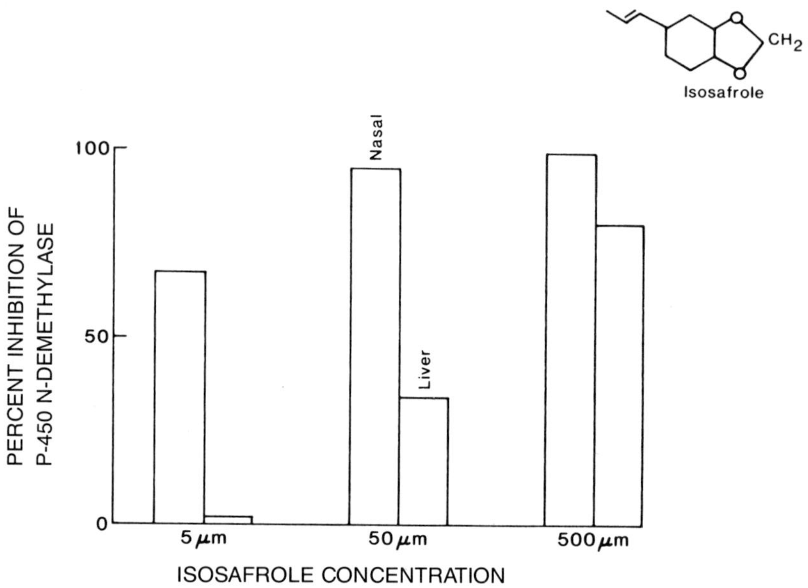

Fig. 4.23. The inhibition of rat nasal and liver cytochrome P_{450}-dependent *N*-demethylase by isosafrole (55).

liver- or lung-derived enzymes (Fig. 4.24). Thus, the use of liver enzymes may cause investigators to miss the potential genotoxicity of inhaled materials in the rat. On the other hand, in the rabbit, both nasal and lung S-9 homogenates, as well as that from liver, activate NPIP (see Fig. 4.24). This indicates that the rat and rabbit would exhibit different tissue susceptibilities to the genotoxic effects of this compound when inhaled. Activation of premutagens by nasal enzymes has been demonstrated for nitrosamines in addition to NPIP and for arylhydrocarbons (23,48).

Summary

All segments of the respiratory tract from the nasal cavity to the periphery of the pulmonary compartment contain enzymes that metabolize xenobiotic compounds. These enzymes are capable of metabolizing some inhaled xenobiotic compounds to products that are less toxic than the inhalant; but, in other cases, the metabolites may be more toxic than the parent molecule. The presence of these enzymes in the respiratory tract indicates that the distribution of potentially toxic metabolites of inhaled material may be different from the distribution after administration by other routes. Thus, the sites susceptible to toxic effects may be altered.

Respiratory tract enzymes can be inhibited or induced by materials administered either systemically or by inhalation. Induction or inhibition of these

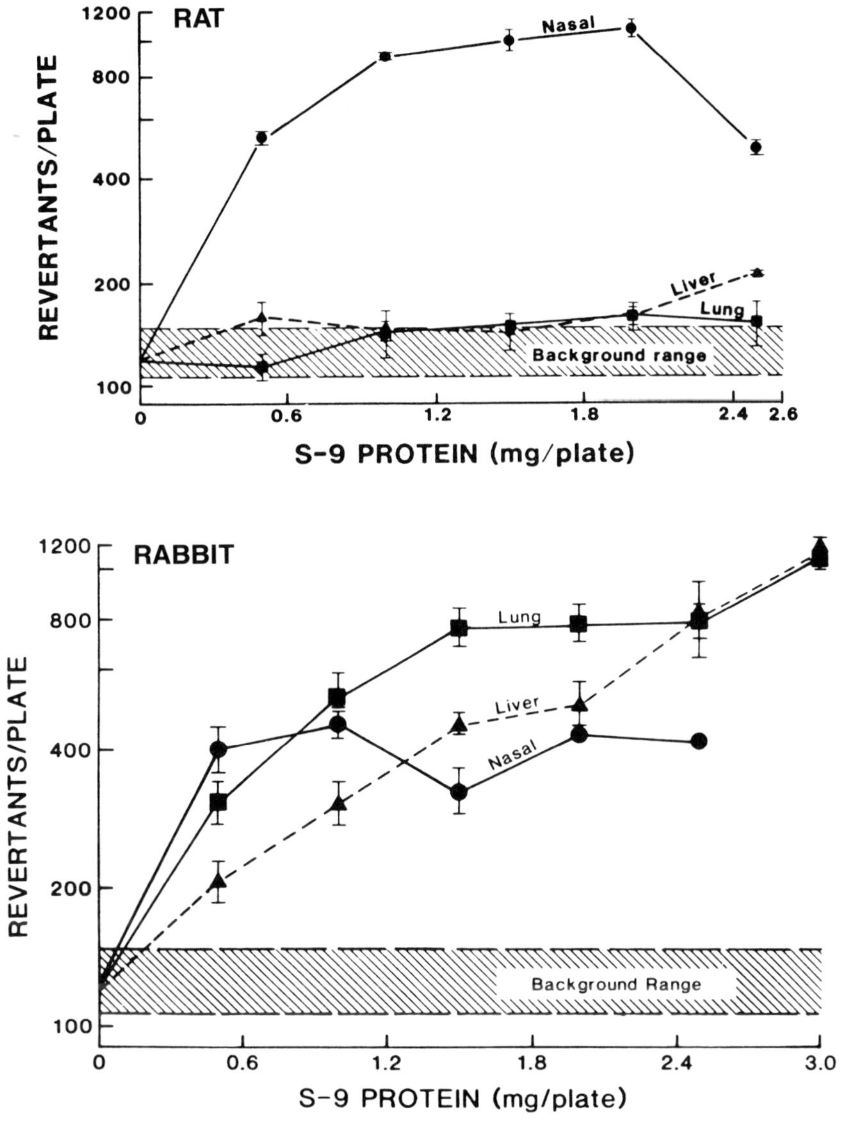

Fig. 4.24. The mutagenic response of TA-100 *Salmonella* to *N*-nitrosopiperidine activated by rat and rabbit nasal, lung, and liver S-9 tissue homogenate (23).

enzymes can alter the toxicity of inhalants. Thus, diet, preadministration of other materials, or the coadministration of a second inhalant may affect the toxicity of inhaled material.

Finally, in standard genotoxicity tests, respiratory tract-derived enzymes can activate chemicals differently than liver enzymes. In some cases, respiratory tract enzymes have a greater capacity to activate than do the liver enzymes. This is an important consideration in examining the cause for site-specific genotoxic effects of inhaled materials.

A variety of experimental results indicate that the respiratory tract metabolizes inhaled materials and that respiratory tract metabolism may have important consequences. Such metabolism may occur not only in the lower respiratory tract but also, to an important degree, in the nasal cavity. An understanding of the chemical transformations of inhalants that occur in the respiratory tract is important to our understanding of the mechanisms of toxicity of inhaled materials in laboratory animals and, ultimately, in humans.

Acknowledgments. This research was supported by the Office of Health and Environmental Research of the Department of Energy under contract DE-AC04-76EV01013 in facilities fully accredited by the American Association for Accreditation of Laboratory Animal Care. I thank Dr. Roger O. McClellan, Dr. Rogene Henderson, Dr. Pat Sabourin, and Dr. James Bond for their thoughtful comments on the manuscript.

References

1. Schlesinger RB (1985) Comparative deposition of inhaled aerosols in experimental animals and man. J Toxicol Environ Health 15:197–214
2. Schlesinger RB (1987) Deposition and clearance of inhaled particles. In: Henderson RF, McClellan RO (eds) Concepts of inhalation toxicology. Hemisphere, Washington DC (in press)
3. Stott WT, McKenna MJ (1984) The comparative absorbtion and excretion of chemical vapors by the upper, lower and intact respiratory tract of rats. Fundam Appl Toxicol 4:594–602
4. Morris JB, Clay RJ, Cavanagh DG (1986) Species differences in upper respiratory tract deposition of acetone and ethanol vapors. Fundam Appl Toxicol 7:671–680
5. Dahl AR, Bechtold WE (1985) Deposition and clearance of a water-reactive vapor, methylphosphonic difluoride (difluoro) inhaled by rats. Toxicol Appl Pharmacol 81:58–66
6. Buckley LA, Jiang XZ, James RA, Morgan KT, Barrow CS (1984) Respiratory tract lesions induced by sensory irritants of the RD50 concentration. Toxicol Appl Pharmacol 74:417–429
7. Giddens WE, Fairchild GA (1972) Effects of sulfur dioxide on the nasal mucosa of mice. Arch Environ Health 25:166–173
8. Miller RR, Ayres JA, Jersey GC, McKenna MJ (1981) Inhalation toxicity of acrylic acid. Fundam Appl Toxicol 1:271–277
9. Buckley LA, Morgan KT, Swenberg JA, James RA, Hamm TE Jr, Barrow CS (1983) Inhalation toxicity of dimethylamine in F-344 rats and B6C3F$_1$ mice. Toxicologist 3(1):24
10. Appleman LM, Woutersen RA, Feron VJ (1982) Inhalation toxicity of acetaldehyde in rats: I, acute and subacute studies. Toxicology 23:293–307

11. Druckrey H, Preussmann R, Ivankovic S, Schmähl D, Afkham J, Blum G, Mennel HD, Müller M, Petropoulos P, Schneider H (1967) Organotrope carcinogene Wirkungen bei 65 verschiedenen *N*-nitroso-Verbindungen on BD-Ratten. Z Krebsforschung 69:103–201
12. Dahl AR, Coslett DS, Bond JA, Hesseltine GR (1985) Exposure of the hamster alimentary tract to benzo(*a*)pyrene metabolites produced in the nose. JNCI 75:135–139
13. Ball LM, Plummer JL, Smith BR, Bend JR (1979) Benzo(*a*)pyrene oxidation, conjugation and disposition in the isolated perfused rabbit lung: role of the glutathione S-transferases. Med Biol 57:298–305
14. Autrup H, Wefald FC, Jeffrey AM, Tate H, Schwartz RD, Trump BF, Harris CC (1980) Metabolism of benzo(*a*)pyrene by cultured tracheobronchial tissues from mice, rats, hamsters, bovines and humans. Int J Cancer 25:293–300
15. Hazleton Laboratories Europe Ltd (1981) The toxicity and carcinogenicity of butadiene gas administered to rats by inhalation for approximately 24 months. Prepared for the International Institute of Synthetic Rubber Producers, New York
16. Huff JE, Melnick RL, Solleveld HA, Haseman JK, Powers M, Miller RA (1985) Multiple organ carcinogenicity of 1,3-butadiene in $B6C3F_1$ mice after 60 weeks of inhalation exposure. Science 227:548–549
17. Gervasi PG, Citti L, Del Monte M, Longo V, Benetti D (1985) Mutagenicity and chemical reactivity of epoxidic intermediates of the isoprene metabolism and other structurally related compounds. Mutat Res 150:77–82
18. Schmidt U, Loeser E (1986) Epoxide of 1,3-butadiene in liver and lung tissue of mouse, rat, monkey and man. In: Kocsis J, Jallow DJ, Witmer CM, Nelson JO, Snyder R (eds) Biological reactive intermediates III. Adv Exp Med Biol 197:951–958
19. Magee PN, Montesano R, Preussmann R (1976) *N*-Nitroso compounds and related carcinogens. In: Searle CE (ed) Chemical carcinogens, ACS monograph 173. American Chemical Society, Washington, pp 491–625
20. Dahl AR (1985) Activation of carcinogens and other xenobiotics by nasal cytochrome P-450. In: Boobis AR, Caldwell J, DeMatteis F, Elcombe CP (eds) Microsomes and drug oxidations. Taylor and Francis, Philadelphia, pp 299–309
21. Brittebo E, Döfberg B, Tjälve H (1981) Estrahepatic sites of metabolism of *N*-nitrosopyrrolidine in mice and rats. Xenobiotica 11:619–625
22. Yang CS, Koop DR, Wang T, Coon MJ (1985) Immunochemical studies on the metabolism of nitrosamines by ethanol-inducible cytochrome P-450. Biochem Biophys Res Commun 128:1007–1013
23. Dahl AR (1985) Mutagenicity of some dialkylnitrosamines, cyclic nitrosamines and *N,N*-diethanolnitrosamine in *Salmonella typhimurium* with rat and rabbit nasal, lung and liver S-9 homogenates. Mutat Res 158:141–147
24. Longo V, Citti L, Gervasi PG (1986) Metabolism of diethylnitrosamine by nasal mucosa and hepatic microsomes from hamster and rat: species specificity of nasal mucosa. Carcinogenesis 7:1323–1328
25. Sabourin PJ, Dahl AR (1985) Distribution of the FAD-containing monooxygenase in respiratory tract tissues. In: Medinsky MA, Muggenburg BA (eds) Annual report LMF-114. National Technical Information Service, US Department of Commerce, Springfield, pp 156–158
26. Tynes RE, Sabourin PJ, Hodgson E (1985) Identification of distinct hepatic and pulmonary forms of the microsomal flavin-containing monooxygenase in the mouse and rabbit. Biochem Biophys Res Commun 126:1069–1075

27. Williams DE, Hale SE, Muerhoff AS, Masters BSS (1985) Rabbit lung flavin-containing monooxygenase. Purification, characterization and induction during pregnancy. Mol Pharmacol 28:381–390
28. Boobis AR, Davies DS (1984) Human cytochromes P-450. Xenobiotica 14:151–185
29. Hadley WM, Dahl AR (1983) Cytochrome P-450-dependent monooxygenase activity in nasal membranes of six species. Drug Metab Dispos 11:275–276
30. Morgan ET, Koop DR, Coon MJ (1982) Catalytic activity of cytochromal P-450 isozyme 3a isolated from liver microsomes of ethanol-treated rabbits. J Biol Chem 257:13951–13957
31. Ding X, Koop DR, Crump BL, Coon MJ (1986) Immunochemical identification of cytochrome P-450 isozyme 3a (P-450_{ALC}) in rabbit nasal and kidney microsomes and evidence for differential induction by alcohol. Mol Pharmacol 30:370–378
32. Boyd MR (1977) Evidence for the Clara cell as a site of cytochrome P-450-dependent mixed-function oxidase activity in lung. Nature 269:713–715
33. Serabjit-Singh CJ, Wolf CR, Philpot RM, Plopper CG (1980) Cytochrome P-450: localization in rabbit lung. Science 207:1469
34. Bogdanffy MS, Randall HW, Morgan KT (1985) Histochemical localization of aldehyde dehydrogenase in the respiratory tract of the Fischer-344 rat. Toxicol Appl Pharmacol 82:560–567
35. Bogdanffy MS, Randall HW, Morgan KT (1985) Histochemical and biochemical detection of carboxyesterase activity in the rat nasal passages. Toxicologist 6:145
36. Dahl AR, Miller SC, Petridou-Fischer J (1987) Carboxylesterases in the respiratory tracts of rabbits, rats and Syrian hamsters. Toxicol Lett 36:129–136
37. Bond JA (1983) Some biotransformation enzymes responsible for polycyclic aromatic hydrocarbon metabolism in rat nasal turbinates: effects on enzyme activities of in vitro modifiers and intraperitoneal and inhalation exposure of rats to inducing agents. Cancer Res 43:4804–4811
38. Vaino H, Hietanen E (1980) Role of extrahepatic metabolism in drug disposition and toxicity. In: Jenner P, Testa B (eds) Concepts in drug metabolism, part A. Dekker, New York, pp 251–284
39. Simon P, Filser JG, Bolt HM (1985) Metabolism and pharmacokinetics of vinyl acetate. Arch Toxicol 57:191–195
40. Dahl AR, Bond JA, Petridou-Fischer J, Sabourin PJ, Whaley SJ (1987) Effects of the respiratory tract on inhaled materials (and vice versa). Fundam Appl Toxicol (in press)
41. Inskeep PB, Guengerich FP (1984) Glutathione-mediated binding of dibromoalkanes to DNA: specificity of rat glutathione S-transferases and dibromoalkane structure. Carcinogenesis 5:805
42. Jakoby WB, Bend JR, Caldwell J (1982) In: Jakoby WB, Bend JR, Caldwell J (eds) Metabolic basis of detoxification: metabolism of functional groups. Academic, New York
43. Pendleton RG, Gessner G, Sawyer J (1980) Studies on lung *N*-methyl-transferases, a pharmacological approach. Naunyn Schmiedebergs Arch Pharmacol 313:263–268
44. Philpot RM, Wolf CR (1981) The properties and distribution of the enzymes of pulmonary cytochromes P-450-dependent monooxygenase systems. In: Hodgson E, Bend JR, Philpot RM (eds) Biochemical toxicology, vol 3. Elsevier, New York, pp 51–76
45. Bond JA, Mauderly JL (1984) Metabolism and macromolecular covalent binding of ^{14}C-1-nitropyrene in isolated perfused and ventilated rat lungs. Cancer Res 44: 3924–3929

46. Baron J, Voigt JM, Whitter TB, Kawabata T, Knapp SA, Guengerich FP, Jakoby WB (1986) Identification of intratissue sites for xenobiotic activation and detoxification. In: Kocsis J, Jollow DJ, Witmer CM, Nelson JO, Snyder R (eds) Biological reactive intermediates III: molecular and cellular mechanisms of action in animal models and human disease. Plenum, New York, pp 119–144
47. Hodgson E, Philpot RM (1973) Interactions of methylenedioxyphenyl (1,3-benzodioxole) compounds with enzymes and their effects on mammals. Drug Metab Rev 3:231
48. Bond JA, Li AP (1982) Rat nasal tissue metabolism of benzo(*a*)pyrene and 2-aminoanthracene to mutagens in *Salmonella typhimurium*. Environ Mutagen 5:311–318
49. ICRP Task Group on Lung Dynamics (1966) Deposition and retention models for internal dosimetry of the human respiratory tract. Health Phys 12:173–207
50. Dipple A (1976) Polynuclear aromatic carcinogens. In: Searle CE (ed) Chemical carcinogens, ACS monograph 173. American Chemical Society, Washington, pp 245–314
51. Malvoisin E, Lhoest G, Poncelet F, Roberfroid M, Mercier M (1979) Identification and quantitation of 1,2-epoxybutene-3 as the primary metabolite of 1,3-butadiene. J Chromatogr 178:419–429
52. Bond JA, Mitchell CE, Li AP (1983) Metabolism and macromolecular covalent binding of benzo(*a*)pyrene in cultured Fischer-344 rat lung type II epithelial cells. Biochem Pharmacol 32:3771–3776
53. Bond JA (1983) Bioactivation and biotransformation of 1-nitropyrene in liver, lung and nasal tissue of rats. Mutat Res 124:315–324
54. Lorenz J, Glatt HR, Fleischmann R, Ferlinz R, Oesch F (1984) Drug metabolism in man and its relationship to three rodent species: monooxygenase, epoxide hydrolase and glutathione S-transferase activities in subcellular fractions of lung and liver. Biochem Med 32:43–56
55. Dahl AR, Brezinski DA (1985) Inhibitors of rabbit nasal cytochrome P-450-dependent hexamethylphosphoramide (HMPA) *N*-demethylase by methylenedioxyphenyl compounds. Biochem Pharmacol 34:631–636

Part II
Methodological Issues in Designing and Conducting Studies with Laboratory Animals

CHAPTER 5

Exposure Facilities and Aerosol Generation and Characterization for Inhalation Experiments

W. Holländer[1]

Introduction

The increasingly stringent requirements of the animal welfare acts (3,57) necessitate a reduction in animal experiments. However, if one is interested in the toxic effects of air pollutants, the in vitro test systems available to date are only of limited value. These studies mostly use undifferentiated (animal) cells which give a poor simulation of the target tissue and its reaction to inhaled materials. On the other hand, the rationale behind animal experiments is to protect human beings from potentially dangerous exposure to pollutants. This means that animal experiments are necessary, because only in well justified cases can experiments occasionally be performed on human volunteers, thus introducing the uncertainties caused by interspecies variability. Since even among rodents the response to the same toxicant may be markedly different (29), the interpretation of animal experiments is a difficult task per se. In addition to the different general sensitivity, changed nose and lung morphology and—in consequence—different inhalability and deposition of the particles may have to be taken into account. If, for instance, the carcinogenicity of nasally deposited wood dust is to be studied, one has to make sure that even the largest wood particles of importance to man will be inspired by the test animals. Hence, before starting the design of exposure facilities and aerosol generators, one has to clearly state the task in hand (acute, subchronic, or chronic exposure) and numerically fix the level of significance to which an effect is to be measured. This will determine the number of animals required. The choice of the animal species, together with the number of animals and the kind of pollutant, determines the operating conditions of exposure facilities and aerosol generation.

As each species has a window of comfort in terms of ambient temperature, relative humidity, and permissible draught in order not to produce artifacts, these data define the conditioning of the exposure chamber air. The aerosol has to be homogeneously mixed with the conditioning air and kept well-mixed until it leaves the chamber.

---

[1]Fraunhofer Institut für Toxikologie und Aerosolforschung, D-3000 Hannover, FRG.

Deposition of Particles in the Respiratory Tract of Humans and Animals

Heyder et al. (22) have published empirical fits to data which describe the experimentally determined human lung deposition in the size range 0.005–12 μm very well. For particles of >0.05 μm, the compartmental depositions in the nose, larynx, bronchi, and alveoli are given. The typical compartmental depositions caused by the main mechanisms diffusion, sedimentation, and impaction can be seen in Fig. 5.1.

Deposition by diffusion and sedimentation depends on the length of time for which a particle remains in situ, rather than on the flow rate, whereas impaction is determined by the latter. Diffusion increases for decreasing particle diameters, while sedimentation and impaction decrease.

Unfortunately, the numerical parameters of the fit embody all the lung morphometric data. Since Heyder et al. did not make an attempt to calculate these parameters from first principles, it is not possible to predict deposition for other lung geometries, which would be required for assessing the relevance of animal inhalation studies to man. Early attempts to calculate compartmental deposition [starting with Findeisen (14)] failed accurately to predict experimental data for various breathing conditions. Recent work, however, has improved on this some-

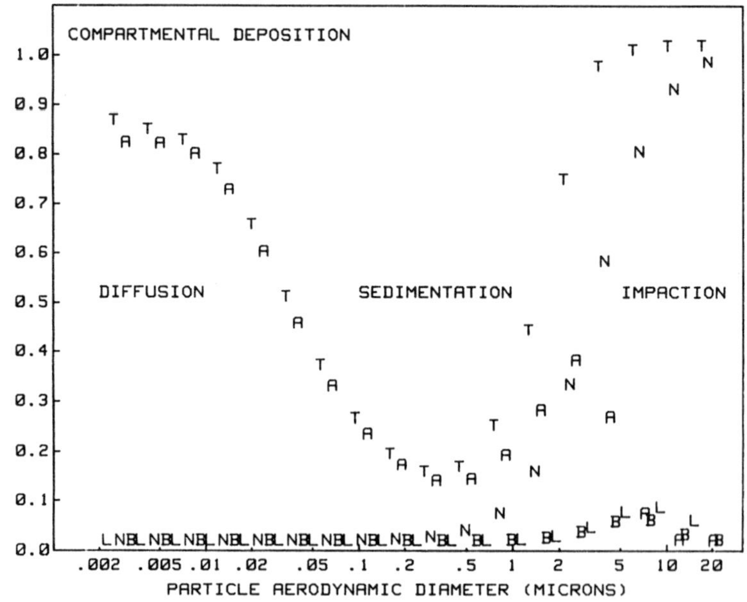

Fig. 5.1. Typical compartmental deposition in the human respiratory tract: *T*, total; *N*, nasal; *A*, alveolar; *L*, laryngeal; *B*, bronchial. Reprinted with permission of the publisher from ref. 18. Copyright 1986 by Elsevier Science Publishing Co., Inc.

what (35,48,66). Whereas human lung morphometry has been known for a long time [e.g., Comroe (9)], data on regional deposition have become available only recently for experimental animals (43).

In assessing the relevance of animal exposure data to man, one must take into account that the metabolic rate of small animals is much higher and therefore the airborne dose per body weight is larger for them than for large animals (19,28). This—at least partially—offsets the short lifespan which may be a limiting factor for carcinogenicity studies.

Exposure Facilities

The design of exposure facilities is primarily determined by the choice of the exposure technique. The upper airways can be bypassed by using an implanted tracheal cannula. This technique has been employed to study the effects of chronic cigarette smoke inhalation. Care must be taken, however, in interpreting results obtained by this method, since lack of air humidification and particle deposition in nose and larynx may radically affect lung behavior.

Oral inhalation is widely used in short-term experiments with human volunteers. A convenient system [described in more detail in (27)] is used, for instance, to determine the deposition of particulate and gaseous components of sidestream smoke. The advantage of this technique lies in the easy administration and measurement of inhaled and exhaled aerosol. However, there are also disadvantages: the obligatory use of a nose clip, and the fact that sedentary mouth breathing is not a normal condition and may exert stress on the test person (or animal). In addition, many animals cannot readily be exposed orally since they are nasal breathers.

In the latter cases, the nose-only exposure technique (Fig. 5.2) is widely used since it avoids ingestion of particles which have deposited upon the pelt or the cage. Also, it prevents the animals from hiding their noses in their own or their cage mates' fur and thus from breathing "filtered" air. Often the animals try to reduce the unwanted exposure by changing their breathing pattern. This requires special equipment when precise dose calculations are needed. If the inhaled volume has to be known for thorough studies, the body holder has to be a plethysmograph. A disadvantage of this is the enormous stress the animals experience in a fixed position; the exposure time must therefore be limited to 1 h, whereas approximately 5 h may be admitted without plethysmograph.

Whole-body exposure is certainly the method of least stress for the animals and is therefore the favored method for chronic studies, but it does have the typical disadvantages avoided by nose-only exposure.

Another problem is the difficulty of maintaining homogeneous temperature, humidity, air velocity, and aerosol distribution in the facility, because of the body heat of the animals and the flow constrictions imposed by the excrement pans. When the animals have to remain in the facility continuously—which may be the

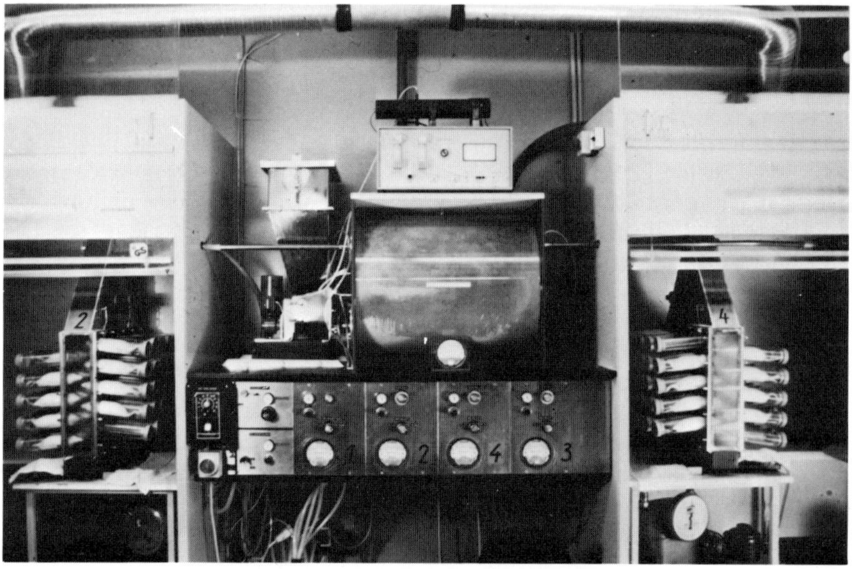

Fig. 5.2. View of the nose-only exposure facility.

case when highly toxic or carcinogenic aerosols or airborne pathogens are used – special measures have to be taken to provide food and water supply and excrement removal.

Design Criteria of Exposure Facilities

Figure 5.3 shows the general scheme of an exposure facility, consisting of the aerosol generator, the output of which is mixed with the conditioning air, together with the inhalation chambers, the sampling and measuring system, and the data acquisition and control unit. Exhaust fans draw the inhalation atmosphere from the generator/air conditioning section through the inhalation chambers. Before releasing the exposure airflow into the environment, exhaust filters remove all toxic substances from the experimental atmosphere. An aerosol/gas sampling and measuring system supplies all of the data necessary for documentation and control of the complete experiment. Any deviations from the set values are used to control aerosol generator and air conditioning.

Before the actual design is undertaken, the pressure relations between the different subunits have to be fixed. Frequently, experiments are performed with specific pathogen-free (SPF) animals. In these cases, preventive methods against contamination by pathogens are required. One precaution is to have overpressure in the inhalation facility relative to its immediate surroundings, but other measures may be necessary too, such as sterile showers and lock boxes for animal

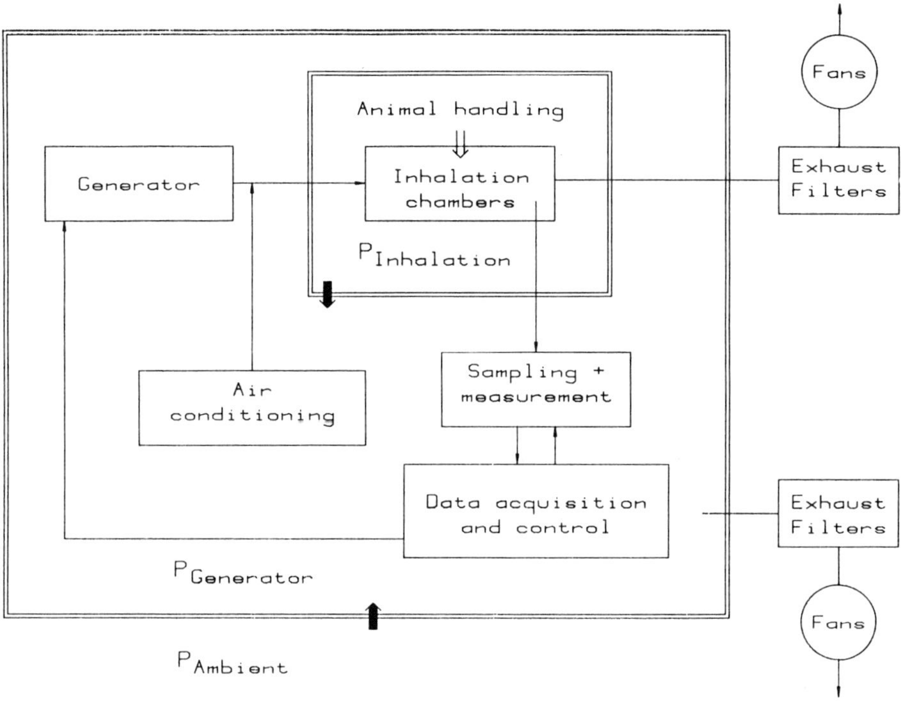

Fig. 5.3. Diagram of an inhalation facility.

handling. On the other hand, the incidental escape of toxic substances into the environment has to be safely excluded. This requires the generation, sampling, and measuring units to operate below ambient pressure. Therefore a suitable pressure relation in the diagram in Fig. 5.3 would be $p_{\text{generator}} < p_{\text{inhalation}} < p_{\text{ambient}}$.

Of course, personnel operating at $p_{\text{generator}}$ have to be protected from toxicants by suitable garments, gas and filter masks, etc., in case of leaks in the generating or inhalation areas. Depending on the nature of the toxic substances the cleaning devices designated as filters in Fig. 5.3 may be wet scrubbers, high-efficiency particulate air filters, charcoal filters, and so on.

To make the whole exposure facility work properly, care has to be taken that the fan characteristics match the cumulative pressure drops in the ducts, bends, filters, etc. Special attention is needed if there are several inhalation chambers in parallel, because any change in the flow resistance of one unit will affect the others. If the flow through the chambers is controlled by valves, the whole system has to be checked after a manipulation on a single valve. The situation is much simpler if active flow control of each inhalation box is available. This may be achieved with individual fans by throttling via their flow rate-pressure drop relationship or by adjusting the voltage of single-phase or the frequency of three-phase blowers. The latter method can be easily and cost-effectively applied in large systems where energy savings offset the higher investment costs.

Since there is a wealth of adequate literature on air conditioning and ventilation (see, e.g., 11,67), listing all the friction factors and pressure drops (of hoses, tubes, fittings, valves, bends, etc.) necessary for properly designing the exposure facility, detailed calculation procedures will not be given here. Flow rates of heavily dustladen air should preferably be measured by devices not seriously affected by dust deposits, such as orifice plates. If the load is very high, regular cleaning intervals have to be assigned and observed. The problems usually start at the inhalation chamber inlet: inside a small distance the aerosol has to be uniformly distributed over the whole cross-section of the chamber. Since it is difficult to achieve turbulent mixing angles wider than 14°, it is necessary to employ sieves if very long conical inlet ducts have to be avoided. Using multiple sieves in series, any desired degree of flow uniformity can be achieved. However, one has to compromise between flow uniformity and particle losses in the sieve stack. A successful approach applied in our institute (see Fig. 5.4) uses diffusors to divert the aerosol in a relatively narrow inlet plenum box in such a way that the pressure available for accelerating the aerosol to the same velocity through the openings in the hole assembly is the same. This can be achieved by proper positioning of the baffles opposite to the inlet tube. The jets from the equally spaced holes merge and the nonuniformity of velocity is evened out over distance. According to measurements by Reichardt [in Schlichting (47)] the jet width $b_{1/2}$ at half center velocity is $0.0848 \cdot x$ where x is the distance from the nozzle exit. Therefore, a maximum velocity variation of 50% is obtained in a dimensionless distance of $x/b_{1/2} = 1/0.0848 \approx 12$. Simple geometrical reasoning shows that $b_{1/2}$ must be equal to the distance between the jets. Better flow uniformity will be observed in larger distances from the hole plate in an empty chamber.

To avoid stagnant vortices which would impair aerosol homogeneity, removal of the air stream through hole plates (as shown in Fig. 5.4) is favored. A great variety of possible flow directions—horizontal, vertical downstream, vertical upstream, and even multi-directional—has been described in the literature. Also, the range of air changes in the inhalation facilities cited in the literature ranges between 6 h^{-1} and 60 h^{-1} (37). Although the connections to the generation and exhaust systems are usually somewhat simpler for vertical air currents, we tend to favor horizontal air flow, because it greatly facilitates animal handling and homogeneous air supply.

So far, only ideal, empty facilities have been considered. The situation is somewhat different in an actual exposure chamber because of the presence of the cages, which act as flow obstacles, and the thermal load generated by the animals, which modifies the flow by buoyancy effects. A suitable dimensionless parameter describing the ratio of buoyancy and inertial forces is the Archimedes number (45)

$$\mathrm{Ar} = h \cdot g \cdot \Delta T / v^2 T$$

where h is chamber height, $(\Delta)T$ is the temperature (difference), g is the gravitational acceleration, and v is the air velocity.

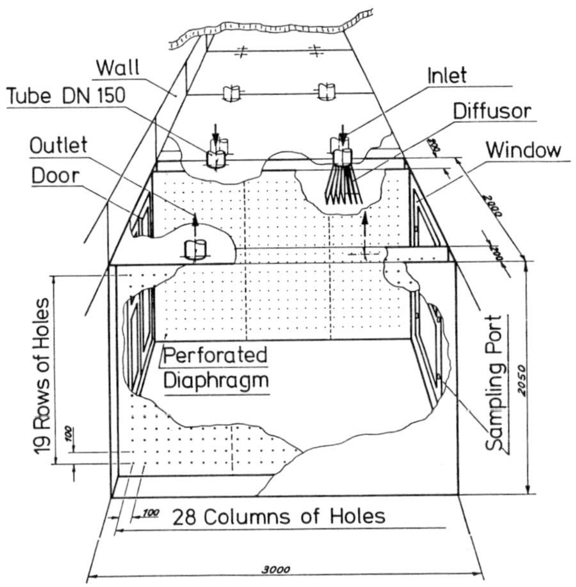

Fig. 5.4. Diagram of a horizontal airflow exposure chamber used at the Fraunhofer Institute, Hannover.

If the inertial forces loose their importance compared to viscous forces, the situation will be described by the Grashof number

$$Gr = h^3 \cdot g \cdot \Delta T/\upsilon^2 T$$

where υ is the kinematic viscosity. Both parameters must be kept within critical values. As an example for an isolated heat source, the average upstream velocity 30 cm above the head of a sitting person is of the order of 15 cm/s (16).

The situation in a cage with horizontal flow and a nearly homogeneous area heat source represented by the animals is different: the average of the vertical velocity component $< w' > = 0$ whereas the root mean square value $< w'^2 > \approx 3$ cm/s, has been determined in an aerosol chamber with stagnant air (Holländer, 1984, unpublished data). The flow pattern can be visualized as mushroom-like parcels of warm rising air interlacing with cool downflowing air (62). Near to the cage rims, where the heat load is reduced, enhanced particle deposition is expected because of the prevalent settling motion and possibly because of vortices induced by the horizontal flow.

Since the settling velocity of 10-µm particles is about 0.3 cm/s and the average horizontal velocity of the order of 1.5 cm/s, losses for larger particles are not negligible, and the spatial aerosol concentration has to be determined under actual operating conditions.

The conclusion following from the above is that the exposure facility has to be designed ad hoc if the experimental boundary conditions do not permit use of one of the established designs (5,7,13,20,23,32,39,54).

Generation of Aerosols

The response of an organism to toxic material depends on the dose, which in the case of inhalation is a function of the mass deposited in the lung. Therefore, the concentration and size distribution of the exposure aerosol must be known and kept constant by the generation technique. Depending on the kind of aerosol under study, the possibility of redispersion of previously collected material has to be taken into account, especially if the particles are not sticky and do not adhere too strongly, which is the case, e.g., for power-plant fly ash. On the other hand, very fine and/or sticky aerosol, like tobacco smoke, has to be produced freshly in order not to be too different from what is encountered in "real life" because of aging effects.

The generation procedure may—and generally will—produce aerosols which are not equivalent in all respects to the desired characteristics. For instance, it may be very difficult to disperse a powder collected from the atmosphere to the same size distribution, because the size dependence of disintegrating shear forces and agglomerating Van der Waals forces makes it very difficult to separate small particles. Often the chemical composition is a function of particle size. This is especially true for condensation aerosols, where small particles are enriched in relatively volatile substances, due to their larger surface. Examples for this finding are given in (17,33,41), although in some cases the situation is more involved (30).

During a dispersion process, charge separation takes place if the work functions of the powder or liquid and the disperser material are different. In most cases, earthing the unit will remove too high excess charges. Nevertheless, the remaining charge may be much higher than the Boltzmann equilibrium charge and could influence lung deposition (38). In this case a radioactive source (e.g., ^{241}Am, ^{85}Kr) may be used to bring the aerosol to thermodynamic charge equilibrium, the condition in which atmospheric aerosol is usually found due to long exposure to ions produced by cosmic rays and natural radioactivity.

In controlling the size distribution of hygroscopic aerosols, it must be remembered that the dry residue mass for a given particle size may depend on the humidity. The latter is therefore an important parameter for the characterization of the aerosol.

For the dispersion of liquids and powders, different physical mechanisms for breaking adhesive forces are employed. One method applicable to both phases is gas injection, which is shown schematically in Fig. 5.5. A ring-shaped nozzle carrying a high-velocity air stream produces a negative pressure differential in its interior which can be used to convey the material to be dispersed from the reservoir to the mixing zone, where the turbulent shear forces are strong enough to overcome viscous and/or adhesive forces of the material to be dispersed. Fig. 5.6 shows the two-stage injector system of Fig. 5.5 with dosing equipment used in an inhalation experiment (31).

For powders, a uniform supply is necessary in all dispersion systems for obtaining constant aerosol concentrations. In the widely known Wright dust feeder,

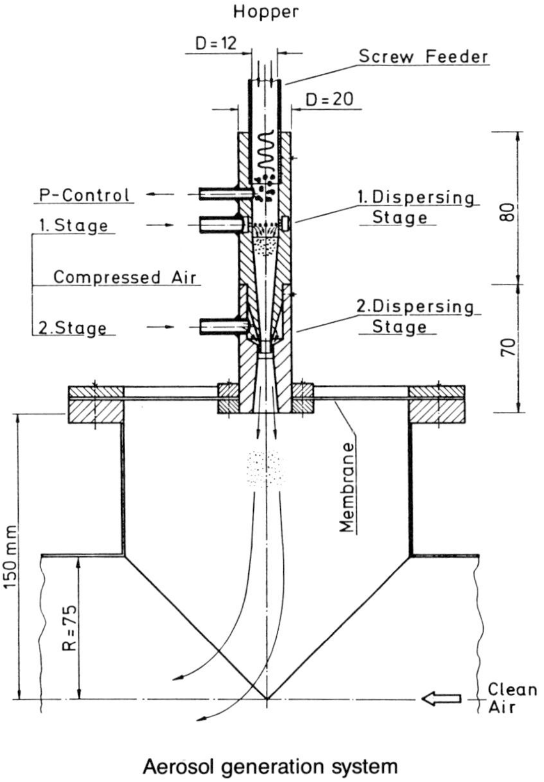

Fig. 5.5. Scheme of the two-stage injector dispersing system.

sintered material is scraped off at a predetermined rate and picked up by the dispersing air. A rotating brush generator which may be useful for inhalation purposes is described in VDI guideline 3491, produced by the Association of German Engineers part 9 (59). It has a piston dosage system into which loose powder must be fed. Homogeneous powder-packing density is of critical importance to constant aerosol concentration. Also, there may be problems with the piston feeder if the powder is prone to sintering. If a concentration monitoring device is included in the generation system, constant output may be easily achieved by controlling the piston feed rate. Other feeding systems have been described which may offer advantages for materials with special properties and mass flow conditions. A different approach to dispersing powders is to form a fluidized bed by forcing gas from below through the dust. Sometimes mechanical oscillations help to disperse the material (52) and to control particle size and concentration to a limited extent.

Most of the methods for dispersing liquids are based on forcing the fluid into thin jets or sheets which then spontaneously disintegrate into droplets due to inherent Rayleigh instability. Although most useful for calibration, due to its

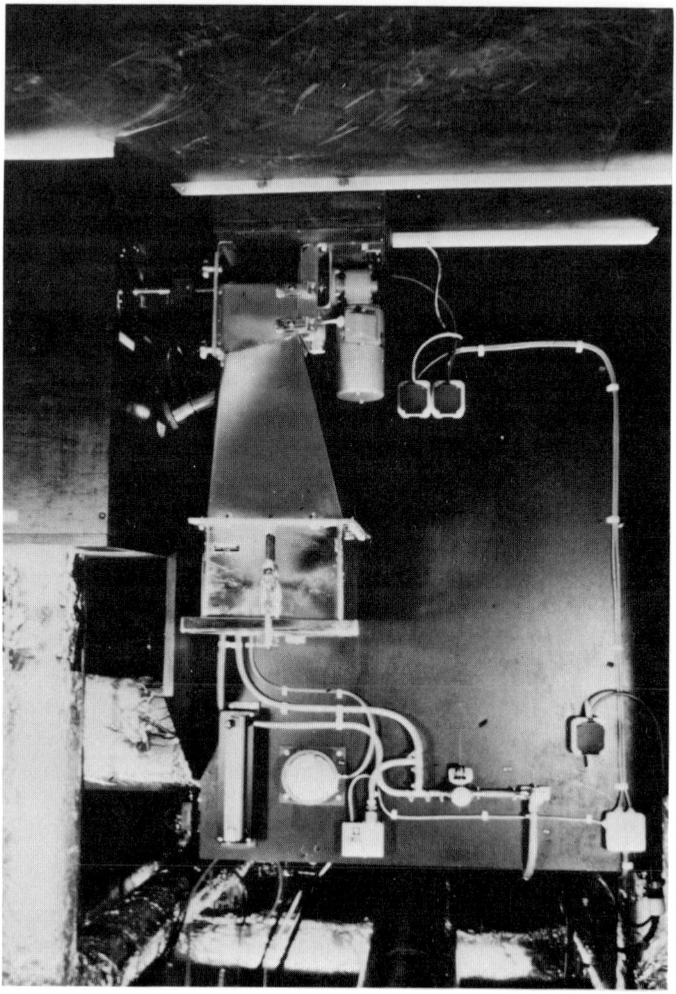

Fig. 5.6. View of the generator including screw feeder, power supply, and injector dispersing system, as shown in Fig. 5.5.

monodisperse output, the Berglund-Liu generator (6) delivers only small aerosol concentrations which do not suffice for most inhalation applications. The spinning-top generator moves the liquid by centrifugal force to the edge of a rapidly rotating disk, where main and satellite droplets form. By properly adjusting rotor speed, liquid feed, and air flow rates, monodisperse or even bidisperse aerosol of fairly high concentration is formed (12,36). In another generator (61), mechanical oscillations of a disk attached to a piezoceramic transducer lead to capillary waves which subsequently disintegrate. The primary size of the fairly uniform droplets is around 40 μm. Although reducing the solution concentration decreases the particle size of the residue, the lowest achievable limit is around 2 μm for particles of well-defined composition, since solvent impurities cannot be ignored in very low solution concentrations. A liquid dispersion method limited by fluid viscosity employs a concave ultrasonic transducer immersed in a fluid in such a way that the converging wave is focused at the surface. The resulting cavitation forces produce a fine, dense, and polydisperse mist. Inhalation devices for asthmatic patients frequently use this principle (60).

Sometimes the liquid serves only as a carrier for solid particles which are left after evaporation of the fluid; a typical example is monodisperse polystyrene latex spheres used for calibration. In this case, the dilution factor, together with the primary droplet size, determines the average number of particles contained in one droplet. In order to avoid multiplets, the latex concentration must be fairly low.

Since generation of particles with liquid or dry dispersion methods becomes increasingly difficult as the required size decreases, a different method based on condensation is usually used for submicron particles. If the airborne vapor concentration C_v of a substance is greater than its saturation concentration C_s, a thermodynamically unstable situation arises which may eventually lead to condensation on foreign particles and/or homogeneous nucleation if the saturation ratio $S = C_v/C_s$ is high enough.

Aerosols from organic substances are often produced in a Sinclair-La Mer generator (50,58). Condensation nuclei produced by evaporating salt from a heated wire are mixed with a well-defined amount of vapor released in the heater section. When the mixture is cooled, C_s is reduced and causes $S > 1$, with vapor condensing on the nuclei as a consequence.

Inorganic materials of very low volatility can be vaporized by an electric ("exploding wire") technique (40). Another method consists in vaporizing a high vapor pressure organic compound of the substance to form the fine aerosol by thermal degradation. For suitably selected compounds the saturation vapor pressure of at least one of the molecular fragments is lower than the actual pressure, so that condensation and eventually nucleation occur.

Homogeneous nucleation has to be suppressed if monodisperse particles of comparatively low concentration ($< 10^6$ cm^{-3}) are needed. This requires careful control of the source rate, which has to match the condensation rate onto the nuclei in order to prevent build-up of very high supersaturation $S \gg 1$, leading to homogeneous nucleation.

In addition to thermal degradation, gas phase and photochemical reactions (55) may be used, as well as radical reactions induced by radioactive sources ["radiolytic aerosols" (44)].

In many cases of practical interest, the aerosol emerges from an incomplete combustion process and is therefore of highly complex chemical composition (cigarette smoke, Diesel exhaust, etc.). Because of the small and sticky particles, and possibility of chemical reactions occurring in collected material, this type of aerosol has to be freshly generated in an original or properly scaled-down device. Photochemical reactions of tropospheric relevance can also be simulated in flow chambers (44). Of course, the whole generation and inhalation facility must be designed with care in order not to distort size distribution and chemical composition in comparison to the system to be simulated.

A method often employed to facilitate in vivo aerosol dose measurement, or even imaging, is labeling with an easily detectable radioactive nuclide. The label must be well attached to the aerosol and not be easily leached by the body fluid. In most cases the parameter which has to be represented by the label is the aerosol mass (because of the biological relevance), but other aerosol parameters can be labeled too. The surface, for instance, can be measured by attached radon daughters.

In some cases, the generation process does not deliver the aerosol with the desired size distribution. Collected dust, for instance, often has an excessive big-particle fraction. Under this condition, the coarse-particle fraction has to be separated by a size discriminating method like an impactor or a channel wheel classifier like the Alpine MZR 20. This instrument allows throughputs of several kilograms per hour and aerodynamic cut diameters down to 5 μm. Sometimes the smaller fraction must not be deposited and has to remain in the airborne state because of the impossibility of subsequent redispersion. Electrostatic classifiers, elutriators, or virtual impactors may serve this purpose. The general principle of such devices consists in a size-dependent force perpendicular to the local fluid motion which separates the particles in the stream according to their size. Before a certain location in the channel wall is reached, all particles not meeting the desired property range (larger or smaller than a certain cutoff point) have been removed. Cascading such devices allows generation of aerosols with a specified size range. If monodisperse particles are needed, they may be extracted through an appropriate window in the channel wall of a differential separating device.

Characterization of Aerosols

For establishing a dose-response relationship in an experiment, first of all the amount of the deposited substance has to be known. This depends on the airborne concentration and chemical composition of the aerosol as well as on its size distribution and other parameters determining the lung deposition. Among these is the electric charge, which attracts particles to the lung tissue by image forces. Also, hygroscopic particles may grow in moist air until equilibrium is reached between vapor pressure reduction according to Raoult's law and vapor pressure increase according to the Kelvin equation. If the particle shape deviates very much from the spherical, deposition may be strongly affected by aerodynamic orientation effects (18). However, for particles other than fibers and flakes this effect probably does not play a great role.

For characterization the particles have to be sampled properly from the generator and/or exposure chamber. Ter Kuile (56) has shown that the criteria for "representative sampling" (sampling efficiencies $>90\%$) are met by the following conditions:

$St_{rep} < 1/16$ (inertial limit)
$Kl_{rep} < 0.01$ (dynamic limit)
$\beta_{rep} < 1/16$ (gravitational limit).

The "inlet" Stokes number $St = v \cdot \tau_p/a$ describes the ratio of the stopping distance of a particle in the velocity field to the characteristic width of the sampling inlet. The stopping distance is determined by the product of the average air velocity at the inlet v and the particle relaxation time τ_p. The corresponding characteristic length is the diameter a of the sampling inlet.

$Kl = \tau_p \cdot u_{sed}/l_{cd}$ is the Levin parameter where l_{cd} is the capture distance and u_{sed} is the particle sedimentation velocity in the earth's gravitational field. The dimensionless number $\beta = u_{sed}/v_{sam}$ compares the sedimentation velocity u_{sed} with the sampling inlet velocity v_{sam}. The inlet has to be designed so as to meet the above requirements when operated with the respective measuring instruments.

The most important factor determining deposition is clearly the mass distribution as a function of particle aerodynamic diameter. Measurement can be accomplished by combining a size-separating technique with a method capable of directly or indirectly measuring mass and gas volume.

The basic procedure of mass determination is by gravimetry, where the aerosol has to be collected on a substrate. From the mass difference before and after collection and the sampling volume, the aerosol concentration in mg/m^3 is obtained. Substrate preparation (conditioning under well-defined temperature and humidity as well as coating to prevent bounce losses) may be required. Since ordinary gravimetry is a tedious procedure, other real-time methods have been developed. They are based on the principle that the resonance frequency of a mechanical oscillator depends on the oscillating mass. In order to obtain good sensitivity, the quality of the oscillator has to be high. This principle was first realized by Sauerbrey (46) with quartz oscillators for the determination of surface films. Aerosol measuring equipment of this kind has been made available by TSI (49). Here the aerosol particles are charged by a needle-to-plane corona discharge and deposited in the center of the oscillator crystal. Recently a method has been developed to produce oscillating quartz filters by heavy ion irradiation and subsequent etching (25).

The sensor of the tapered element oscillating microbalance (TEOM; Fig. 5.7) is a thin, hollow, glass cylinder which carries a small filter on top through which the aerosol is pumped. Increasing filter mass reduces the resonance frequency of the glass cylinder set into transversal oscillations by an alternating electric field (64).

In addition to these methods for direct mass measurements, other techniques based on different physical principles are used. For instance, the β-attenuation method measures the ionization in a reference and a measuring chamber produced by the electrons penetrating a reference and the dustladen filter (34,51). A slight but nonnegligible influence of the atomic weight on the specific attenuation has to be taken into account for different β energies.

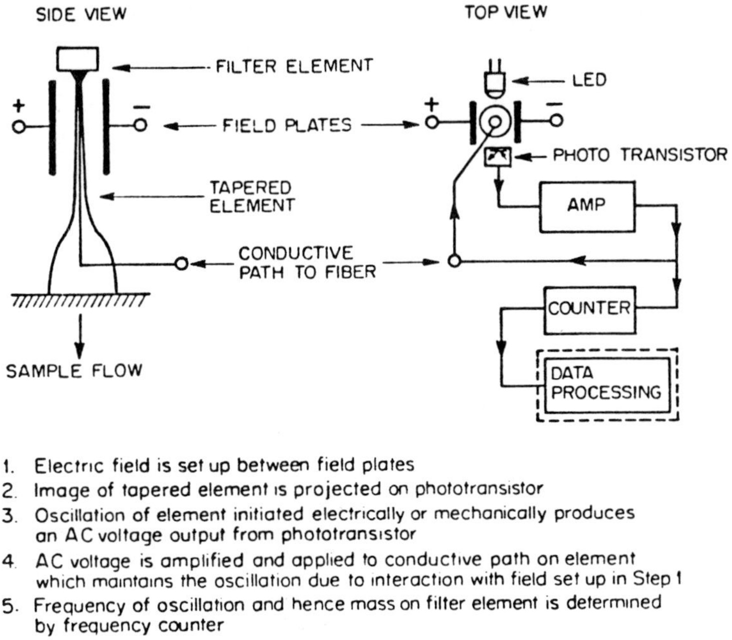

Fig. 5.7. Schematic representation of the Tapered element oscillating microbalance (TEOM) operation.

Depending on the aerosol, a variety of element- or compound-specific methods like γ-spectroscopy, AAS, ICP, XRF, HPLC, GC/MS, electron microprobe, etc., can be employed efficiently. For brevity, these analytical methods will not be discussed in detail.

The most common aerosol size separating and collecting device is the cascade impactor. The aerosol is accelerated in a long nozzle which helps the particles to acquire the gas velocity. In the stagnation flow developing near the impaction plate, however, the particles cannot follow the streamlines because of their inertia and impact onto the collecting substrate. Deposition is characterized by the dimensionless Stokes number already encountered among the sampling criteria.

Because of the discontinuous separating characteristics of impactors, they cannot resolve monodisperse particles. Centrifuges do cope with this requirement because the particle deposition location is a smooth function of aerodynamic diameter.

Centrifuges as well as impactors have been equipped with quartz mass sensors (53), which allows real-time monitoring. This is a very important aspect if online control of the generator system is desired.

In many cases, direct mass monitoring is not required to maintain constant generator output. Optical particle counters and the aerodynamic particle sizer (TSI APS 3300 (63)] provide number distributions as a function of optical (or

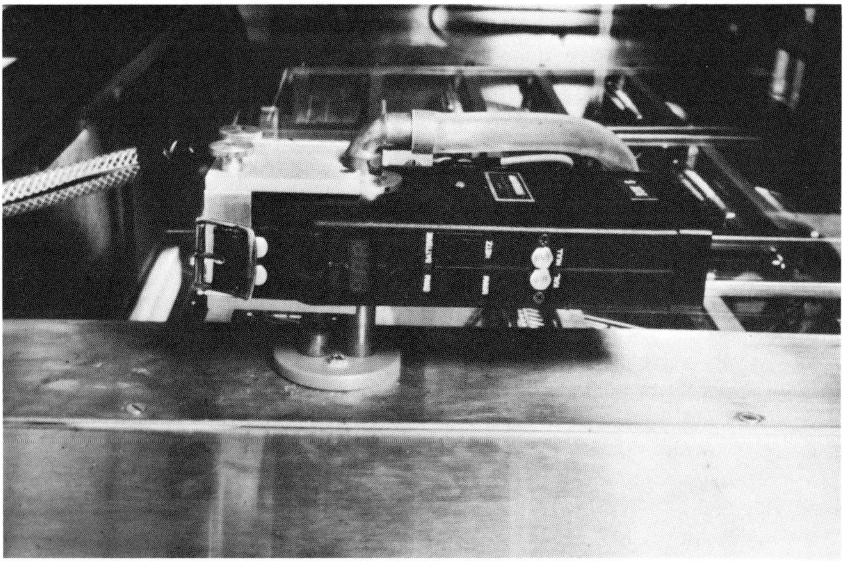

Fig. 5.8. TM Digital scattered light monitor as real-time generator controller.

aerodynamic) size. In most cases this information suffices as input parameters for a sensible generator control strategy (8). Even the simpler information as to the light attenuation or scattering from a particle collective may suffice for this purpose. Instruments based on this method measure the particles either collected on a filter [e.g., the Palas Filterfotometer (26)] or in the airborne state [e.g., Hund TM Digital (4)]. An example for real-time chamber concentration monitoring is shown in Fig. 5.8. The combination of diffusion battery/electrostatic classifier with a condensation nucleus counter provides particle number distributions as a function of diffusion/electrical mobility diameter in a semi-online manner only, because the measurement takes about 2 min and requires an inversion routine to obtain the distribution from a series of measurements.

Since a complete account of the numerous particle measuring methods is clearly beyond the scope of this paper, the following references provide a representative list of useful methods (1,2,15,21,24).

Conclusions

Full coverage of all topics which have to be addressed in inhalation experiments is clearly impossible in such a short overview. Probably the most useful introductory books are Phalen's monograph (42) and Willeke's symposium volume (65), which contain a wealth of references on more specialized problems.

References

1. Lundgren DA, Harris S Jr., Marlow WH, Lippmann M, Clark WE, Durham MD (eds) (1979) Aerosol measurement. University Presses of Florida, Gainesville
2. Marple VA, Liu BY (eds) (1983) Aerosols in the mining and industrial work environments, vol 1: Fundamentals and status; vol 2: Characterization; vol 3: Instrumentation. Ann Arbor Science, Ann Arbor.
3. Animal Welfare Act of 1970 (Public Law 91–579; 7 US Code 2121 et seq.); Regulations found in the code of federal regulations, title 9: Animals and animal products, chap 1, subchap A (May 1972)
4. Armbruster L, Breuer H (1983) Dust monitoring and the principle of on-line dust control. In: Marple VA, Liu BY (eds) Aerosols in the mining and industrial work environments, vol 3, pp 689–699
5. Bell KA, Avol EL, Bailey RM, Kleinman MT, Landis DA, Heisler SL (1980) Design operation and dynamics of aerosol exposure facilities for human subjects. In: Willeke K (ed) Generation of aerosols and facilities for exposure experiments. Ann Arbor Science, Ann Arbor, pp 475–492
6. Berglund RN, Liu BYH (1973) Generation of monodispersal aerosol standards. Environ Sci Technol 7:147–153
7. Carpenter RL, Barr FP, Leydig RL, Rajala RE (1979) Microprocessor-controlled inhalation system for repeated exposure of animals to aerosols. Rev Sci Instrum 50:560
8. Chen BT, Crow DJ (1986) Use of an aerodynamic particle sizer as a real-time monitor in generation of ideal solid aerosols. J Aerosol Sci 17:963–972
9. Comroe JH (1968) Physiologie der Atmung. Schattauer, Stuttgart
10. Drew RT, Laskin S (1973) Environmental inhalation chambers, In: Gray WI (ed) Methods of animal experimentation, vol. IV. Academic, New York, pp 1–41
11. Eck B (1978) Technische Strömungslehre, Bd. 1: Grundlagen, Bd. 2: Anwendungen. Springer, Berlin, Heidelberg, New York
12. Eisner AD, Martonen TB (1986) Simultaneous production of two monodisperse aerosols with a spinning top instrument. In: Schikarski W, Fissan H, Friedlander SK (eds) Aerosols: Formation and reactivity. 2nd International Aerosol Conference, Berlin. Pergamon, Oxford, pp 1049–1052
13. Ferin J, Leach LJ (1980) Horizontal airflow inhalation exposure chamber. In: Willeke K (ed) Generation of aerosols and facilities for exposure experiments. Ann Arbor Science, Ann Arbor, pp 517–524
14. Findeisen W (1935) Über das Absetzen kleiner, in der Luft suspendierter Teilchen in der menschlichen Lunge bei der Atmung. Pflügers Arch 236:367–379
15. Liu BYH (ed) (1976) Fine particles, Academic, New York
16. Finkelstein W, Fitzner K, Moog W (1973) Messungen von Raumluftgeschwindigkeiten in der Klimatechnik. Heiz Lüft, Haustech No 3:17–23
17. Fisher GL (1980) Size-related chemical and physical properties of power plant fly ash. In: Willeke K (ed) Generation of aerosols and facilities for exposure experiments. Ann Arbor Science, Ann Arbor, pp 203–214
18. Gallily I, Schiby D, Cohen AH, Holländer W, Schless D, Stöber W (1986) On the inertial separation of nonspherical aerosol particles from laminar flows. I. the cylindrical case. Aerosol Sci Technol 5:267–286
19. Guyton AC (1947) Measurement of the respiratory volumes of laboratory animals. Am J Physiol 150:70–77

20. Hackney JD, Linn WS, Buckley RD, Pedersen EE, Karuza SK, Law DC, Fischer DA (1975) Experimental studies on human health effects of air pollutants. I. Design considerations, Arch Environ Health 30:373
21. Dennis R (ed) (1976) Handbook on aerosols Technical Information Center, Energy Research and Development Administration, NTIS, Springfield
22. Heyder J, Gebhart J, Rudolfs G, Schiller CF, Stahlhofen, W (1986) Deposition of particles in the human respiratory tract in the size range 0.005–15 μm. J Aerosol Sci 17:811–825
23. Hinners RG, Burkart JK, Contner GL (1966) Animal exposure chambers in air pollution studies. Arch Environ Health 13:609
24. Holländer W (1981) The measurement of dust properties. In: VDI-Berichte 429 Schwebstoffe und Stäube—Analytische und technische Aspekte. Kolloquium Nürnberg 1981. VDI, Düsseldorf, pp 35–57
25. Holländer W, Pape E, Plachky M, Vater P, Brandt R (1986) Aerosol mass determination with nuclear track filters from quartz crystals. J Aerosol Sci 17:859–871
26. Hollander W, Schörmann J, Stöber W, Mönig FJ, Schwarzer N (1981) Sensitive integrated and timeresolved aerosol measurement by means of light-transmission changes of metal-coated Nucleporefilters (Filter-Fotometer). Environ Sci Technol 15:471–473
27. Holländer W, Stöber, W (1986) Aerosols of smoke, respiratory physiology and deposition. Arch Toxicol Suppl 9:74–87
28. Hörnicke H (1969) Atmung und Gaswechsel. In: Handbuch der Tierernährung, vol. I, part 3. Paul Parey, Berlin, pp 298–332
29. Ishinishi N, Koizumi A, McClellan, RO, Stöber W (eds) (1986) Carcinogenic and mutagenic effects of Diesel engine exhaust. Elsevier, Amsterdam. (Proceedings of the international satellite symposium on toxicological effects of emissions from Diesel engines, Tsukuba)
30. Jenkins RW, Stöber W (1979) Chemical variability of mainstream cigarette smoke as a function of aerodynamic particle size. J Aerosol Sci 10:355–362
31. Koch W, Lödding H, Oenning G, Muhle H (1986) The generation and the measurement of dry aerosols in large-scale inhalation experiments. J Aerosol Sci, 17:499–504
32. Leach LJ, Spiegl CJ, Wilson RH, Sylvester GE, Lauterbach KE (1959) A multiple chamber exposure unit designed for chronic inhalation studies. Am Ind Hyg Assoc J 20:13–21
33. Linton RW, Williams P, Evans CA Jr, Natusch DFS (1977) Determination of the surface predominance of toxic elements in airborne particles by ion microprobe mass spectrometry and Auger electron spectrometry. Anal Chem 49:
34. Macias ES, Husar RB (1976) A review of atmospheric particulate mass measurement via the beta attenuation technique. In: Liu BYH (ed) Fine particles. Academic, New York, pp 536–564
35. Martonen TB, Miller FJ (1986) Dosimetry and species sensitivity: Key factors in hazard evaluation using animal exposure data. J Aerosol Sci 17:316–319
36. May KR (1949) An improved spinning top homogeneous spray apparatus. J Appl Phys 20:932–938
37. McFarland HN (1976) Respiratory toxicology. In: Hays WJ Jr (ed) Essays in Toxicology. vol 7, Academic, New York, pp 121–154
38. Melandri C, Tarroni G, Prodi V, De Zaiacomo T, Formignani M, Lombardi CC (1983) Deposition of charged particles in the human airways. J Aerosol Sci 14:184–186

39. Moss OR (1981) A chamber providing uniform concentration of particulates for exposure of animals on tiers separated by catch pans. In: Drew RT (ed) Inhalation chamber technology. Brookhaven National Laboratory, Upton, NY, BNL Formal Report No 51318
40. Müller W (1959) The development of an electric-wire explosion studied with the help of a Kerr-cell camera. In: Chance WG, Müller HK (eds). Exploding wires. Plenum, New York, pp 201–214
41. Ondov JM, Ragaini RC, Biermann AH (1979) Emissions and particle-size distributions of minor and trace elements at two western coal-fired power plants equipped with cold-side electrostatic precipitators. Environ Sci Technol 13:946–953
42. Phalen, RF (1984) Inhalation studies: Foundations and techniques. CRC Press, Boca Raton
43. Raabe OG, Al-Bayati MA, Teague SV, Rasolt A (1985) Regional deposition of inhaled monodisperse coarse and fine aerosol particles in small laboratory animals. Presented at the Sixth international symposium on inhaled particles, Cambridge, UK, September 2–6, 1985
44. Raes F, Janssens A (1984) Combined photolytic and radiolytic aerosol formation in a SO_2-NO_2-air mixture. In: Versino B, Angeletti G (eds) Physico-Chemical Behaviour of Atmospheric Pollutants. Proceedings of the Third European Symposium held in Varese, Italy, 10–12 April 1984. Reidel, Dordrecht, pp 364–372
45. Regenscheit B (1970) Die Archimedes-Zahl. Kennzahl zur Beurteilung von Raumströmungen. Gesund Ing 91:170–177
46. Sauerbrey G (1959) Verwendung von Schwingquarzen zur Wägung dünner Schichten und zur Mikrowägung. Z Phys 155:206–222
47. Schlichting H (1965) Grenzschicht-Theorie. Braun, Karlsruhe
48. Schum M, Yeh HC (1980) Theoretical evaluation of aerosol deposition in anatomical models of mammalian lung airways. Bull Math Biol 42:1–15
49. Sem GJ, Daley PS (1979) Performance evaluation of a new piezoelectric aerosol sensor. In: Lundgren DA, Harris S Jr, Marlow WH, Lippmann M, Clark WE, Durham MD (eds) Aerosol measurement. University Presses of Florida, Gainesville, pp 672–686
50. Sinclair D, La Mer VK (1949) Light scattering as a measure of particle size in aerosols. The production of monodisperse aerosols. Chem Rev 44:245–267
51. Spohr F (1986) Einsatzmöglichkeiten der radiometrischen Staubmeßtechnik. Chemie-Technik 15:110–113
52. Spurny KR (1980) Fiber generation and length classification. Generation of aerosols and facilities for exposure experiments. In: Willeke K (ed) Generation of aerosols and facilities for exposure experiments. Ann Arbor Science, Ann Arbor, pp 257–298
53. Stöber W, Mönig FJ, Flachsbart H, Schwarzer N (1980) Design and performance of an aerosol mass distribution monitor. EPA-600/2-80-053. Office of Research and Development USEPA, Research Triangle Park, NC
54. Stuart BO, Willard DH, Howard EB (1971) Studies of inhaled radon daughters, uranium ore dust, Diesel exhaust and cigarette smoke in dogs and hamsters. In: Walton WH (ed) Inhaled Particles, vol III. Unwin, Old Woking, England, p 543
55. Takahashi K, Kasahara M, Itoh M (1975) A kinetic model of sulfuric acid aerosol formation from photochemical oxidation of sulfur dioxide vapor. J Aerosol Sci 6:45–55
56. Ter Kuile WM (1979) Comparable dust sampling at the workplace. Delft, TNO (TNO Report F 1699 September 1979)

57. Tierschutzgesetz: Erstes Gesetz zur Änderung des Tierschutzgesetzes. Bundesgesetzblatt Teil 1, Z 5702 A, Nr. 42, 22.8.1986, S. 1309
58. VDI-Handbuch (1981) Herstellungsverfahren für Prüfaerosole. Aerosolgenerator nach Sinclair und La Mer. VDI 3491, Bl 4, Ausgabe 12/80
59. VDI-Richtlinien (1984) Messen von Partikeln Herstellen von Prüfaerosolen mittels eines Bürstendosierers, VDI 3491, Bl 9, Entwurf
60. VDI-Richtlinien (1984) Messen von Partikeln, Herstellung von Prüfaerosolen unter Verwendung von Ultraschallzerstäubern. VDI 3491, Bl 11, Entwurf
61. VDI-Richtlinien (1986) Herstellen von Prüfaerosolen unter Verwendung von Kapillarwellengeneratoren. VDI 3491, Bl 14, Entwurf
62. Van Dyke M (1982) An Album of Fluid Motion. Parabolic, Stanford, CA
63. Wilson JC, Liu BYH (1980) Aerodynamic particle size measurement by laser-Doppler velocimetry. J Aerosol Sci 11:139–150
64. Whitby R, Gibbs R, Johnson R, Hill B, Shimpi S, Jorgenson R (1982) Real-time Diesel particulate measurement using a tapered element oscillating microbalance. SAE Technical Paper 82 0463. International Congress and Exposition, Detroit, Michigan, 22–26 February 1982
65. Willeke K (ed) (1980) Generation of aerosols and facilities for exposure experiments. Ann Arbor Science, Ann Arbor
66. Yu CP, Xu GB (1986) Predictive models for deposition of Diesel exhaust particulates in human and rat lungs. Aerosol Sci Technol 5:337–347
67. Zoebl H, Kruschik J (1982) Strömung durch Rohre und Ventile. Tabellen und Berechnungsverfahren zur Dimensionierung von Rohrleitungssystemen, 2nd ed. Springer, Vienna, New York

CHAPTER 6

Different Methods Used in Acute and Subchronic Inhalation Studies of Potential Lung Irritants, with Particular Attention to Lung Function Measurements

J. Pauluhn[1]

Introduction

Inhalation toxicity studies are carried out on either a vapor or an aerosol form of a potential lung irritant, depending on its physicochemical properties. Owing to the frequently high reactivity of locally irritant vapors with the moisture contained in air expired by the test species, the possibility of a secondary change of the test substance in the inhalation chamber atmosphere cannot be excluded. This factor must therefore be taken into account both in the analytical characterization of the test atmosphere and in the choice of the mode of exposure.

Investigation of the toxic action of potential lung irritants in vapor and aerosol form can be carried out qualitatively and quantitatively on the basis of several parameters. In the present work we consider the diagnostic value of lung function tests carried out on rats exposed acutely to thionyl chloride (vapor) and on rats exposed acutely and subchronically to an isocyanurate aerosol. Thionyl chloride is a typical upper respiratory tract irritant; the isocyanurate was investigated as an example of the less reactive potential lung irritants. Owing to the aerosol size, the isocyanurate is deposited in the lower respiratory tract. A comparative evaluation is made of investigations of the lung mechanics based on conventional inhalation toxicity parameters, such as the relationship between lung weight and body weight, the intoxication symptoms (irritation of the mucosal membranes), or histological examination of the respiratory tract.

Method of Exposure

The isocyanurate investigated is a relatively viscous substance with a low vapor pressure, so that inhalation toxicity studies can only be carried out on its aerosol form. In order to achieve exposure of all the potential target structures of the respiratory tract in the test species, an aerosol with a mass median aerodynamic diameter (MMAD) of approximately 1.5 μm is generated (13). The polydisper-

[1]Department of Toxicology, Bayer AG, D 5600 Wuppertal 1, FRG.

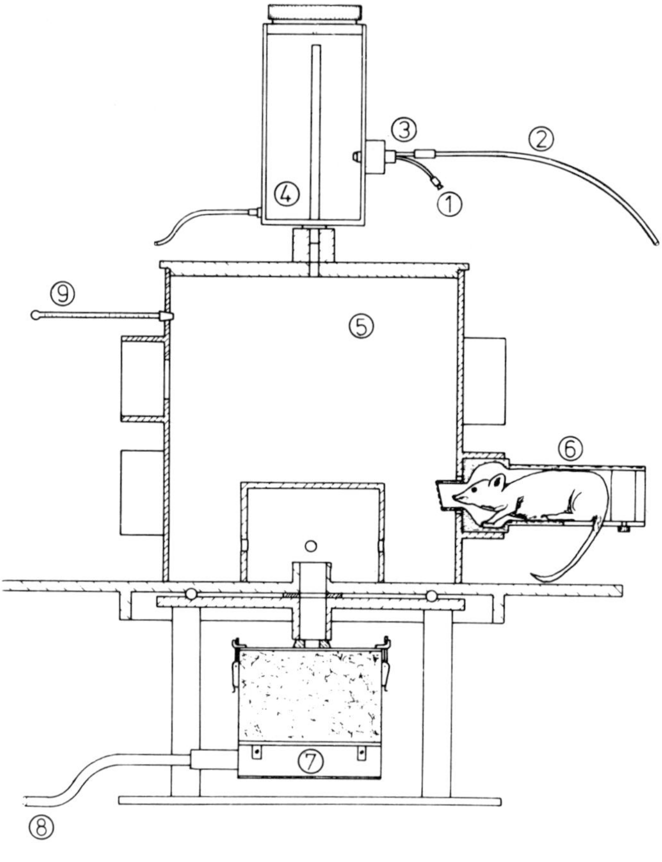

Fig. 6.1. Inhalation chamber with an aerosol generation system. 1, Feed of spray solution by an infusion pump; 2, compressed air (10 l/min); pressure approx. 600 kPa; 3, two-component nozzle (Rhema Labortechnik); 4, separator (baffle); 5, inhalation chamber; 6, rat in exposure tube; 7, cotton-wool filter (adsorbent); 8, suction (vacuum system) with hygrometer; 9, thermometer.

sity of the aerosol is described in terms of the geometric standard deviation σ, and is approximately 1.6.

Fig. 6.1 gives a representative example of a head/nose inhalation chamber for inhalation toxicity studies on an aerosol. The baffle principle of the preseparator increases the yield of inhalable aerosol (15), and allows larger particles to be separated.

Test substances that react easily with the humidity of the test atmosphere, e.g., thionyl chloride, are investigated in the inhalation chamber illustrated in Fig. 6.2. The flow dynamics of the head/nose inhalation chamber prevent the exhaled air from mixing with the primarily generated test atmosphere. This is achieved by the provision of separate routes for the inlet and outlet of the test atmosphere.

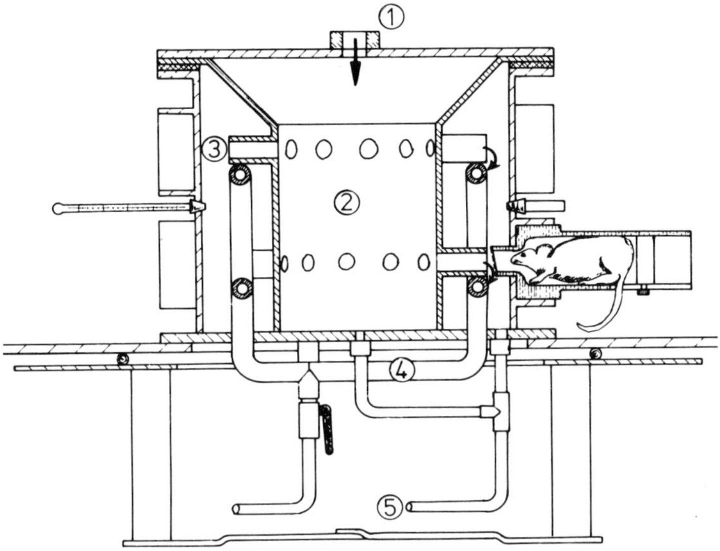

Fig. 6.2. Inhalation chamber for reactive test substances. 1, Test material inlet; 2, inner inhalation chamber (overpressure system); 3, exposure zone; 4, underpressure system; 5 scrubbing system.

Samples are collected from the respiratory area of the rats under virtually isokinetic conditions. Moisture-determined decomposition products are of no analytical or toxicological significance in the determination of the test substance concentration. A similar flow principle is used in the V-shaped Lovelace and Battelle inhalation chambers (3).

Characterization of the Test Atmosphere

An aerosol should have the maximal inhalability for the test species in question. Aerosols are characterized by the test substance concentration and aerosol mass distribution. The method of sample collection of the test atmosphere should, as far as this is technically feasible, exclude anisokinetic sampling errors. Only then can a representative characterization of the test atmosphere be ensured with different suction velocities and geometries of different experimental arrangements.

In view of the relatively small volume of the inhalation chamber (about 10–20 litres), an air supply rate of about 10 l/min, a sampling rate of not less than 8 ml/s and not more than 80 ml/s is aimed at for air samples. Approximately 30% of the supplied air escapes through the exposure tubes.

The tolerance limits for sampling probe diameters can be calculated according to generally accepted recommendations (1,4,9) in such a way that a representative characterization of the test atmosphere is also possible under anisokinetic sample collection conditions.

Under the experimental conditions described, a polyethylene glycol E 400 (PE) aerosol was produced using the aerosol generation technique illustrated in Fig. 6.1 (nominally 10,000 μl PE/m³ air, 10,000 μl ethanol/m³ air). In this aerosol, which is often used as an inert vehicle substance, 99% of the particles are in the size range of approximately 0.5–7.4 μm (MMAD 1.4 μm, σ about 1.4). Taking the above-mentioned sample collection criteria into account, the sampling probe radius can be calculated as follows (1):

$$5\left(\frac{F\tau}{4\pi}\right)^{1/3} \leq r_p \leq \left(\frac{F}{g\tau\pi}\right)^{1/2}/5$$

F = 8–80 cm³/s
τ = $1.0 \times 10^{-6} - 1.7\ 10^{-4}$ s
g = 980 cm/s²
r_p = probe radius (in cm)

The probe diameters (D_p) for particles with aerodynamic diameters of 0.5–7.4 μm were calculated by the above equation for the extreme sampling rates of 8 and 80 ml/s and are presented in Table 6.1. Thus, under the specified conditions, it is possible to ensure representative sample collection even under anisokinetic sampling conditions if the internal diameter (D_p) of the probe is 1.3 ± 0.3 cm.

The particle characteristics of the PE aerosol in the breathing zone of the rats were analyzed on the basis of a particle number distribution (TSI-APS 3300 aerodynamic particle sizer with 2 dilution stages, TSI Model 3200). The technical details of this measurement and dilution system have been discussed by Remiarz and Johnson (14). The mass-related particle analysis was done with the aid of a Berner 8-stage cascade impactor with cut-off diameters of 0.12, 0.25, 0.49, 0.90, 1.85, 3.96, 7.42, and 14.8 μm. Punched out aluminum foil was used as the impaction medium.

The TSI laser velocimeter allows a real-time analysis of the particle number distribution. The results of the particle analysis are then available immediately after sample collection. The laser velocimeter correlates the number of particles showing a defined transit time over a specified distance with the aerodynamic

Table 6.1. Calculation of D_p

Sampling rate		Calculated probe diameter (cm)				
$F_{0.5}$	8:	0.09	<	D_p	<	20.4
	80:	0.19	<	D_p	<	64.5
$F_{7.4}$	8:	0.48	<	D_p	<	1.6
	80:	1.0	<	D_p	<	4.9

particle diameter. The result is therefore a number-related particle distribution, described by the number median aerodynamic diameter (NMAD) and the geometric standard deviation σ. In order to relate the NMAD with the mass-related concentrations determined and the cascade impactor analyses, the NMAD is converted into MMAD by the following equation (4):

$$\ln(\text{MMAD}) = \ln(\text{NMAD} \times \text{density}) + 3(\ln(\sigma))^2$$

The aerosol generation system shown in Fig. 6.1 produces a (mass-based) monomodal aerosol distribution. The monomodality is checked by plotting the frequency distribution graphically.

In theory, particles can be precipitated in the dilution system of the TSI laser velocimeter. However, a check of the recovery rate for a PE aerosol showed that, taking into account the above boundary conditions (mass of 99% of the particles ≤ 7.4 µm; adequate probe diameter), the recovery rate is high. An NMAD of 0.92 µm was used as a starting point for the calculation.

Calculation of particle volume:

$$\begin{aligned} \text{Equation: } 4/3\pi r^3;\ r &= 0.46 \times 10^{-4} \text{ cm } (r = \text{NMAD}/2) \\ &= 4/3\pi(0.46 \times 10^{-4})^3 \\ \text{Particle volume} &= 0.41 \times 10^{-12} \text{ cm}^3 \end{aligned}$$

Calculation of particle mass:

$$\begin{aligned} \text{Equation: Volume} \times \text{Density; PE density} &= 1.13 \times 10^3 \text{ mg/cm}^3 \\ &= 0.46 \times 10^{-9} \text{ mg/particle} \\ 1 \text{ mg/m}^3 &= 2.17 \times 10^9 \text{ particles/m}^3 \\ &= 2170 \text{ particles/cm}^3 \end{aligned}$$

Calculation of nominal number of particles in the test atmosphere:

$$\begin{aligned} 10{,}000 \text{ µl PE/m}^3 &= 11{,}300 \text{ mg PE/m}^3 \text{ air} \\ 11{,}300 \text{ mg PE/m}^3 &= 25 \times 10^6 \text{ particles/cm}^3 \end{aligned}$$

In calculations of the nominal number of particles in the test atmosphere it is a prerequisite that the solvent (ethanol) is quantitatively evaporized on nebulization.

Figure 6.3 shows the test substance concentrations determined analytically in the respiration area of the rats against the nominal concentrations. The various test substances were dissolved in the PE-ethanol vehicle and nebulized in the system illustrated in Fig. 6.1.

As can be seen from Fig. 6.3, the generation efficiency is approximately 14% on nebulization of various test substances (in all cases 10,000 µl PE/m^3, 10,000 µl ethanol/m^3; nebulization of spray solutions of different concentrations); in other words, approximately 3.5×10^6 particles/cm^3 would be expected, assuming adequate sample collection and alignment of practice with theory (boundary conditions: relatively monodisperse distribution, quantitative evapo-

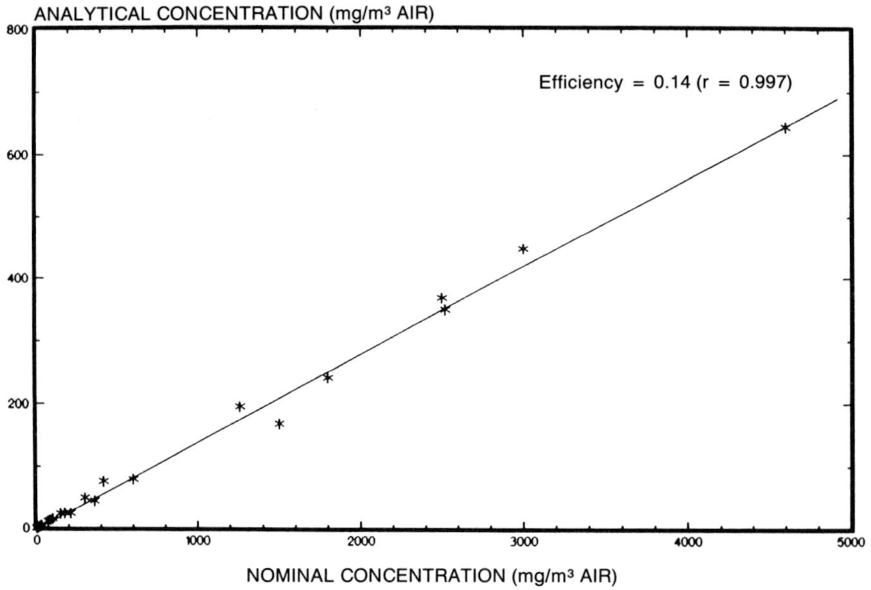

Fig. 6.3. Efficiency of PE aerosol generation. Analytical vs. nominal concentration. Vehicle: 20,000 μl/m³ air.

ration of ethanol during aerosol generation, no effect of the test substance on the density of the PE vehicle). The individual results of the particle number determinations (TSI) with the PE aerosol were in the range of approximately 2.4×10^6–4.6×10^6 particles/cm³ test atmosphere. The boundary conditions used in the above equations to calculate the particle characteristics have therefore been confirmed experimentally.

As can be seen from Fig. 6.4, irrespective of the properties of the test substance, the concentration investigated, and the aerosol characterization method used, there are no concentration-dependent changes in the MMAD in the investigations presented in Fig. 6.3. It can be seen from Table 6.2 that the MMAD calculated on the basis of the NMAD correlates to the required degree of accuracy with the MMAD values found directly on the cascade impactor, irrespective of whether a PE aerosol at a high concentration or a isocyanurate aerosol at a comparatively low concentration was investigated. The fact that the σ values were greater with the Berner cascade impactor is due to the lower resolution of the impactor in comparison with the TSI system.

Comparative concentration determinations with the Berner cascade impactor and filter analyses did not reveal any essential differences in the mass concentrations. Wall losses in the impactor system can therefore be disregarded. The two physically different measuring methods thus yield consistent results. The rats exposed under the conditions described underwent a series of lung function tests. The method and the results of these tests are described below.

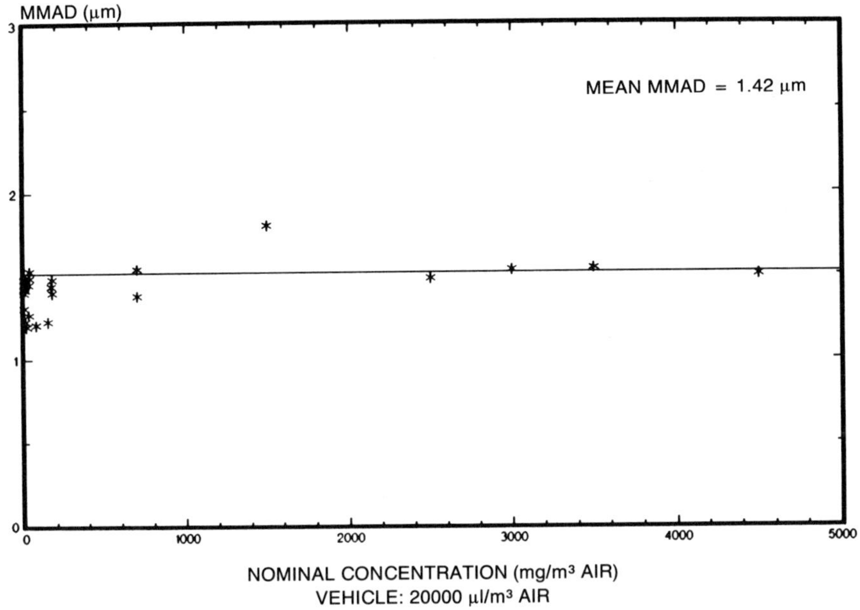

Fig. 6.4. Concentration dependence of the MMAD.

Lung Function Tests

The lung function tests and the calculations of corresponding lung function parameters were carried out with a Pulmonary Mechanics Computer Model 6 (Buxco Electronics, CT, USA).

The rats were anesthetized with approximately 2.5 ml of 10% hexobarbital (Evipan-Natrium, Bayer AG) solution/kg body weight, administered by the intraperitoneal route. In the pulmonary function the optimal depth of anesthesia was one at which the rats had a respiration rate of some 90 ± 20/min.

Table 6.2. Comparison of the MMAD and σ values calculated from cascade impactor and TSI laser velocimeter studies

Substance and system	MMAD (µm)	σ
Isocyanurate (+10% acetone)[a]		
TSI APS 33	1.5	1.3
Berner Impactor	1.5	1.6
20 000 µl vehicle PE/m³ air		
TSI APS 33[b]	1.4	1.4
Berner Impactor	1.4	1.9

PE: polyethylene glycol – ethanol
[a]Actual concentration: 0.4–3–25 mg/m³ air
[b]2 dilution steps (TSI Model 3200)

The measurements were done in a whole-body flow plethysmograph. The air flows were determined from the pressure difference across a 400-mesh wire gauze (diameter 2 cm), measured with a differential pressure transducer mounted on the plethysmograph wall (MP 45 $\pm$ 2 cmH_2O, Validyne, Northridge, CA, USA).

The transpulmonary pressure was measured with the aid of an orotracheal catheter (stainless steel, internal diameter 1.8 mm, length 55 mm) and an esophageal catheter filled with water (PVC, external diameter 1.7 mm, length 160 mm), using a Statham P23 pressure transducer (Statham, Hato Ray, Puerto Rico). The orotracheal catheter was inserted into the rat trachea noninvasively under visual control using a laryngoscope, and the esophageal catheter was introduced, avoiding air bubbles, under pressure control into the esophagus parietalis (maximal esophageal pressure). The catheter was positioned (phase and amplitude check) with the aid of an oscillograph (Honeywell UV recorder, Model 1895).

The dynamic compliance (C_{dyn}; ml/cm H_2O) and the lung resistance (*Res*; cm H_2O/ml/s) were calculated according to the method of Amdur and Mead (2) on a Buxco analog computer.

Before the flow-volume measurement the rats were hyperventilated for a short time until apnea was induced. At a transpulmonary pressure of 20 cm H_2O the slow, forced inspiration phase changed over to rapid forced expiration (expiration against a subatmospheric pressure of -30 cm H_2O). The mean mid-expiratory flow (MMEF; ml/s) and the peak expiratory flow (PEF; ml/s) served as the measurement parameters. The quasistatic compliance (C_{stat}) was calculated from the graphically determined slope ($\Delta V/\Delta P$) of the pressure-volume curve, which was maintained by slow, forced expiration at pressure intervals of 2 cm H_2O. This arrangement was also used to determine the total lung capacity (TLC; ml), the residual volume (*RV*; ml), and the vital capacity (VC; ml).

Acetylcholine Provocation Test

The acetylcholine aerosol was produced with the aid of a DeVilbiss aerosol generator (10 L air/min). The aerosol was passed through a hot zone (120°C) and a drying tube packed with silica gel (7,12). This resulted in a very fine-particle aerosol with an NMAD of approximately 0.9 μm. In the region of the orotracheal catheter opening the acetylcholine concentration was around 590 mg/m^3 air. The provocation substance was acetylcholine hydrochloride, 25% acetylcholine chloride in Levatit water (Aldrich Chemical Co., Steinheim, FRG).

After an adaptation phase of approximately 3 min provocation was carried out for a total of 5 min, with simultaneous measurements of Res and C_{dyn}. The stability and the reproducibility of the "provocative atmosphere" were measured continuously with a TSI light-scattering photometer (TSI Respiratory Aerosol Monitor Model 5150). In this test the difference in lung resistance before and after provocation was determined (ΔRes) (7,12).

Measurement of Functional Residual Capacity (FRC)

The FRC was measured in a completely closed plethysmograph (V = constant) according to the recommendations of Palecek (11). The FRC value was calculated from the following equation:

$$FRC = (P_b - PH_2O - \Delta P_{ao})/\Delta P_{ao} \times \Delta V - V_t,$$

in which:

P_b = barometric pressure (mm Hg)
PH_2O = vapor pressure of water at 37°C (= 47 mm Hg)
ΔP_{ao} = pressure change in the orotracheal catheter (mm Hg)
ΔV = volume change in the plethysmograph during the measurement of the orotracheal catheter pressure (measurement in mm Hg and conversion into ml)
V_t = dead volume = 1.25 ml.

The methods of lung function studies and the interpretation of the lung function parameters were in accordance with the recommendations of Drazen (6), Diamond and O'Donnell (5), Likens and Mauderly (8), and Palecek (11).

The arrangement used for the lung function tests is shown in Fig. 6.5. The inhalation chamber shown in Fig. 6.2 was used for the studies with thionyl chloride. The rats were head-nose exposed for 4 h to thionyl chloride vapor at concentrations of 63, 403, and 1596 mg/m³ air, and lung function tests were then carried out on the 1st and 14th days of observation. Immediately after the end of exposure the rats exposed to 63 mg/m³ air showed transient hyperemia of the visible nasal mucous membranes. Exposure to 403 mg/m³ air gave rise to blood-stained nasal discharge, respiratory difficulties, and mucosal irritation. In the group exposed to 1596 mg/m³ air these symptoms persisted until the end of the 14-day observation period. All three concentrations were tolerated without any fatalities.

The lung function tests carried out on rats acutely exposed to thionyl chloride are depicted in Fig. 6.6; C_{stat} and C_{dyn} remained unchanged. The decrease of the specific compliance ($C_{spec} = C_{stat}$/FRC) in the rats exposed to 1596 mg/m³ air is regarded as being in a causative relationship with an increase in FRC. The increased lung resistance (Res) and the reduced MMEF and PEF values point to an elevation of the central and upper airways resistance. The increase in the airways resistance (Res, MMEF, and PEF) established during the 14-day observation period suggests inflammatory processes in the upper airways. No particular effects were observed in the acetylcholine provocation test (ΔRes).

The finding that only in the rats exposed to 1596 mg/m³ air was there a toxicologically significant increase in the flow resistances can be traced back to nasal respiration in rats. It was only when a threshold concentration had been reached that the airways situated distal to the nasopharyngeal region were also damaged. Under the conditions of this investigation (use of an orotracheal catheter), the flow changes in the nasopharyngeal region could not be determined.

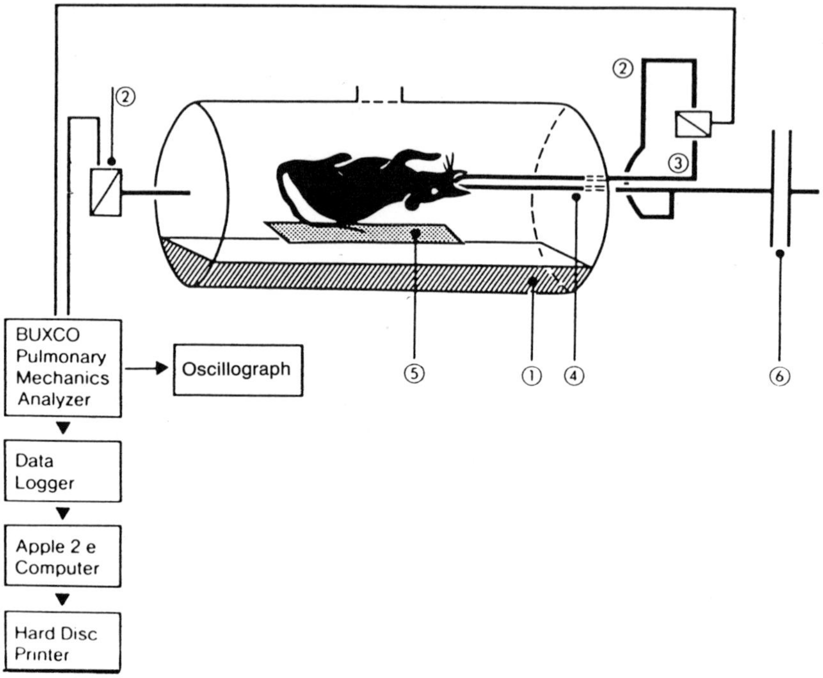

Fig. 6.5. Arrangement used for the lung function tests. 1, Whole-body flow plethysmograph (Buxco Electronics); 2, validyne differential pressure transducer; 3, esophageal catheter; 4, orotracheal catheter; 5, insulation material; 6, feed of acetylcholine aerosol.

The lung function studies with rats exposed acutely to an isocyanurate aerosol (MMAD 1.5 μm, σ 1.6) yielded the following results: rats exposed to 11 mg/m³ air showed a temporary reddening of the visible nasal mucous membranes. In the 65 mg/m³ group dyspnea was also observed after the exposure, and blood-stained noses in the 118 mg/m³ group.

From the 65 mg/m³ concentration upwards there was a concentration-dependent decrease in C_{stat} and C_{spec}, in MMEF, and in PEF. The changes in C_{dyn}, Res, and ΔRes were of no toxicological significance. The most important results of the lung function tests are summarized in Table 6.3. The most distinct concentration-dependent change occurred in C_{spec}. Investigation of this most sensitive parameter on the 8th and 14th days of observation revealed clear signs of recovery (Fig. 6.7). These results lead to the conclusion that the isocyanurate aerosol produces functional changes mainly in the peripheral regions of the lungs. Normalization of the most sensitive parameter C_{stat} or C_{spec} within the observation period indicates that the changes could be causally connected with functionally increased liquid transudation into the alveolar interstitium.

The same lung function tests were carried out on rats exposed subchronically to the isocyanurate (head-nose exposure each working day for 13 weeks; 0, 0.4,

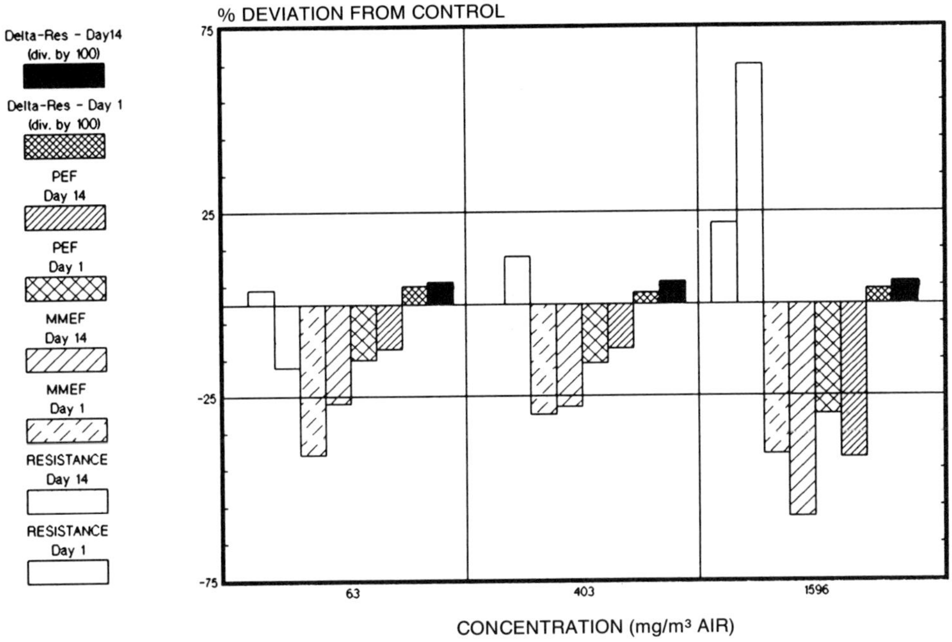

Fig. 6.6. Flow resistance.

3, and 25 mg/m³ air): some results are presented in Fig. 6.8. The relationship between the lung weight and the body weight is illustrated in Fig. 6.9. All findings essential for the evaluation of the lung function are summarized in Table 6.4, from which it will be seen that the increase in lung weight is the most sensitive parameter. Histological examinations gave no indication of any changes in the nasopharyngeal cavity or in the pulmonary airways. Focal proliferations were determined only in the lungs of animals exposed to 25 mg/m³.

Table 6.3. Isocyanurate: acute 1 × 4 h exposure; measurement on 1st observation day

Parameter		air	11	65	118
			(mg/m³ air)		
C_{dyn}	(ml/cm H_2O)	0.29	0.27	0.27	0.25
C_{stat}	(ml/cm H_2O)	0.61	0.56	0.42	0.31
C_{spec}	(ml/cm H_2O/ml)	0.15	0.12	0.09	0.06
Res	(cm H_2O/ml/s)	0.23	0.23	0.20	0.23
MMEF	(ml/s)	64	63	53	51
PEF	(ml/s)	76	76	71	70
TLC	(ml)	10.5	10.4	9.3	8.5
FRC	(ml)	4.0	4.6	4.9	5.2

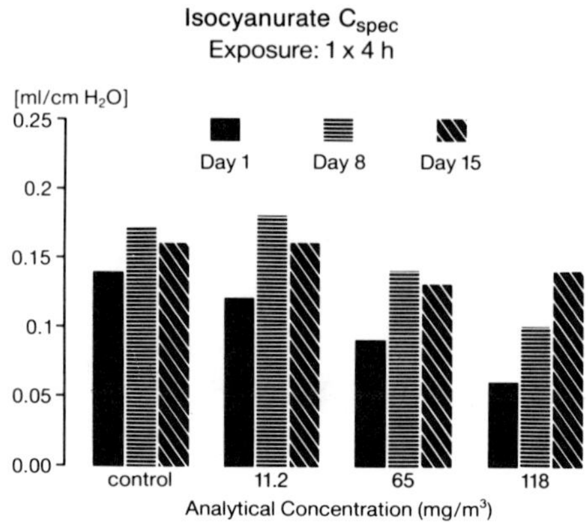

Fig. 6.7. Isocyanurate, acute inhalation.

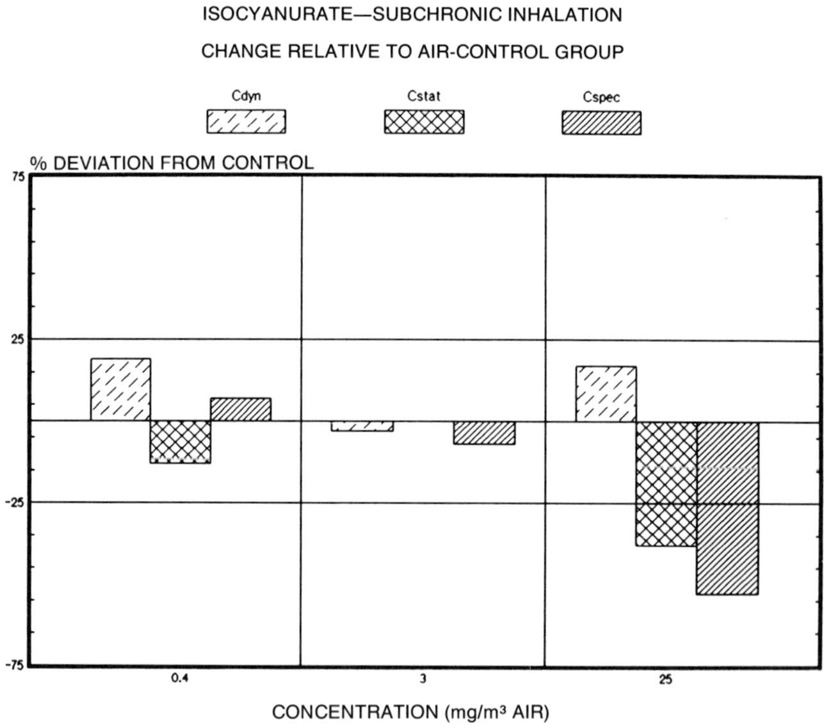

Fig. 6.8. Static, dynamic, and specific compliance.

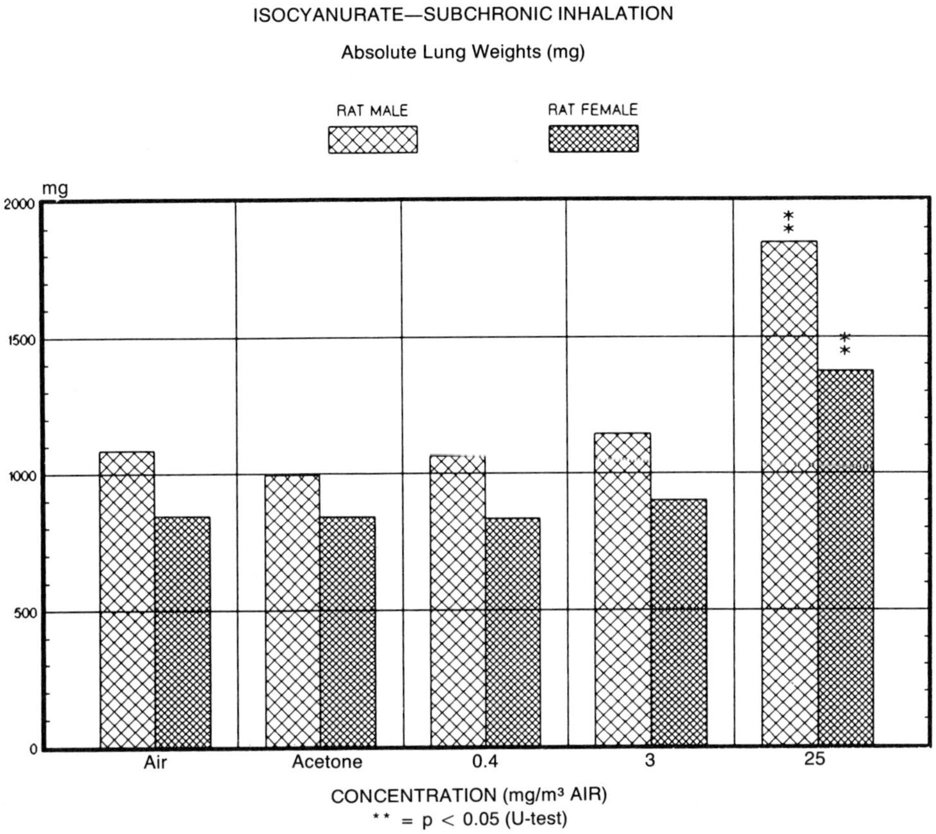

Fig. 6.9. Lung weights.

Like the results of the acute exposure studies, lung function tests revealed the presence of obstructive changes in the region of the peripheral airways. The increased lung weights can be traced back to increased liquid transudation into the interstitium with drainage via the lymph (10). This is regarded as the primary cause of the reduced compliance (C_{stat}).

An elevated concentration-dependent reactivity of the bronchial muscles to acetylcholine aerosol was not observed in either the acutely or the subchronically exposed rats.

The results of this work show that lung function tests carried out within the framework of inhalation toxicity investigations allow reliable conclusions to be drawn about pathophysiological lung alterations even with small numbers of animals. However, in the acetylcholine provocation test no particular diagnostic value could be established either in the rats exposed to thionyl chloride vapor (upper respiratory tract) or in those exposed to a fine-particle isocyanurate aerosol, although in an investigation of cholinesterase inhibitors as positive

Table 6.4. Isocyanurate, subchronic inhalation

	0.4	3 (mg/m³ air)	25
C_{dyn}	n	n	n
C_{stat}	n	n	− (−38%)
C_{spec}	n	n	− (−58%)
Res	n	n	n
MMEF	n	n	− (−37%)
PEF	n	n	n
TLC	n	n	n
VC	n	n	− (−38%)
RV	n	n	+ (+60%)
Lung weight	n	n	+ (+85%)[a]
Histology	n	n	focal proliferations

n, normal.
[a]based on male rats.

substances (12) a concentration-dependent bronchoconstrictive activity of acetylcholine aerosol had been ascertained.

In respect of the determination of the no-observable-effect level, lung function tests on this scale have proved to be no more sensitive than the conventional parameters, e.g., lung-weight determinations or histological examinations of the respiratory tract. However, these investigations of the lung mechanics do show that lung function tests permit a deeper insight into pathophysiological lung alterations. They are therefore useful for describing the nature and the localizations of lung damage together with the resulting secondary reactions. Lung function tests can also contribute to saving experimental animals, since the same animals can be used repeatedly, owing to the noninvasive nature of the technique.

References

1. ACGIH (American Conference of Governmental Industrial Hygienists) (1978) Air sampling instruments for evaluation of atmospheric contaminants, 5th ed. ACGIH, Cincinnati, p F1-F11
2. Amdur MO, Mead J (1958) Mechanics of respiration in unanesthetized guinea pigs. Am J Physiol 192:364–368
3. Cannon WC, Blanton EF, McDonald KE (1983) The flow-past chamber: An improved nose-only exposure system for rodents. Am Ind Hyg Assoc J 4:923–928
4. Dennis R (1976) Handbook of aerosols. Technical Information Center, Energy Research and Development Administration, pp 110–114
5. Diamond L, O'Donnell M (1977) Pulmonary mechanics in normal rats. J Appl Physiol 43:942–948

6. Drazen JM (1984) Physiological basis and interpretation of indices of pulmonary mechanics. Environ Health Perspect 56:3–9
7. Heinrich U, Wilhelm A (1984) Lung function tests on hamsters and rats using the whole body plethysmograph. In: Grosdanoff P, Bass R, Hackenberg U, Henschler D, Müller D, Klimisch H-J (eds) Problems of inhalatory toxicity studies. Munich, MMV Medizinische Verlag, pp 255–266 (BGA Schriften 5)
8. Likens SA, Mauderly JL (1979) Respiratory measurements in small laboratory animals: A literature review. Lovelace Biomedical & Environmental Research Institute
9. Lundgren D, Calvert S (1967) Aerosol sampling with a side port probe. Am Ind Hyg Assoc J 28:208–215
10. Nieman GF (1985) Current concepts of Lung-Fluid Balance. Resp Care 30:1062–1076
11. Palecek F (1969) Measurement of ventilatory mechanics in rats. J Appl Physiol 27:149–156
12. Pauluhn J, Machemer L, Kimmerle G (1987) Effects of inhaled cholinesterase inhibitors on bronchial tonus and on plasma and erythrocyte acetylcholin esterase activity in rats. Toxicology 46:177–190
13. Raabe OG (1982) Deposition and clearance of inhaled aerosols. In Witschi H, Nettesheim P (eds) Mechanisms in respiratory toxicology, vol 1. CRC Press, Boca Raton, pp 27–68
14. Remiarz RJ, Johnson EM (1984) A new diluter for high concentration measurements with the aerodynamic particle sizer. TSI Q 10(1):7–12
15. Tillery MI, Woody GO, Ettinger HJ (1976) Generation and characterization of aerosols and vapors for inhalation experiments. Environ Health Perspect 16:25–40

CHAPTER 7

Chronic Inhalation Toxicity Studies: Protocols and Pitfalls

P.E. Morrow[1] and R. Mermelstein[2]

Introduction

Long-term toxicity testing by the inhalation route is not a simple undertaking. The design, implementation, interpretation, and financial cost of long-term toxicity testing necessitate thorough preparation and assembly of an extensive preliminary toxicity data base. Such studies should only be considered when prechronic (short-term) investigations raise concern about the consequences of long-term inhalation of the material under consideration, or when regulatory requirements mandate them.

The objectives of a chronic inhalation study should be clearly defined at the outset, and the associated endpoints to be evaluated should be specified in the test protocol. Because of the long time requirements of chronic inhalation studies in two species and at several exposure levels, which may exceed 5 years, as well as the tremendous cost, estimated to be near $3–5 million per compound, the importance of careful and comprehensive planning cannot be overemphasized. Contingency planning, consideration of unlikely events, definition of circumstances under which intervention or modification of the test plan may be required, are essential elements of the preparatory tasks of such an investigation.

In the planning of a chronic inhalation study, there is a temptation to be all-inclusive and forget that there is a limit to the number of questions which can be addressed in a single study. Such a desire should be carefully balanced because, as the number of subsidiary questions or subsets of investigations increases, so does the possibility of making errors and endangering the principal objectives of the study. As with any investigation, some elements of the chronic inhalation study are essential, while others may be best characterized as "information nice to have." By definition, the principal part of a chronic inhalation study is the one dealing with the animals exposed to the test material over their life span and the subsequent histopathological examination of the various organs and tissues.

[1]University of Rochester, Rochester, NY 14642, USA.
[2]Xerox Corporation, Rochester, NY 14644, USA.

In a chronic inhalation study, the respiratory system should be the focus of histopathological evaluation, but the other organs should not be ignored. At intervals, some animals should be sacrificed in order to examine carefully their organs and thereby provide early warning of the onset of adverse developments. Other essential elements of the chronic inhalation study are the periodic performance of clinical laboratory tests and determinations of the actual amount of test material in the respiratory system, especially the lung. Optional parts of the study include determinations of the clearance kinetics of the test material and measurement of various biochemical (e.g., urinary mutagenicity, hydroxyproline, connective tissue determinations, etc.) and immunological parameters. The prechronic study results or other information on the test material will frequently provide additional guidance as to what is essential and what is ancillary information.

In this paper we describe some major components of chronic inhalation study design, especially those that we believe are of special importance and often prone to produce problems in either conducting the investigation or interpreting the results. Our selection is derived mainly from our personal experience and it should not be considered as constituting a comprehensive coverage of this challenging and complex topic. It is clear that advances in any scientific field are only made when difficulties and problems are recognized and there is an atmosphere of free exchange of discussion and ideas.

Study Design Considerations

Prechronic Studies

Acquisition of preliminary toxicology information from one or more prechronic inhalation studies (e.g., 13-week) is a prudent and necessary prerequisite to the long-term investigation. Prechronic studies should be designed to provide information on the exposure concentrations to be used and demonstrate that all of the procedures, protocols, and assays intended for use in the chronic study are operating well. In this manner, experimental problems can be identified and corrected and nonessential procedures eliminated without jeopardizing the success of the chronic study.

Some difficulties associated with the setting of exposure levels for chronic inhalation toxicity studies have been discussed in detail (23). The test material should be evaluated at four prechronic exposure levels spanning a range of 1–1.5 orders of magnitude in order to enable the detection of nonlinear effects. The prechronic exposure levels should not result in an overload effect; with limitations, this condition may be acceptable during the later stages of the chronic inhalation study. This matter will be more fully discussed later in this presentation. A chronic toxicity evaluation requires testing of the material of interest at three exposure levels in two test species over their life span. To provide for continuity between the prechronic and chronic studies, it is helpful if at least one of the exposure concentration levels is the same in both prechronic and chronic investigations.

Characterization of the Test Material

A prerequisite of the chronic inhalation study is a comprehensive and careful physical and chemical characterization of the material under consideration. Stability of the material under the conditions of the study should be established or demonstrated. Independent of the physical characteristics of a material, be it a gas, liquid or a particle, the aerosolization and maintenance of a stable aerosol concentration are critical aspects of the chronic study which should be addressed in the prechronic investigations.

The Exposure System

The design and operations of large-scale inhalation systems have been reviewed by several authors (7,31). Many systems, e.g., Rochester, use vertical flow chambers for whole-body inhalation experiments. Others depend on horizontal flow chambers such as those used at the Fraunhofer Institute, or on Hazelton (Moss) chambers which combine horizontal and vertical flow. For certain special experiments, when the test material is highly toxic or radioactive, or its supply is limited, exposure by the nose-only route is usually preferred, but with chronic exposure this is difficult. An account of the methodology used for chronic nose-only exposure of laboratory animals to inhaled fibrous aerosols has been published (32).

Independent of the nature of the exposure system used, the aerosol distribution of the test material at the various exposure concentrations used should be established and periodically verified. Small differences in the temporal and spatial distribution of the aerosol in the multitiered inhalation exposure chambers can be compensated for by periodic rotation of the animals, and can thereby achieve more uniform exposures and lung depositions of the test material (11,38).

Selection of the Animal Model

The selection of the most appropriate test animal model for an inhalation study is not a simple matter. The advantages and disadvantages of different species have been carefully reviewed by Hakkinen and Witschi (9).

The principles of animal extrapolation and their use in risk assessment have been discussed by Calabrese (5) and in a recent publication (21). Considerations of respiratory tract absorption, interspecies differences in the anatomy of the tracheobronchial tree, particle deposition, mucus flow patterns and the role of scaling factors are discussed.

Among 169 chemicals under evaluation by the National Toxicology Program (NTP) during fiscal year 1984, only 10% of these chronic investigations used the inhalation route (27). The two rodents most frequently used in carcinogenesis studies, and on which reasonable baseline data on history, survival, and growth pattern information are available, are the B6C3F1 mouse and the F344 rat (6). Detailed information on the history of body weight gain, survival, and incidence of various types of neoplasia in the F344 rat has also been published (33). However, information is not readily available on organ weight development in either of these two widely used experimental test animals. Substantial information on the spontaneous tumors and common diseases in two colonies of Syrian hamsters has been published (29). Several different strains of viral antibody-free mice and rats are commercially available, but there is only limited availability of high quality hamsters on the commercial market currently. These considerations suggest that F344 rats and either B6C3F1 mice or hamsters are most frequently used in chronic inhalation investigations.

Animal Health and Management

Constant monitoring and evaluation of the health status of the animals is essential for a successful investigation. The minimum test requirements are defined in the various regulatory guidelines (EPA and OECD GLP Guidelines) (28). Serial sacrifice procedures, followed by microscopic examination of at least the respiratory system, provide an ongoing view of the effects, if any, of the test material on the animals.

The use of animals to test hypotheses, evaluate the safety of materials, and train scientists and physicians, carries with it obligations and responsibilities. These have been codified in professional standards and legislative requirements. Among the key requirements are the need to provide adequate nutrition and housing, minimize pain and suffering during procedures, and establish review groups to evaluate the proposed use of the animals. An obvious requirement for a responsible scientific investigation is the use of the minimum number of test animals required to achieve the objective of the study.

Quality research results are dependent upon healthy and well-maintained animals. Infection, disease, malnutrition and injuries may confound the experimental results and thus complicate the interpretation of the investigation. Procurement and proper maintenance of specific pathogen-free, viral antibody-free test animals are essential elements of a high quality investigation. The importance of maintaining the separation of animals from various sources and of possibly diverse health status should be obvious. As the chronic inhalation investigation progresses, the proper care and maintenance of the test animals becomes even more important. Decisions to terminate a study due to serious illness or other complicating factors may be relatively easy during the early stages of an investigation, but become difficult and very costly as the study progresses. Thus, it is advisable to consider the possibility of such developments before the implementation of the study and make adequate preparations for dealing with such an event.

Data Management and Quality Assurance

The ability to evaluate the status of the investigation on an ongoing basis is one of the important challenges during the performance of a chronic inhalation study. A tremendous amount of data is generated during the course of the study, and its transformation to meaningful information for the investigator is not a trivial matter. Consider the data collected on just one animal during the chronic inhalation study. During the first 3–4 months body weight is generally recorded weekly. During most of the course of the investigation such measurement may be made monthly, while near the end of the study more frequent measurements may be warranted in order to provide an early warning of possible body weight loss and onset of more serious processes. Some of the other routine measurements during the life of the test animal include food consumption, clinical chemistry and hematology (25–40 parameters). Following death or sacrifice of the test animal, observations on perhaps a dozen tissues and organs must be made and histopathological findings need to be recorded.

In large chronic inhalation studies, the availability of sufficient numbers of high quality animals is a frequent constraint. A solution sometimes employed is the sequential start of the study in two or three installments. Scheduling of the various activities, generating workplans for the diverse technical personnel in such a case becomes an even more complex task than usual.

With the availability of low-cost computing capacity numerous laboratory tasks have become automated, and personal and minicomputers are frequently used in various laboratory applications. Perhaps more suited for chronic inhalation studies are larger integrated systems, capable of accommodating, integrating, and transforming data from several different subinvestigations and providing various types of outputs. Analyses of data, tabulation of results, and preparation of reports are some of the more useful features of most of these systems. Among the currently available commercial systems are Xybion (Xybion Medical Systems Corp., Cedar Knolls, NJ), used by Battelle, Geneva and Lovelace ITRI, Albuquerque, and Datatox (Instem Computer Systems Stone, Stoffs, ST15 0LT UK), used at the Fraunhofer Institute. Detailed evaluation of these data management systems is beyond the scope of this paper and the knowledge of the authors.

A chronic inhalation study, whether it is performed for scientific or regulatory purposes, usually becomes a critical part of a health or safety assessment. This probability demands that the study be performed in such a way that the results are valid. The best way to assure this objective is through a comprehensive quality assurance program which includes, but is not limited to, the laboratory selection, staff evaluation, study design, test material characterization, test animal selection and monitoring, observation of performance of various procedures and protocols, documentation of results, and publication. The design, construction, maintenance, and proper operation of a large inhalation facility is expensive. An even more challenging task is the recruitment and continued professional development of competent staff. The creation and maintenance of the "correct conditions" for a quality investigation represent a complex task which requires the expertise of numerous disciplines. A recent conference explored some of these issues and covered various US and international regulatory requirements with emphasis on Good Laboratory Practice requirements, but the special requirements of inhalation studies were not discussed in any detail (14).

Setting Exposure Levels

"In order to establish a quantitative dose-response relationship at the critical site, one must first estimate how much of the inhaled aerosol is initially deposited and at what sites within the respiratory system, how rapidly and to what degree the deposited particles are cleared from the respiratory tract and lungs, and finally, what fraction of the retained material reaches the critical site within the lungs or other parts of the body to produce damage or in case of a therapeutic agent, initiate a beneficial response" (10).

Although Professor Hatch's admonitions were directed at particle exposures, they apply equally well to gas and vapor exposures. Anyone with experience in inhalation toxicology will nod appreciatively at his remarks, but few will claim that these tenets of quantitative inhalation toxicology are widely applied.

The initiation of toxicity testing, largely by NTP, within the last decade, has dramatized our failure to make inhalation toxicology a more quantitative science. Toxicity testing, insofar as airborne toxicants are concerned, developed by relying on exposure levels and failed to recognize the distinctions between exposure concentrations, intake, deposition, retention, and dose. Unfortunately, regulatory agencies have adopted this same posture on an international scale.

Doubtlessly, the use of exposure levels was initially based on its simplicity, but now the experience of toxicity testing has vividly demonstrated that this simplification produced difficult problems in experimental design and the interpretation of experimental findings. Our thinking in inhalation toxicology has become equally fuzzy: witness our use of the term "dose" to describe exposure level.

Dosimetry

What is dose? To the toxicologist, dose ideally describes the time integral of effective concentration of a material present at the effector site. Consequently, we are generally unable to measure the true dose and must settle for some form or relation of dose.

The physician describes dose as the "administered dose," which more or less corresponds to intake. The radiation biologist describes "radiation dose" as the energy absorbed (deposited) in a tissue or organ; at other times radiation dose must be expressed as the time integral of energy deposition in an organ, and thus closely resembles a true dose. Obviously, these are only a few examples of how the term "dose" is used.

Figure 7.1 shows a schematization of the relationships between exposure concentration (C), intake (delivery) rate (I), deposition (D), and retention (R): the

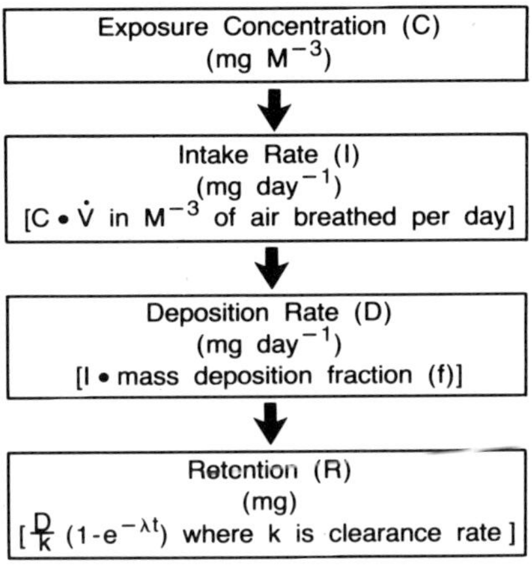

Fig. 7.1. Exposure–dose relationships. In this representation, the relation between dust exposure concentration, dust intake, dust deposition and dust retention is simply depicted. Dose corresponds closely to retention, as described in the text, but all of these levels of dosimetric information have been used, with varying degrees of success, as surrogates for the true toxicological dose.

last being the closest to true dose. This depiction indicates that there is a succession of factors which lie between exposure concentration and dose, any one or combination of which can behave both as a dose determinant and a dose estimator. It follows from this that the likelihood of exposure level being a good estimator of dose is undependably small.

Since we find the true dose to be such an elusive measurement, what should we seek instead? In pragmatic terms, we should start with some level of information which is as closely related to dose as possible and work our way "backwards" to establish exposure levels. This is obviously the reverse of what we have been doing.

How do we select and obtain the starting information? The answer can vary according to the level of confidence desired, the size of the study and related issues. In general, the answer is the same: the closer the information is to the dose estimation, the better it will serve to estimate the exposure level.

For many materials which are found to have limited retention in the lungs, an estimate of intake ($V \cdot C$) or better, of deposition ($V \cdot C \cdot f$) may be sufficient, where C is the exposure concentration, V the total volume of air breathed and f is the mass deposition fraction. If the material is retained for weeks, months, or years in the lungs or in some associated tissues, e.g., pulmonary lymph nodes, then the dose approximation of $D/K\ (1 - e^{\lambda\ t})$ may suffice, where $(1 - e^{\lambda\ t})$ is the appropriate retention function of the material at the target site and D/K represents the fraction of the steady-state lung burden achieved, where D is the deposition rate in mg day^{-1} and K is the clearance rate in mg day^{-1} (see Fig. 7.1).

Why is this a better approach than starting with the exposure concentration and estimating this same level of information? Obviously, the estimation process is identical in its assumptions and experimental requirements. As already mentioned, the answer arises from the need to limit lung burdens or lung dose. From this perspective, we derive what is reasonable as an exposure level.

What is technically achievable in producing airborne dust levels does have some limitations, but one can easily vary airborne levels from micrograms to grams per cubic meter, a factor of 10^6 or more; consequently the aerosol production limitation is small. The range of concentrations that is feasible encompasses both realistic levels of the material in the ambient or workplace environment, and the range of experimental levels required for inhalation studies.

Dust Overload Concept

What evidence supports the need for a lung burden or dose limitation? In a recent publication (23) the concept of dust overloading was reviewed. In this paper we will cite only two examples. Bolton et al. (2) reported on their experience with rats exposed chronically to International Union Against Cancer (UICC) amosite. They found that rats with >1.5 mg lung burden of amosite showed a significant prolongation of pulmonary retention at a time when the typical long-term pathologic effects of amosite were absent. In the animals with prolonged amosite retention, the main histologic feature was dustladen macrophages. The second example we will cite is a study reported by Muhle and coworkers with a plastic copolymer acrosol (25,26). The retention of this plastic dust, which appears to be relatively benign, was shown to be similarly prolonged when lung levels in the rat exceed a few milligrams. Microgram quantities of a special monitoring aerosol of $^{59}Fe_2O_3$ were given by nose-only administration to these dust-exposed rats at various times. At low lung burdens, the exposed animals cleared Fe_2O_3 at the same rate as sham-exposed control animals, viz., with an approximately 65-day half-time. However, when the pulmonary retention of the copolymer dust constituted a few milligrams, its retention became prolonged and the Fe_2O_3 clearance was concurrently slowed (>100 days).

How the absolute lung burden of a dust can affect its pulmonary retention is depicted for a hypothetical case in Fig. 7.2.

The studies with dust overloads described, as well as those with diesel particles (19,36,37), coal dust (16), and quartz (15), all indicate that when lung dust levels exceed several milligrams per gram of lung tissue, there is a decrease in lung clearance which approaches a complete cessation. Concomitantly, the build-up rate of dust in the lung becomes much faster and more linear, reflecting the absence of dust removal (Fig. 7.3).

Associated with this reduction of dust clearance are various kinds of lung injury. In the last regard, dusts which have been regarded historically as relatively innocuous, usually on the basis of high-level, short-term studies, e.g., TiO_2, have produced fibrosis and tumors (17), whereas dusts with an established toxicity, e.g., α-quartz, have produced atypical pathologic endpoints. For example, Groth

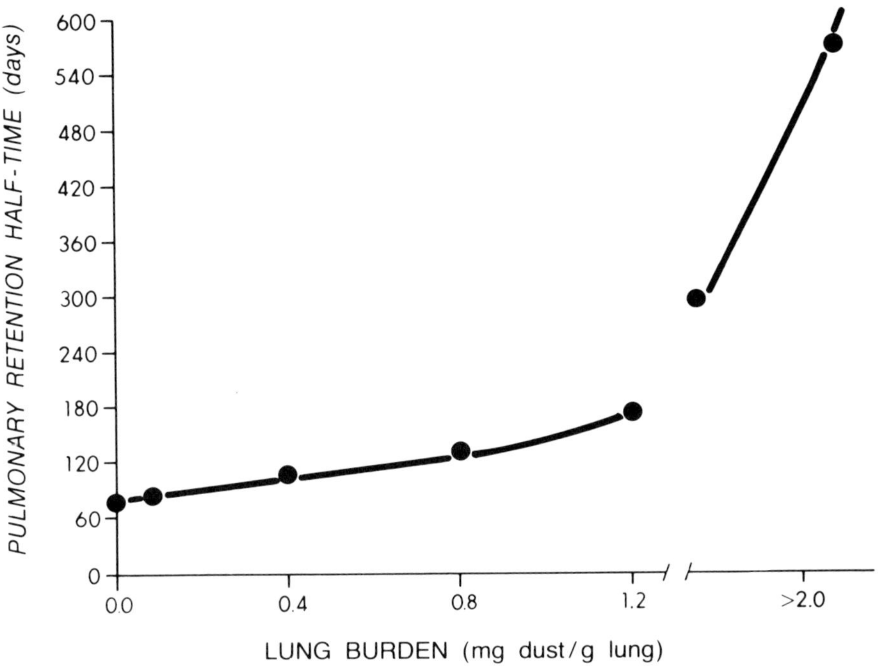

Fig. 7.2. Pulmonary dust burden and retention. Using a hypothetical case where the lung burden of a persistently retained dust is increased in absolute amounts, this depiction suggests that during a chronic study, serial retention measurements will tend to give longer retention half-times. This progressive increase in retention half-times will become unexpectedly rapid and disproportionate if the effects of dust overloading are induced by excessive burdens.

et al. (8) and Holland et al. (13) both showed that in the overloaded lung, quartz became tumorigenic. Brand (4) indicated on independent grounds that there is likely to be a "foreign body" tumorigenic effect of excessive amounts of dusts in the lungs.

At this time, the overload effect seems to be nonspecific, and applies primarily to dusts which are persistently retained in the lungs. The effect is indicative of abnormal pulmonary clearance with dust-laden macrophages accumulating in the air spaces. Presently, we believe lung dust levels of approximately 1–5 mg g^{-1} lung tissue produce the overload effects in the F344 rat. Data for other test species are, unfortunately, very limited.

After reviewing the available information on the dust overload concept, we have concluded that both a prospective and a retrospective examination of the phenomenon are in order on the basis of composite dust volume rather than on the dust mass. This simply means that we hypothesize that the volumetric amount of dust available for phagocytosis is the significant factor in dust over-

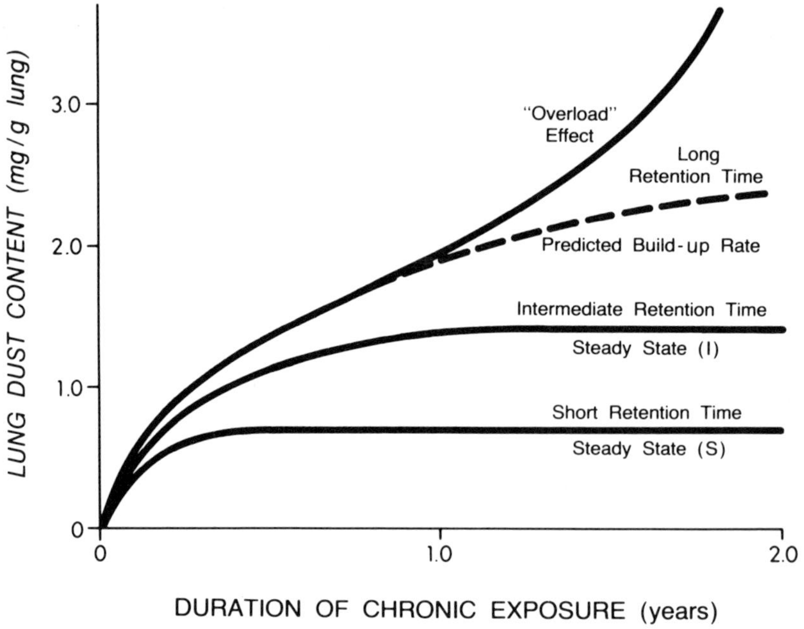

Fig. 7.3. Build-up rates of lung dust during chronic inhalation exposures. In the hypothetical examples of dust build-up rates given, we can assume that the rate of dust deposition (D) is constant for three different dusts. For example, if $D = 0.0160$ mg day^{-1} in all cases, and the short, intermediate and long retention half-times were assumed to be 7, 30, and 140 days, respectively, the estimated maximal or steady-state lung burdens would be approximately 0.16, 0.70, and 3.2 mg, respectively, with the last case being capable of producing dust overloading in lungs of the F344 rat and a modification of build-up kinetics to a faster, more linear rate, similar to that depicted.

loading; consequently a correction should be made in comparing dust of high and low density. For example, TiO_2, where ρ, the density, is 4.3, would require about 4.3 times the mass of carbon (ρ=1.0) to produce overloading. This type of volume-related analysis might be refined further by looking for particle number and size effects, again excluding particle density. These speculations all depend upon phagocytosis being the critical element in the overload concept and stand in distinction to more conventional toxic responses where the mass of the material is important.

Exposure Level Estimations

Given that we do not want to exceed (except possibly at one chronic exposure level) a dust level greater than 2 mg dust g^{-1} lung, then it is straightforward to calculate the airborne dust concentration which will produce this level on a chronic exposure basis.

Two examples follow. In the first case, we will assume the mass median aerodynamic diameter (MMAD) of the test dust is 2.5 μm. By prechronic testing, the rat appeared to deposit 5% of the dust breathed in the deep lungs, the retention half-time for the material appeared to be approximately 30 days, and the value of $\lambda = 0.693/30$ days or 0.0231 day^{-1} and $K = \lambda$ (lung content, R). Since a 30-day retention half-time is relatively short, the rats will reach a steady-state lung burden, where $D/K \simeq 1$, after approximately 6 months.

The desired steady-state lung burden, R_{SS}, was chosen to be 2 mg; therefore, with a steady-state lung burden, 0.0231 day^{-1} (2 mg) or 0.045 mg day^{-1} is the steady-state clearance rate (K_{SS}), which must be equal to the deposition rate per day (D). Since a rat breathes about 0.45m^3 day^{-1}, where the exposure day is taken to be 300 min (300 min × 0.15 1 min^{-1})/1000 1 m^{-3}, the amount of dust deposited can be estimated from the 5% deposition fraction. The amount must be equivalent to 0.05 ($\dot{V}C$) where $\dot{V}$ = 0.045 m^3 day^{-1}. Thus, C(0.00225 m^3 day^{-1}) must equal 0.045 mg day^{-1}; this occurs when C, the exposure concentration, is 20 mg m^{-3}. A reasonable chronic study exposure protocol, therefore, might utilize dust levels of 28 mg m^{-3}, 8.0 mg m^{-3}, and 2.2 mg m^{-3}, for example.

If, in the foregoing example, the retention half-time for the dust had been found to be about 120 days instead of 30 days, the 2-year exposure study would just be long enough to achieve a steady-state burden (approximately 6 retention half-times or 720 days). Since λ = 0.0058 day^{-1} in this case, the steady-state clearance rate (K_{SS}) is estimated to be 0.0115 mg day^{-1} with a 2-mg lung burden (0.0058 day^{-1} • 2 mg). Now the product C(0.00225 m^3 day^{-1}) must equal a deposition rate (D) of 0.0115 mg day^{-1} and an exposure concentration of 5.1 mg m^{-3}. For this circumstance, the selection of exposure concentrations in the chronic study would have to be reduced to perhaps 8.0, 2.0, and 0.5 mg m^{-3}, respectively.

With a different particle size, there would be a different mass deposition fraction. A 1% rat-respirable fraction would raise the foregoing exposure concentrations by a factor of 5, for example, so it is readily apparent that exposure concentrations could vary 100-fold, with reasonable distinctions in the MMAD and retention half-times.

Use of Small-Particle Enrichment

Frequently, the chronic inhalation toxicity of a material or complex mixture in the form of a dust needs to be evaluated, but only part of it is respirable by either humans or the test animal. In order to avoid excessive exposure concentrations and needless transportation of large quantities of material through the inhalation facility, enrichment of the small particle fraction of the test material is a useful solution. The following example will serve as an illustration.

Suppose that the MMAD of a test material is 10.0 μm, its human respirable fraction according to the American Conference of Governmental Industrial Hygienists (ACGIH) criteria is 2.0%, and in prechronic testing the deposited fraction in the F344 rat is about 0.2%. It is desired to evaluate the toxicity of the dust at 5 mg m^{-3} rat-respirable concentration. This means that the total dust concentration would be 2500 mg m^{-3} (5 mg m^{-3}/0.002). However, if the dust is enriched in rat-respirable content from 0.2% to 12% the total dust concentration required in the chamber is reduced to 42 mg m^{-3}, a much more reasonable concentration of material to manage. This presumably could be achieved by reducing the MMAD to 1.0 μm (30).

The inhalation toxicology of the "enriched dust" is established from the observations of its biologic effects, if any, on the various parts of the respiratory system and a knowledge of its particle size characteristics. For a safety assessment, the human respirable fraction of the enriched dust can be calculated by reference to the United Kingdom Medical Research Council (MRC) or ACGIH curves (20) which can be related to the original test material. In the foregoing case, the 60-fold increase in rat-respirable fraction produces a 30-fold increase in the percentage respirable in man. In terms of the original test material this is equivalent to about 5 times the nuisance dust Threshold Limit Values in the occupational setting (1).

Considerations of Dust Deposition and Retention

The examples of using prechronic exposure information to establish exposure levels presented above could have utilized information from deposition models for the F344 rat (30) and for man (12,24). At the very least, prechronic experimental findings should be routinely checked against the predictions of such models to be certain that they are in reasonable agreement and not suspect as the deposition value for the material has a dominant role in determining the exposure levels chosen.

Pulmonary clearance and retention of particulate matter, both experimental data and mathematical models, have been the topic of several reports (12,24,34). Depending on the characteristics of the test material, it may be phagocytosed, dissolved, transformed, or remain unchanged while resident in the lungs. The quantitative allocation of these different processes to dust clearance has rarely been determined (22).

Even without detailed mechanistic information on dust removal, a prolongation of dust retention is clearly not limited to dust overloading, a concept which has been stressed in this presentation. There are features to dust overloading which tend to distinguish it from compartmental effects, clearance by dissolution, and cytotoxic actions of the dust (22). Dust overloading appears to be uniquely associated with accumulation of dustladen macrophages, and the rapid induction of a general type of dust disposition, injury pattern, and lung dust burden (23). Although the pulmonary macrophage is believed to be central to the overload phenomenon, possible toxicological alterations in macrophage function due to inhaled materials are far more extensive than considered in this presentation (3). Moreover, we do not know to what extent macrophage removal varies with different materials (22), but in terms of other known clearance mechanisms, it must be considered crucial to the host defense system.

Since the dust prolongation factors cited are not mutually exclusive, a moderate and progressive increase in retention half-times in a chronic inhalation study can be expected even when excessive dust burdens are absent. This tendency is depicted in Fig. 7.2.

In any case, the pulmonary burden of the test material should be determined periodically, preferably three or four times during and at the end of the chronic inhalation study. Such determinations can be sometimes accomplished by tagging a portion of the test material with a tracer material and making the appropriate measurement. For a comprehensive assessment of the test material, its clearance and retention, behavior as a function of exposure concentration should be followed. Since such determinations frequently require a sacrifice of the test animals, alternative procedures involving surrogate materials are commonly used. Well characterized materials whose pulmonary behavior is reasonably well known and which are available with a suitable radioactive tag are widely used. As already mentioned, iron oxide with a ^{59}Fe tag, whose clearance is believed to be macrophage-mediated (18), has been extensively applied (25,26). Polystyrene microspheres in various sizes and having different radioactive tags are commercially available (e.g., 3M Corp.). Also, gallium oxide particles and ^{134}Cs-fused aluminosilicate particles have been used at the Inhalation Toxicology Research Institute in Albuquerque (35,36).

Conclusions

We are pleased to note that efforts to develop more definitive guidelines for prechronic and chronic inhalation testing are currently under consideration. It appears that many, if not all, of the design considerations (and potential pitfalls) discussed in this presentation are under discussion by the Toxicology Design Review Committee on behalf of the United States National Toxicology Program (Toxicology Design Review Committee, personal communication, 1987), and possibly by others, but it is premature to contemplate what and when changes will be promulgated. In the meantime, we hope that our perceptions of conducting chronic inhalation studies and recommendations for changes will reduce some of the attendant risks and miscalculations which encumber the investigator. We believe they will concomitantly provide both those in the regulatory arena and investigators with a clearer insight to the needs of and problems inherent in chronic inhalation study protocols. Careful consideration of these factors should enhance the probability of a successful outcome to the chronic inhalation study. Successful in this context means acquisition of the desired, valid information.

References

1. American Conference of Governmental Industrial Hygienists (1981) Documentation of threshold limit values for substances in workroom air, American Conference for Governmental Industrial Hygienists, Cincinnati

2. Bolton RE, Vincent JH, Jones AD, Addison J, Beckett ST (1983) An overload hypothesis for pulmonary clearance of UICC amosite fiber inhaled by rats. Br J Ind Med 40:264–272
3. Brain JD (1986) Toxicological aspects of alteration of pulmonary macrophage function. Ann Rev Pharmacol Toxicol 26:547–565
4. Brand KG (1986) Fibrotic scar cancer in the light of foreign body tumorigenesis. In: Goldsmith D, Winn D, Shy C (eds) Silica, silicosis and cancer. Praeger, New York, pp 281–286
5. Calabrese EJ (ed) (1983) Principles of animal extrapolation. Wiley, New York
6. Cameron TP, Hukman RL, Kornreich MR, Tarone RE (1985) History, survival and growth patterns of B6C3F1 mice and F344 rats in the National Cancer Institute carcinogenesis testing program. Fundam Appl Toxicol 5:526–538
7. Drew, RT (1985) The design and operation of systems for inhalation exposure of animals. In: Witschi HP, Brain JD (eds) Toxicology of inhaled materials. Springer, Berlin Heidelberg New York, pp 3–22
8. Groth DA, Stettler LE, Platek SF, Lai JB, Burg JR (1986) Lung tumors in rats treated with quartz by intratracheal instillation. In: Goldsmith D, Winn D, Shy C (eds) Silica, silicosis and cancer. Praeger, New York, pp 243–263
9. Hakkinen PJ, Witschi HP (1985) Animal models. In: Witschi HP, Brain JD (eds) Toxicology of inhaled materials. Springer, Berlin Heidelberg New York, pp 96–114
10. Hatch TF (1964) Dose-response relationship. In: Hatch TF, Gross P (eds) Pulmonary deposition and retention of inhaled aerosols. Academic, New York, pp 3–5
11. Hemenway DR, Sylwester D, Gale PN, Vacek P, Evans JN (1983) Effectiveness of animal rotation in achieving uniform dust exposures and lung dust deposition in horizontal flow chambers. Amer Ind Hyg Assoc J 44:655–658
12. Heyder J, Gebhart J, Heigwer G, Roth C, Stahlhofen W (1973) Experimental studies of total deposition of aerosol particles in the human respiratory tract. J Aerosol Sci 4:191–208
13. Holland LM, Wilson JS, Tillery MI, Smith DM (1986) Lung cancer in rats exposed to fibrogenic dusts. In: Goldsmith D, Winn D, Shy C (eds) Silica, silicosis and cancer. Praeger, New York, pp 267–279
14. Hoover BK, Baldwin JK, Uelner AF, Whitmire CI, Davies CL, Briston DW (eds) (1984) Managing, conduct, and data quality of toxicology studies. Princeton Scientific, Princeton
15. Klosterkotter W, Buneman G (1961) Animal experiments on the elimination of inhaled dusts. In: Davies CN (ed) Inhaled particles and vapours. Pergamon, Oxford, pp 327–337
16. Le Bouffant L (1971) Influence de la nature des poussières et de la charge pulmonaire sur l'expuration. In: Walton WH (ed) Inhaled particles, vol 3. Unwin, Old Woking, pp 227–237
17. Lee KP, Trochimowicz HJ, Reinhardt CF (1985) Pulmonary response of rats exposed to titanium dioxide (TiO_2) by inhalation for two years. Toxicol Appl Pharmacol 79:179–182
18. Lehnert BE, Morrow PE (1985) Association of ^{59}iron oxide with alveolar macrophages during alveolar clearance. Exp Lung Res 9:1–16
19. McClellan RO (1986) Health effects of diesel exhaust: a case study in risk assessment. Am Ind Hyg Assoc J 47:1–13
20. Mercer TT (1973) Respirable activity samplers. In: Mercer TT (ed) Aerosol technol-

ogy in hazard evaluations. Academic, New York, pp 284–315

21. Miller FJ, Menzel DB (eds) (1984) Fundamentals of extrapolation modeling of inhaled toxicants. Hemisphere, New York
22. Morrow PE (1973) Alveolar clearance of aerosols. Arch Int Med 131:101–108
23. Morrow PE (1986) The setting of particulate exposure levels for chronic inhalation toxicity studies. J Amer Coll Toxicol 5:533–544
24. Morrow PE, Yu CP (1985) Models of aerosol behavior in airways. In: Moren F, Newhouse MT, Dolovich MB (eds) Aerosols in medicine: principles, diagnosis and therapy. Elsevier, Amsterdam, pp 149–191
25. Muhle H, Bellman B, Heinrich U (1987) Overloading of lung clearance of experimental animals to particles. In: Walton WH (ed) Inhaled particles, vol 6. Pergamon, Oxford (in press)
26. Muhle H, Bellmann B, Creutzenberg O, Kilpper R, Mermelstein R (1987) Pulmonary deposition, retention and clearance of a pigmented polymer in rats. This volume
27. National Toxicology Program (1985) Fiscal Year 1985 Annual Plan, NTP-85-055. US Department of Health and Human Services. Washington DC, pp 105–113
28. Phalen RF (1984) Regulations and guidelines. In: Phalen RF (ed) Inhalation studies: Foundations and techniques. CRC Press, Boca Raton, pp 243–256
29. Pour P, Mohr U, Cardesa A, Althoff J, Kmoch N (1976) Spontaneous tumors and common diseases in two colonies of Syrian hamsters. II. Respiratory tract and digestive system. J Natl Cancer Inst 56:937–948
30. Raabe OG, Al-Bayati MA, Teague SV, Rasolt A (1987) Regional deposition of inhaled monodisperse coarse and fine particles in small laboratory animals. In: Walton WH (ed) Inhaled particles, vol 6. Pergamon, Oxford (in press)
31. Schreck RM, Chan TL, Soderholm SC (1981) Design, operation and characterization of large volume exposure chambers. In: Leong BKJ (ed) Inhalation toxicology and technology. Ann Arbor, Ann Arbor, pp 29–56
32. Smith DM, Ortiz LW, Archuleta RF, Spalding JF, Tillery MI, Ettinger HJ, Thomas RG (1980) A method for chronic "nose-only" exposures of laboratory animals to inhaled fibrous aerosols. In: Leong BKJ (ed) Inhalation toxicology and technology, Ann Arbor, Ann Arbor, pp 89–105
33. Solleveld HA, Haseman JK, McConnell EE (1984) Natural history of body weight gain, survival, and neoplasma in the F344 rat. J Natl Cancer Inst 72:929–940
34. Valberg PA (1985) Determination of retained lung dose. In: Witschi HP, Brain JD (eds) Toxicology of inhaled materials. Springer, Berlin Heidelberg New York, pp 57–94
35. Wolff RK, Kanapilly GM, Gray RH, McClellan RO (1984) Deposition and retention of aggregate ^{67}Ga-203 particles in beagle dogs, Fischer-344 rats and CD-1 mice. Am Ind Hyg Assoc J 45:377–381
36. Wolff RK, Henderson RF, Snipes MB, Mauderly JL, McClellan RO (1985) Particle clearance and accumulated lung burdens in rats. Am Assoc for Aerosol Research, abstracts of annual meeting, Albuquerque, New Mexico, p 9P11
37. Wolff RK, Henderson RF, Snipes MB, Griffith WC, Mauderly JL, Cuddihy RG, McClellan RO (1987) Alterations in particle accumulation and clearance in lungs of rats chronically exposed to diesel exhaust. Fundam Appl Toxicol 9:154–166
38. Yeh HC, Newton GJ, Barr EB, Carpenter RL, Hobbs CH (1986) Studies of the temporal and spatial distribution of aerosols in multi-tiered inhalation exposure chambers. Am Ind Hyg Assoc J 47:540–545

CHAPTER 8

Carcinogenicity Protocols

R.A. Griesemer[1]

Inhalation is the most important route of exposure to carcinogens. Some of the substances found to be carcinogenic for humans by this route are listed in Table 8.1. Everyone will recognize tobacco smoke, asbestos, and radon as important public health concerns.

For several of these substances [bis(chloromethyl)ether, mustard gas, vinyl chloride] evidence for carcinogenicity was found first in experimental animals, but for the majority the discovery came from epidemiologic studies. The emphasis on epidemiologic studies reflects the importance of identifying the etiologic agents of respiratory cancers and the difficulties of doing so through animal experiments. Inhalation bioassays in animals are relatively insensitive as compared to bioassays by other routes of exposure. They are also expensive, costing about 3.5 million U.S. dollars per assay at present (for two species, three dosage levels). It is not surprising, therefore, that the recent literature on occupational causes of respiratory cancer contains more than four times as many citations for epidemiologic studies as for animal studies (45). For perspective, of the last 128 substances tested by one of the world's largest bioassay programs, the U.S. National Toxicology Program, only ten substances had been assayed by the inhalation route (Table 8.2), and many of these had had prior indications of carcinogenicity by other routes of exposure.

But inhalation bioassays are not the only way to identify respiratory carcinogens. In this chapter I will briefly present alternate methods and suggest a practical approach to testing for respiratory carcinogenicity.

Before proceeding, however, it is necessary to recall that animal bioassays for carcinogenicity might be designed to fulfill more than one purpose (Table 8.3) and that the design of the bioassay has to be adjusted accordingly. For example, if the sole purpose is to detect carcinogenic activity, the sensitivity of the test is greatest when all the dosed animals are assigned to a single high dosage group. Once carcinogenic activity has been demonstrated, subsequent dose-response studies require multiple dosage groups with the majority in the range of observed

---

[1]Biology Division, Oak Ridge National Laboratory, Oak Ridge, TN 37831, USA.

Table 8.1. Some human respiratory carcinogens[a]

Chemicals and groups of chemicals	
	Asbestos
	Chloromethyl ethers
	Chromium compounds
	Mustard gas
	Tobacco smoke
	Vinyl chloride
Industrial processes and occupational exposure	
	Boot and shoe manufacture and repair
	Furniture and cabinet making
	Nickel refining
	Underground hematite mining (with exposure to radon)

[a] Adapted from Merletti et al. (19) with permission.

effects. In practice a compromise is often attempted in which two or three closely spaced dose levels are employed to detect carcinogenicity and concurrently to learn something about dose-response relationships. This approach has the advantage that dose-related trends in response may give supporting evidence for causal relationships. Among the disadvantages are that only a small portion of the dose-response curve will be revealed and at greater expense (each additional dosage group in a long-term inhalation bioassay adds about 500,000 U.S. dollars to the cost). Moreover, the majority of substances assayed can be expected to be non-carcinogenic (unless there is prior suspicion from other data) and extensive dose-response studies would be unproductive.

The discussion that follows will concentrate on one purpose of animal bioassays, the assay of previously untested substances for carcinogenic activity in the

Table 8.2. U.S. national toxicology program recent inhalation bioassays

Substance tested	Report number and date[a]
1,2-Dibromo-3-chloropropane	206 March, 1982
1,2-Dibromoethane	210 March, 1982
Propylene oxide	267 March, 1985
Propylene	272 November, 1985
1,3-Butadiene	288 August, 1984
Dichloromethane (methylene chloride)	306 January, 1986
Tetrachloroethylene (perchloroethylene)	311 August, 1986
Methyl methacrylate	314 October, 1986
Ethylene Oxide	326 Draft[b]
1,2-Epoxybutane	329 Draft[b]

[a] National Toxicology Program Technical Report Series, USDHHS.
[b] Unpublished draft.

Table 8.3. Purposes of animal bioassays for carcinogenicity

1.	Detect carcinogenic activity
2.	Establish dose-response relationships
3.	Investigate mechanisms of action
4.	Evaluate preventive or therapeutic measures

respiratory tract. The major assay methods to be discussed are listed in Table 8.4 and have been reviewed by Nettesheim and Griesemer (24). Regrettably, space does not permit recognizing all the many important publications in this field.

Animal Bioassays for Carcinogenicity

General Design Considerations

The primary purpose of carcinogenicity bioassays is to determine whether exposure to a test substance alters the pattern of tumor development in that species. In principle, the experiments are designed and conducted in such a way that the only experimental variable is the administration of the test substance and thus the differences in tumor responses between dosed and control animals can be attributed to the test substance.

The basic requirements for long-term assays for carcinogenicity are described in Supplement 2 to the *IARC Monographs on the Evaluation of the Carcinogenic*

Table 8.4. Bioassay methods for respiratory carcinogenicity

Animal bioassays
Inhalation
Intratracheal instillation
Intrapleural injection
Nonrespiratory routes of exposures
Localized site bioassays
Intrapulmonic injection
Intrabronchial mucosal injection
Intrabronchial pellet
Tracheal lavage
Heterotopic tracheal transplants
Short-term in vivo assays
Mouse lung adenoma assay
Preneoplasia
Early biochemical markers
In vitro assays
Fetal lung transformation assays
In vivo/in vitro assays

Risk of Chemicals to Humans (47) and its revision (49). These sources also contain references to a number of guidelines proposed by individuals and organizations from several countries. Another recent source is the *Handbook of Carcinogen Testing* (20). Statistical considerations for design and analysis are described in Gart et al. (7).

In a typical animal bioassay for carcinogenicity (Table 8.5), animals of both sexes of two rodent species are randomly assigned to one or more exposure groups or to concurrent control groups of about 50 animals each. The test substance is administered at high but tolerated dose levels for the majority of the animals' lives and the animals are examined for visible or palpable tumors until death (or sacrifice). At death evaluation is made of the location and types of tumors, the incidence of tumors, the degrees of malignancy, and the causes of death. A comparison is then made between the tumor patterns in dosed vs control animals with adjustments for differences in survival times, competing causes of death, etc.

Some of the more important design considerations are listed in Table 8.6. Even without details, this partial listing gives some indications of the complexity of designing long-term or lifetime animal bioassays. Among the deficiencies and pitfalls revealed by retrospective analysis of many bioassays are: group sizes too small or dose levels too low to detect effects, incomplete recording of the eventual resolution of clinical signs, intercurrent outbreaks of infectious diseases, nonuniform dissection and sampling at necropsy, unjustified grouping of diagnoses for evaluation, incomplete recording of multiple lesions per site or in paired organs, difficulties in dissociating effects on target sites from background cancers, unequal survival times among groups of animals requiring age-adjusted analyses, and unjustified substitution of historic for matched control animals.

Inhalation Bioassays

Inhalation exposures are of two types, commonly referred to as whole-body and nose-only exposures. Each poses some special problems. Whole-body exposures in chambers, where the animals are in an atmosphere containing the test substance, require uniform mixing of the chamber air and unimpeded access of air to each animal (see also Holländer, *this volume*). From among the many design considerations (Table 8.7) two illustrative examples are multiple versus single animals per cage and the use of mesh or solid cages. The number of animals per

Table 8.5. Elements of a typical carcinogenicity bioassay

Both sexes of two species of rodents
Animals randomized into dosed and control groups of about 50 animals/group
Test substances administered for most or all of the animals' lives
One dose level the highest that can be tolerated without interfering with the experiment
Tumor response evaluated clinically and pathologically
Analysis for differences in tumor patterns from controls

Table 8.6. Some design considerations for carcinogenicity bioassays

Test substance
Technical grade or pure
Extent of effort to characterize impurities
Stability in storage and under assay conditions
Toxicologic properties of vehicles or solvents used
Animals
Selection of species and strains
Genetic constitution. Inbred or outbred
Method of randomization
Age at start of bioassay
Disease status
Husbandry
Type of caging and cleaning agents
Bedding type and contaminants
Food and water and contaminants
Caloric intake level
Use of insecticides
Light/dark cycles
Potential for cross-contamination with other assays
Protocol
Single or multiple generations
Route of exposure
Dose level selection and spacing
Frequency and duration of exposure
Group sizes
Thoroughness of clinical examinations
Thoroughness of necropsy examinations
Rationale for serial or terminal sacrifices
Sampling for histopathology
Data handling and analysis
Quality assurance
Retention of records and public accessibility to primary data

cage and the presence of bedding are important not only for the piling-up of animals and possible filtration of air through fur or bedding but also for possible changes in the local environment from exhaled air and from ammonia and other gases from the excreta. Also important considerations are stresses related to group dynamics or conversely to absence of contact with other individuals. Individually housed rodents tend not to live as long as those housed in groups. Mesh cages permit better air circulation than solid sided cages but might contribute to ulcers on the feet if attention is not given to mesh size and smoothness of construction. With wire-bottom cages the possibility of vitamin K deficiency and other nutritional disorders through decreased opportunity for normal coprophagia is a concern. In one experiment with C57B1/6 mice, for example, the

Table 8.7. Some design considerations for inhalation bioassays

Test substance	
	How generate an aerosol
	Dynamic or static delivery
	How to maintain a steady concentration
	Loss to chamber walls (and to food) and stability
	Make-up air composition, flow rate, temperature
	Sampling during exposure
Facilities and equipment	
	Chamber or nose-only exposure design and venting
	Air mixing/stratification within chamber
	Mesh or solid caging
	How conduct physical examinations in chambers
	How to feed and water during exposure
	How to safely clean the chamber and equipment
Exposure conditions	
	5–6 h, 5 days/week to simulate occupational exposure
	22 h, 7 days/week to simulate maximal environmental exposure (fivefold difference)
	Single or group housing
	Type of bedding, if any
	Mix sexes/species within a chamber
	Humidity and ammonia controls
Animals	
	Modulation of breathing patterns
	Tissue tolerance or adaptation
	Tumor types expected
	Tumors at distant sites
	Intercurrent infectious diseases

median survival time was 102 weeks in wire cages and 127 weeks in solid cages with bedding, presumably for nutritional reasons (26).

Nose-only exposure is designed to avoid contamination by the test substance of the fur and the cage environment, in order to diminish oral exposure from the active grooming that follows each period of inhalation exposure. The method has the additional advantage of requiring less test substance but major disadvantages are the requirement for special apparatus, the labor involved in handling the animals, and the stresses introduced by handling and confinement. Moreover, some contamination of the fur of the head is unavoidable.

Whether whole-body or nose-only exposures are used, measurements of exposure doses to the respiratory tissues and to the digestive tract are necessary. For example, particle clearance by the mucociliary escalator typically results in swallowing of most of particulate test materials (see Cuddihy, this volume). After repeated or prolonged exposures, induced lesions such as foci of inflammation or squamous metaplasia might appreciably alter the amounts of test material delivered to the tissues as well as the tissue distribution and clearance or retention. The possible influence of Sendai virus infections (a common latent rodent infection that characteristically causes cell fusions) in the process of carcinogenicity has not been fully evaluated as yet but apparently may be either facilitory or inhibitory (27).

Many other design considerations could be mentioned. Inhalation of irritating substances such as tobacco smoke or formaldehyde results in changes in breathing patterns that are more pronounced in mice and hamsters than in rats (see also Mauderly, this volume), thus altering respiratory rates and minute volumes and the doses to the target tissues. Rodents are obligate nose-breathers, differing from humans who typically breathe partly through their mouths when forced to inhale irritant substances. The airway configurations of experimental animals and humans differ, particularly in regard to nasal scrolling, laryngeal bending, angles of bronchial branching, and pulmonary lobulation. For these and other considerations including body size and comparative metabolism (see also Dahl, *this volume*), exposure assessments cannot rely entirely on the concentrations of the test substance in the inspired air.

Comparisons of respiratory tumor types among animal species also deserve mention here (see also Mohr and Dungworth, *this volume*). Inhalation bioassays in mice typically produce pulmonary adenomas and bronchioalveolar carcinomas, of which the latter have a counterpart in humans. In rats and Syrian hamsters, all the types of respiratory tumors found in humans have been produced except for the small cell lung cancer for which only two reports were found. In one report, two such tumors were produced in hamsters given diethylnitrosamine subcutaneously at birth (23). In the other report, 20 of 100 rats given BaP with Fe_2O_3 intratracheally developed small cell lung cancers (2), presumably related to retention of large particles. No small lung cell cancers have been reported from inhalation bioassays, even with tobacco smoke. A recent abstract, however, indicates that a model system has now been developed to produce pulmonary endocrine tumors (34).

It should be emphasized that the respiratory tract may serve both as a portal of entry as well as a target site for carcinogens. Whenever possible, the resulting tumor patterns should be established for the entire body.

Limitations of Inhalation Bioassays

The major limitation of inhalation bioassays for carcinogenicity is their relative insensitivity. To begin with, animal bioassays in general are not very sensitive. Even with group sizes of 50 and low background incidences of tumors at the target site(s), one can only detect increases in tumor incidences of about 10% or more. Increasing the group sizes to several hundred animals each increases the sensitivity relatively little (7). To maximize the potential to detect a carcinogenic effect, therefore, the animals in the highest dosage group are customarily administered the largest amount they can tolerate without interfering with their ability to grow and develop and to survive long enough to be at risk of late-developing tumors.

Inhalation studies, however, are often limited too by the doses that can be delivered. In some instances the test materials cannot be generated at high concentrations or are unstable or explosive. Sometimes the test materials are rapidly absorbed and are more acutely toxic by the inhalation route than by other routes such as the oral route where substances are diluted by the gastrointestinal contents, absorbed gradually, and perhaps detoxified by the microflora and the animals' digestive processes. In addition, inhaled test substances are distributed across a very large surface area in the lung rather than concentrated at potential target sites. Moreover, the common practice of employing exposure periods of 5–6 h per day, 5 days per week results in exposure for about 18% of the time (30 h per week), with considerable time for recovery and tissue repair between exposure periods.

Whether or not the low dosages relative to the amounts that can be administered by other means account entirely for the limited successes, the collective experience to date has been that the inhalation route is a relatively insensitive way to assay carcinogens in animals (16). For tobacco smoke, for example, Dontenwill (5) was able to produce laryngeal neoplasms in hamsters but few or no lung tumors after considerable experimentation. Lung tumors were produced in one study, in 7 of 80 rats (4) but success required manipulation of the smoking schedule to increase the doses by gradually adapting the animals to the acute toxic effects, by allowing recovery periods between cigarettes, and by lifetime exposure. If tobacco smoke had not been incriminated already as a carcinogen and if the usual bioassay methods had been applied, it is doubtful that a positive result would have been obtained with tobacco smoke in the lungs of rodents. In contrast, the carcinogenicity of tobacco smoke condensates is readily demonstrated by intrapulmonary injection (3) or by application to the skin of mice. For asbestos, lung tumors have been produced in rodents by inhalation but much greater tumor responses have been obtained by intratracheal or intrapleural instillations.

Intratracheal Instillation

Another approach that is particularly useful for particulate suspensions is to instill the test substance directly into the trachea where much of the inoculum is then aspirated into the airways. In a typical bioassay, the test substance is suspended in a gelatin-saline solution or adsorbed to a carrier such as carbon or ferric oxide particles to prolong the retention in the lung. The inoculum is injected through the larynx of anesthetized hamsters or rats into the trachea in volumes of about 0.1 ml. Weekly injections are made for about 15 weeks and the animals are then observed for tumor development. The reference standard is BaP-Fe_2O_3 in the Syrian hamster (30,31) which produces pulmonary carcinomas in a dose-related way in less than a year.

The intratracheal instillation method is the easiest and most convenient way to assay for respiratory carcinogenicity although it is obviously not applicable to gases and vapors. Any animal species can be used. Of great advantage are the bypassing of the nasal filter and the opportunity to give large quantities of inoculum. Because of its ease and simplicity, there are about 100 reports in the literature of the use of this assay method. Among the disadvantages are that the inoculum is not as evenly distributed as by inhalation and the doses to the tissues are somewhat difficult to quantitate as compared to localized site bioassays (below) (see also Cuddihy, *this volume*).

Space does not permit discussion of variations on this theme, such as the use of permanent tracheostomies or tracheal cannulas. An untried method possibly worth mention, however, is intranasal administration. Anesthetized rodents, because they are obligate nose breathers, inhale liquids dropped on the external nares and no other manipulation is required.

Intrapleural Injection

Injections into the pleural cavity can be made transmurally or through thoracotomies. As the target tissue by this route of exposure is the pleural mesothelium, this method has been used mostly for asbestos and other fibers. A variety of asbestos samples administered by the intrapleural injection method produced a high incidence of mesothelial sarcomas in a relatively short time in rats and hamsters (37,38,44). Hueper and Payne (12,13) also produced mesothelial sarcomas within 12–14 months in the pleura of 60%–70% of rats exposed to chromium compounds by the intrapleural route, but no tumors with the same substances administered by the inhalation or intratracheal methods.

Nonrespiratory Routes of Exposure

Administration of test substances by a variety of nonrespiratory routes such as oral, dermal, or systemic may produce tumors in the respiratory tract if the ultimate carcinogen reaches or forms in respiratory tissues. Urethan, for example, produces lung tumors in mice after a variety of routes of administration including intraperitoneal, transplacental, and intratracheal. Diethylnitrosamine given subcutaneously produces large numbers of respiratory tract tumors (mostly benign) in Syrian and European hamsters and in mice (21,22). No special methods are required with any of the systemically administered carcinogens, just the usual systematic, thorough study of the respiratory tract.

Localized Site Bioassays

Repeated applications of measured amounts of test substances to predetermined localized tissue sites permits more precise estimates of the doses to the target tissues, better definition of the susceptibilities of tissue types to cancer induction, and more certain attribution of cancer formation at that site to the application of the test substance.

The methods that have been used include direct intrapulmonic injection, transfixation of carcinogen-impregnated thread, intrabronchial pellet implants, intrabronchial mucosal injection, lavage of a localized area of trachea, and exposure of heterotopic tracheal transplants [reviewed by Nettesheim and Griesemer (24)]. Space permits only brief descriptions of three of the methods that appear more useful for carcinogenicity bioassays.

Direct Intrapulmonic Injection

Injections can be made directly into the lung through the chest wall or under direct visualization through a thoracotomy. In this assay, the test material, typically suspended in melted wax such as beeswax, is injected into the lung where the wax pellet hardens and provides sustained local release of the test substance. Tumors may form around the pellet or at distant sites.

This method has not been widely applied as yet but has been useful for evaluating cigarette smoke condensates (CSC). In one such study (3), invasive and metastasizing carcinomas formed locally in the lungs of 42% of rats given 67 mg CSC and pulmonary carcinoma formed with concentrations as low as 1 mg CSC. The release rates of the constituents of CSC from beeswax pellets have been reported (29). The method has several disadvantages, however. A surgical procedure is required to ensure placement of the pellet in the lung. The test material dislodges tissue and is warm or hot at the time of injection depending on the melting temperature of the wax vehicle used. Sarcomas that occasionally form around the pellet may be more analogous to physical state carcinogenesis.

It is not likely that this method will have wide application but where vehicles with suitable release rates for the substance in question are known, this assay system should be considered.

Tracheal Lavage

This method developed by Schreiber (33) utilizes a syringe-catheter assembly with double tubing that permits lavage of a localized area (5 mm) of the trachea in an anesthetized animal. In the one published series of studies, 1% *N*-nitroso-*N*-methylurea in either citrate buffer or in 10% ethanol in water applied to the tracheas of Syrian hamsters for 5–8 s, two times per week, for 15 weeks produced 100% carcinomas at the site of topical application in the trachea (33,51).

The potential of this method has not been fully explored. It has the advantages of preselection of target site and well defined carcinogen exposure. For test substances that are water soluble this assay method has considerable promise.

Heterotopic Tracheal Transplants

Rodent tracheal, bronchial, and pulmonary tissues can be successfully transplanted to syngeneic or immunosuppressed hosts. A tracheal transplant assay system has been developed in which entire rat or hamster tracheas are transplanted to subcutaneous sites in syngeneic hosts (8,14). Carcinogens can be introduced by injection or by implantation of pellets into the lumen and the progress of tumor development can be followed by exfoliative cytology and biopsy or by serial harvest of tracheas and subsequent in vitro culture or histopathologic examination of the tissues. The reference standard carcinogens are benzo(a)pyrene (25) and 7,12-dimethylbenzanthracene (9), which produce invasive tracheal carcinomas in as little as 2 months.

In further development of the model, it has been found possible to denude the rodent trachea by physical or enzymatic means and to repopulate the epithelial lining with tracheal or bronchial cells from another species including humans (1,39) or to transplant human bronchus to immunosuppressed rodents (10). It is now possible, therefore, to assay test substances directly on human respiratory epithelium. Another development has been the creation of stomata to the skin at both ends of the transplanted trachea which permits the flow-through of gases such as formaldehyde (35).

This assay method has successfully demonstrated the carcinogenicity or cocarcinogenicity of asbestos and nickel compounds as well as polycyclic hydrocarbons (42,43,50). Although more extensive validation studies are desirable, the assay method appears sufficiently developed and standardized for widespread application. Its disadvantages of labor intensiveness and the single type of airway tissue employed are offset by the specificity of the target tissue, the increased accuracy of measurement of exposure doses to a defined target cell population, the rapidity of tumor response, and the relatively low cost as compared to inhalation bioassays.

Short-Term In Vivo Assays

To avoid the expense of long-term or lifetime animal biopsies and to obtain bioassay results more quickly, four types of shorter bioassays have been developed for various organ systems. One type depends on the ability to detect the time to onset of tumor formation visually (e.g., skin), by palpation (e.g., breast, spleen), or by exfoliative cytology (e.g., cervix). Although the respiratory organs may seem inaccessible, they lend themselves to radiographic examination, to exfoliative cytology, and to bronchoscopic examination, all underutilized techniques in respiratory bioassays. A second type of shorter bioassay is based upon the more rapid production of tumors at body sites with normally high background tumor incidences, as revealed by serial sacrifices (e.g., the mouse lung adenoma assay). The third group of bioassays depend on the detection of preneoplastic lesions biochemically or histologically (e.g., liver, bladder) shortly after carcinogen administration. Progress in this respect in the respiratory system is lagging behind that in other organ systems. A fourth possible type of shorter in vivo assay takes advantage of pretreatment of the target tissue with a subcarcinogenic dose of a carcinogen followed by administration of the test substance. One might consider as a screening technique, for example, applying DMBA or NMU to the larynx or a single intratracheal instillation of BaP, followed by the test material by a convenient route.

Mouse Lung Adenoma Assay

This method, developed into an assay by Shimkin and Stoner (36), takes advantage of the fact that the appearance of pulmonary adenomas which occur spontaneously in some strains of mice can be enhanced by administration of carcinogens. In a typical assay, groups of weanling Strain A mice are administered the test substance once or repeatedly by a convenient route. Four to six months later the animals are killed and the lung tumors counted. Counts of the visible nodules on the pleural surfaces correlate well with counts of all the tumors in cleared lungs simplifying the measurement of results. Urethan-induced lung tumors serve as a positive reference control.

The results of a number of assays have revealed that 50 of 93 (54%) carcinogens and 7 of 23 (30%) noncarcinogens were active in the mouse lung adenoma assay (28). All the substances detected as active by the assay were genotoxic in other assays. The relatively large proportion of false negative assays may be attributed in part to the requirement that the carcinogen must reach the target tissues. The comparative data base of carcinogens and noncarcinogens obtained from animal bioassays (which are seldom replicated) might also contain errors of categorical assignments. In any case, the rate of false negatives is sufficiently high to indicate that the mouse lung adenoma assay might best be used for screening compounds prior to selection for inhalation or other assays. One might also question what is being measured in this assay, tumor induction or accelerated development of spontaneous lesions (see also Witschi, this volume and Witschi (46)).

Early Markers of Neoplasia

In other organs, notably liver, kidney and urinary bladder, considerable progress has been made in delineating a plausible sequence of biochemical and structural changes between the administration of the carcinogen and the formation of carcinomas (49). The usefulness of the detection of lesions such as biochemically altered foci of cells in the liver parenchyma as short term assays for carcinogenicity is very promising but not yet established. Because the majority of the lesions do not progress to invasive carcinoma and the changes have not yet been proven to be related or sequential, it could be argued that many or all of the lesions are not relevant to subsequent carcinogenesis. Nevertheless, the finding of such lesions either earlier or at greater incidence in dosed animals as compared to matched control animals should be considered for the present as strongly suggestive of carcinogenicity and therefore as a useful screening assay for substances that are active in the early stages of carcinogenicity.

Relatively little progress has been made in this direction in the respiratory system, however. Part of the difficulty can be attributed to the many more tissue types in various parts of the respiratory system (stratified, olfactory, mucociliary, endocrine, glandular, alveolar) which can give rise to either the nodular sequence of tumor formation characteristically found in solid parenchymal organs or the flatter dysplastic sequence of changes characteristic of the epithelial lining of tubular organs. Another difference from liver is the more rapid cell turnover in the respiratory tract that makes more difficult the synchronization of cells, the uniform application of agents that cause hyperplasia, the recognition of selective resistance to carcinogens, and the evaluation of the pathogenetic sequence on quantitative grounds. The same general approaches used in the liver could be applied to parts of the respiratory tract, however, as Witschi and associates (46) have illustrated for the alveolar epithelium of the mouse with butylated hydroxytoluene. One might suppose that histochemical markers for pulmonary endocrine cells in particular will emerge as early markers of neoplasia, but endocrine tumors of the lung are not the predominant tumor type that forms in experimental animals from carcinogen exposure.

New assay methods may soon appear, however. One direction with promise is the recent proliferation of discoveries of monoclonal antibodies that have affinities for different respiratory cell types and to some extent for tumor cell types. Another is that some of the gene products (particularly growth factors) from the unstable developing cell clones may someday become useful screening tools for preneoplasia. Or perhaps the detection of amplification, expression, mutation, or altered regulation of oncogenes might serve as the basis for bioassays. All have promise.

Speculation aside, very early biochemical markers for neoplasia in the respiratory system do not yet exist. The cytological changes that occur a little later during the progression of the neoplastic process, however, are useful indicators of preneoplasia in animals just as they are in humans (32).

In Vitro Assays

Cell Transformation Assays

In the respiratory system, in vitro epithelial cell transformation assays present the same opportunities and limitations as in other organ systems. Enough is known now about the nutrient requirements of various respiratory epithelial cells to suggest that several assays are possible and only require standardization and validation with a battery of test substances. For example, primary cultures of rat tracheal epithelium survive in culture for short periods without replication, but after carcinogen exposure (e.g., BaP, DMBA, MMNG), the surviving cells undergo morphologic alteration and can be subpassaged (6,15,18,39), making "immortalization" an assay endpoint. With additional passage, the ability of subclones to grow in soft agar emerges and eventually (in some clones) transplantability into animals with subsequent benign or malignant growth. Similar in vitro transformation assays can be performed also with human bronchial epithelial cells (11). The endpoints measured can be expanded by application of cytogenetic or molecular genetic techniques. One limitation of this general approach is that the cells may not be capable of metabolizing some carcinogens to an active form. An important advantage, however, is the opportunity to introduce selective pressures or promoting agents to enhance the expression of effects, not only to reduce the time to obtain results but also to evaluate the effects of combined treatments on late-stage carcinogenesis. The altered growth capacity of cells exposed in vitro to carcinogens provides a rapid, inexpensive screening assay.

In Vivo/In Vitro Assays

The metabolic limitation of in vitro assays can be avoided by administering the test substance to the whole animal. At intervals following animal exposure, cell and organ cultures can be initiated and studied (40,41) as in the preceding paragraph. Various manipulations can be applied in vitro such as glutamate deficiency (17) to select for tumor clones. Finally, the cells can be reintroduced into an animal to learn their biological behavior under in vivo conditions.

A variant of this assay is the exposure of a pregnant animal to the test substance with the subsequent in vitro culture of fetal respiratory tissues to disclose evidence of transformation. This assay awaits further investigation.

Bioassay Strategy

If carcinogenicity bioassays are required by a governmental regulatory agency, inhalation bioassays may be unavoidable. On the other hand, if one only wishes to know whether a substance has carcinogenic activity, there are simpler and cheaper approaches.

First, enough information might be at hand from bioassays and experiments conducted by other routes of exposure, so that retesting by the respiratory route is not needed. Extrapolations from one route of exposure to another have their limitations but much of the uncertainty can be reduced by pharmacokinetic studies that measure the doses to the target tissues following different modes of administration. Moreover, if the test substance or its active metabolites is widely distributed in the body after uptake, the route of exposure lessens in importance.

If respiratory bioassays are still required, I suggest starting, for particulate suspensions or liquids, with the intratracheal injection method in rats or hamsters (Table 8.8). A very large dose can be given in 5–15 weekly administrations and the animals observed without additional treatment for a year or until they show signs of illness. Concurrently, a small, intratracheal exposure experiment could be conducted with monitoring by exfoliative cytology and with serial sacrifices at about monthly intervals for 3 months or so, to detect preneoplastic lesions histologically and for subsequent in vitro culture to detect subculturability. For fibers, consideration should be given to bringing them into contact with meso-

Table 8.8. Bioassay strategy

A. For particulates, fibers, and liquids		
Steps		
	1. Extrapolation from other exposure routes	
	2. Additional pharmacokinetic studies	
	3a. Intratracheal instillation	
		≥ 1 year
		Histopathology
	4a. Intratracheal	
		Concurrent with step 3a
		90-day serial sacrifice
		Exfoliative cytology
		Histopathology
		In vitro subculturability
	5. Inhalation bioassay	
		(Last step)
B. For gases, mists, smokes, and vapors substitute		
	3b. Flow-through tracheal transplants	
		Exfoliative cytology
		Histopathology
		In vitro subculturability
	4b. Inhalation	
		Concurrent with step 3b
		90-day serial sacrifice
		Exfoliative cytology
		Histopathology
		In vitro cultivability

thelial tissues by intrapleural inoculation. For gases or vapors, a small, short serial sacrifice study by the inhalation route could be conducted. Properly designed for two species, this experiment could fulfill the requirements of the subchronic toxicity test that would be needed if a long term bioassay is indicated and could also provide information about the nature and location of biologic effects in relation to dose. A cheaper but technically demanding approach for gases is the flow-through tracheal transplant method where exfoliative cytology could be added easily to the histologic and cell culture end points.

The mouse lung adenoma assay is not recommended for routine use because of the high false negative error rate but may be a useful screening technique when it can be demonstrated that the test substance reaches the lung.

Summary

Carcinogenicity protocols for respiratory routes of exposure do not differ in principle from those for other exposure routes. In practice, however, inhalation bioassays in animals require special attention to exposure monitoring and to possible environmental alterations in respiratory function. The temptation to reduce costs through smaller group sizes, fewer concentration levels, early sacrifice intervals, or deletion of chamber-control groups must be avoided.

Because inhalation bioassays are cumbersome and expensive, few substances have been tested adequately by this means in spite of the importance of the respiratory tract as a portal of entry for environmental and occupational chemicals. Moreover, inhalation bioassays are relatively insensitive for detecting carcinogens. Alternate exposure modes that have been developed include direct injections into the lung parenchyma, the pleural or mediastinal cavities, or into the bronchial mucosa; intratracheal instillations; repeated topical applications to localized sites by lavage or into heterotransplanted tracheas; and systemic administration. The most commonly used respiratory carcinogenicity assays other than inhalation are intratracheal instillations in Syrian hamsters and parenteral administration in strain A mice. The induction of lung tumors in strain A mice is a useful screening test but has a high rate of false negative results.

Efforts to develop short-term in vivo assays based on biochemical markers of early foci or through two-stage protocols have lagged behind the progress in other organ systems. Prospects for in vivo/in vitro assays are promising but require validation.

A tiered approach to carcinogenicity testing in the respiratory system is proposed, with inhalation bioassays as the last tier. If carcinogenic activity is not found by this means, the data should provide substantial evidence for the lack of carcinogenicity to experimental animals. If, on the other hand, carcinogenic activity is demonstrated, the data will provide a rational basis for subsequent investigations of the conditions under which carcinogenicity might be expressed (the next step in health hazard assessment).

Acknowledgment. Research for this paper was sponsored by the Office of Health and Environmental Research, US Department of Energy, under contract DE-AC05-840R21400 with the Martin Marietta Energy Systems, Inc.

References

1. Baba M, Klein-Szanto AJP, Trono D, Obara T, Yoakum GH, Masui T, Harris CC (1987) Preneoplastic and neoplastic growth of xenotransplanted lung-derived human cell lines, using deepithelialized rat tracheas. Cancer Res 47:573–578
2. Blair WH (1974) Chemical induction of lung carcinomas in rats. In: Karbe E, Park JF (eds) Experimental lung cancer: carcinogenesis and bioassay. Springer, Berlin Heidelberg New York, pp 199–206
3. Dagle GE, McDonald KE, Smith LG, Stevens DL (1978) Pulmonary carcinogenesis in rats given implants of cigarette smoke condensate in beeswax pellets. JNCI 61:905–910
4. Dalby WE, Nettesheim P, Griesemer R, Caton JE, Guerin MR (1980) Chronic inhalation of cigarette smoke by F344 rats. JNCI 64:383–390
5. Dontenwill W, Chevalier H-J, Harke H-P, Lafrenz U, Reckzeh G, Schneider B (1973) Investigations on the effects of chronic cigarette-smoke inhalation in Syrian golden hamsters. JNCI 51:1781–1832

6. Fitzgerald DJ, Kitamura H, Barrett JC, Nettesheim P (1986) Analysis of growth fractions and stem cell compartments in transformed rat tracheal epithelial cell colonies. Cancer Res 46:4642–4649
7. Gart JJ, Krewski D, Lee PN, Tarone R, Wahrendorf J (1987) Statistical methods in cancer research, vol III: The design and analysis of long-term animal experiments. IARC, Lyon (Scientific Pub., 79)
8. Griesemer RA, Kendrick J, Nettesheim P (1974) Tracheal grafts. In: Karbe E, Park JF (eds) Experimental lung cancer: carcinogenesis and bioassay. Springer, Berlin Heidelberg New York, pp 539–547
9. Griesemer RA, Nettesheim P, Martin DH, Caton JE (1977) Quantitative exposure of grafted rat tracheas to 7,12-dimethylbenz(a)anthracene. Cancer Res 37:1266–1271
10. Harris CC (1976) Chemical carcinogenesis and experimental models using human tissues. Beitr Pathol 158:389–404
11. Harris CC (1987) Human tissues and cells in carcinogenesis research. Cancer Res 47:1–10
12. Hueper WC, Payne WW (1959) Experimental cancers in rats produced by chromium compounds and their significance to industry and public health. Am Ind Hyg Assoc J 20:274–288
13. Hueper WC, Payne WW (1962) Experimental studies in metal carcinogenesis. Arch Environ Health 5:51–68
14. Kendrick J, Nettesheim P, Hammons AS (1974) Tumor induction in tracheal grafts: a new experimental model for respiratory carcinogenesis studies. JNCI 52:1317–1325
15. Kitamura H, Fitzgerald DJ, Li L-A, Barrett C, Nettesheim P (1986) Morphological characterization of transformed colonies in rat tracheal epithelial cell cultures exposed to carcinogen. Cancer Res 46:4631–4641
16. Laskin S, Sellakumar A (1974) Models in chemical respiratory carcinogenesis. In: Karbe E, Park JF (eds) Experimental lung cancer: carcinogenesis and bioassay. Springer, Berlin Heidelberg New York, pp 7–19
17. Marchok AC, Huang SF, Martin DH (1984) Selection of carcinogen-altered rat tracheal epithelial cells preexposed to 7,12-dimethylbenz[a]anthracene by their loss of a need for pyruvate to survive in culture. Carcinogenesis 5:789–796
18. Marchok AC, Huang SF, Martin DH, Johnston WW (1986) Progression-linked properties of specific-lesion cell populations from 7,12-dimethylbenz[a]anthracene-exposed rat tracheal implants. Carcinogenesis 7:1165–1173
19. Merletti F, Heseltine E, Saracci R, Simonato L, Vainio H, Wilbourn J (1984) Target organs for carcinogenicity of chemicals and industrial exposures in humans: a review of results in the IARC monographs on the evaluation of the carcinogenic risk of chemicals to humans. Cancer Res 44:2244–2250
20. Milman HA, Weisburger EK (eds) (1985) Handbook of carcinogen testing. Noyes, Park Ridge, New Jersey
21. Mohr U (1970) Effects of diethylnitrosamine in the respiratory system of Syrian golden hamsters. In: Nettesheim P, Hanna MG, Deatheridge JW (eds) Morphology of experimental respiratory carcinogenesis. USAEC Division of Technical Information, Oak Ridge, pp 255–265
22. Montesano R, Saffiotti U (1968) Carcinogenic response of the respiratory tract of Syrian golden hamsters to different doses of diethylnitrosamine. Cancer Res 28:2198–2210
23. Montesano R, Saffiotti U (1970) Carcinogenic response of the hamster respiratory tract to single subcutaneous administrations of diethylnitrosamine at birth. JNCI 44:413–417

24. Nettesheim P, Griesemer RA (1978) Experimental models for studies of respiratory tract carcinogenesis. In: Harris CC (ed) Pathogenesis and therapy of lung cancer. Dekker, New York, pp 75–188
25. Nettesheim P, Griesemer RA, Martin DH, Caton JR (1977) Induction of preneoplastic and neoplastic lesions in grafted rat tracheas continuously exposed to benzo(a)pyrene. Cancer Res 37:1272–1278
26. Nettesheim P, Hanna MG, Doherty DG, Newell RF, Hellman A (1970) Effects of chronic exposure to artificial smog and chromium oxide dust on the incidence of lung tumors in mice. In: Hanna MG, Nettesheim P, Gilbert JR (eds) Inhalation carcinogenesis. USAEC Division of Technical Information, Oak Ridge, pp 305–317
27. Peck RM, Eaton GJ, Peck EB, Litwin S (1983) Influence of Sendai virus on carcinogenesis in strain A mice. Lab Anim Sci 33:154–156
28. Pereira MA, Stoner GD (1985) Comparison of rat liver foci assay and strain A mouse lung tumor assay to detect carcinogens: a review. Fund Appl Toxicol 5:688–699
29. Rubin IB, Guerin MR (1977) Chemical evaluation of the beeswax pellet implantation bioassay model for studies of environmental carcinogens. JNCI 58:641–644
30. Saffiotti U, Montesano R, Sellakumar AR, Cefis F, Kaufman DG (1972) Respiratory tract carcinogenesis in hamsters induced by different numbers of administration of benzo(a)pyrene and ferric oxide. Cancer Res 32:1073–1081
31. Saffiotti U, Montesano R, Sellakumar AR, Kaufman, DG (1972) Respiratory tract carcinogenesis induced in hamsters by different dose levels of benzo(a)pyrene and ferric oxide. JNCI 49:1199–1204
32. Schreiber H, Saccomanno G, Martin DH, Brennan L (1974) Sequential cytological changes during development of respiratory tract tumors induced in hamsters by benzo(a)pyrene-ferric oxide. Cancer Res 34:689–698
33. Schreiber H, Schreiber K, Martin DH (1975) Experimental tumor induction in a circumscribed region of the hamster trachea: correlation of histology and exfoliative cytology. JNCI 54:187–197
34. Schuller HM, Witschi HP (1987) A novel in vivo model for the induction of carcinoids and small cell cancer of the lung, Toxicologist 7:19
35. Shiba M, Marchok AC, Klein-Szanto AJP (1983) An open-ended rat tracheal implant model: toxic effects of formaldehyde on the respiratory epithelium. Toxicol Lett 16:241–248
36. Shimkin MB, Stoner GD (1975) Lung tumors in mice: Application to carcinogenesis bioassay. In: Klein G, Weinhouse S, Haddow A (eds) Advances in cancer research, vol 21. Academic, New York, pp 1–58
37. Smith WE, Hubert DD (1974) The intrapleural route as a means for estimating carcinogenicity. In: Karbe E, Park JF (eds) Experimental lung cancer: carcinogenesis and bioassay. Springer, Basel Heidelberg New York, pp 92–101
38. Stanton MF, Wrench C (1972) Mechanisms of mesothelioma induction with asbestos and fibrous glass. JNCI 49:797–821
39. Terzaghi M, Klein-Szanto AJP (1980) Differentiation of normal and cultured preneoplastic tracheal epithelial cells in rats: importance of epithelial mesenchymal interactions. JNCI 65:1039–1048
40. Terzaghi M, Nettesheim P (1983) Combined in vivo-in vitro studies of neoplastic development in rat respiratory tissues. In: Reznik-Schuller HM (ed) Comparative respiratory tract carcinogenesis, vol 2. CRC, Boca Raton, pp 189–197
41. Terzaghi M, Nettesheim P, Riester L (1982) Effect of carcinogen dose on the dynamics of neoplastic development in rat tracheal epithelium. Cancer Res 42:4511–4518

42. Topping DC, Nettesheim P, Martin DH (1980) Toxic and tumorigenic effects of asbestos on tracheal mucosa. J Environ Pathol Toxicol 3:261–275
43. Topping DC, Nettesheim P (1980) Two-stage carcinogenesis studies with asbestos in Fischer 344 rats. JNCI 65:627–630
44. Wagner JC, Berry G (1969) Mesotheliomas in rats following inoculation with asbestos. Br J Cancer 23:567–581
45. Weiss W (1986) Oncology overview. Selected abstracts on potential occupational causes of cancer. I. The respiratory tract. National Technical Information Service, Springfield
46. Witschi, HP (1983) Enhancement of tumor formation in mouse lung. In: Slaga TJ (ed) Mechanisms of tumor promotion, vol 1. Tumor promotion in internal organs. CRC, Boca Raton, pp 71–89
47. WHO/IARC (1980) IARC Monographs on the evaluation of the carcinogenic risk of chemicals to humans, suppl. 2. Long-term and short-term screening assays for carcinogens: a critical appraisal. IARC, Lyon
48. WHO/IARC (1982) IARC Monographs on the evaluation of the carcinogenic risk of chemicals to humans, suppl 4. Chemicals, industrial processes and industries associated with cancer in humans. IARC, Lyon
49. WHO/IARC (1987) IARC Monographs on the evaluation of the carcinogenic risk of chemicals to humans. Long-term and short-term screening assays for carcinogens: a critical appraisal. IARC, Lyon (Scientific Pub. No. 83)
50. Yarita T, Nettesheim P (1978) Carcinogenicity of nickel subsulfide for respiratory tract mucosa. Cancer Res 38:3140–3145
51. Yarita T, Nettesheim P, Williams ML (1978) Tumor induction in the trachea of hamsters with *N*-nitroso-*N*-methylurea. Cancer Res 38:1667–1676

Part III
Interpretation of Toxicokinetic Studies with Airborne Toxicants

CHAPTER 9

Interspecies Dosimetry of Reactive Gases*

F.J. Miller,[1] J.H. Overton,[1] T.R. Gerrity,[1] and R.C. Graham[2]

Introduction

The development of dosimetry models that can provide a description of the uptake and distribution of inhaled compounds throughout the body is an integral component of the risk assessment process. The availability of such models allows for more informed judgments of potential risk from human exposure since toxicological data obtained in a variety of animal species using different exposure regimens can be compared to humans on the basis of dose delivered to the target site. This also enables information from studies that are comparable, from a delivered dose perspective, to be assessed collectively, thereby increasing the likelihood that the interpretation of the toxicological results will be correct. Knowledge of the respiratory tract dosimetry of inhaled reactive gases is particularly important since due to their reactivity, they often bind to target sites within the respiratory tract, causing toxicity.

Interspecies dosimetric comparisons of reactive gases must be approached using a model conceptualization that incorporates the major factors affecting the uptake of the gas. Among these factors are respiratory tract morphology, route, rate, and depth of breathing, physicochemical properties of the gas, the physical processes governing gas transport, and the physical and chemical properties of the liquid lining and tissue of the airways and gas exchange units. These various factors interact in a complex manner to determine dose and must be considered in developing mathematical dosimetry models.

---

*The research described in this article has been reviewed by the Health Effects Research Laboratory, U.S. Environmental Protection Agency and approved for publication. Approval does not signify that the contents necessarily reflect the views and policies of the Agency nor does mention of trade names or commercial products constitute endorsement or recommendation for use.

[1]U.S. Environmental Protection Agency, Health Effects Research Laboratory, Research Triangle Park, NC 27711, USA.

[2]Northrop Services Inc., Environmental Sciences, Research Triangle Park, NC 27709, USA.

Despite the difficulties in developing physiologically based mathematical dosimetry models, their desirability is without question. Experimental data on the uptake of reactive gases is limited, in part due to needing to use radiolabeling or isotopic ratio mass spectroscopy techniques to determine delivered dose to specific target sites. Even as improved methods become available for use in experimental studies of the regional dosimetry of reactive gases, there are many exposure scenarios for which it is not practical to obtain experimental data. This does not minimize the need to obtain more experimental measurements of gas uptake. On the contrary, experimental data are critically needed for validation and refinement of theoretical dosimetry models, as well as for determining health effects.

Typically, the proportion of the total toxicological data for inhaled pollutants represented by epidemiological and human clinical studies is small compared to the proportion available from studies using animals. This imbalance stems from the nature and inherent limitations of epidemiological and human clinical studies. Because of confounding variables, it is difficult for epidemiological investigations to quantitatively identify pollutants and the exposure patterns which cause disease. Clinical studies cannot employ chronic exposures and usually require the use of noninvasive techniques, thereby greatly limiting the assessment of potential effects in man. In contrast, animal studies can provide a fuller evaluation of disease since a wide range of concentrations, exposure regimens, pollutants, and biological endpoints can be employed. However, quantitatively relating effective pollutant exposure concentrations in animals to those for man is difficult. Realizing that the ultimate use of experimental or theoretical absorption data is to allow concentration-response curves to be converted to dose-response curves for the purposes of intra- and interspecies comparisons of toxicological results, mathematical dosimetry models are needed to facilitate the process. Thus far, modeling efforts for reactive gases have primarily focused on ozone (1–8), although some modeling of the uptake of formaldehyde (9) and nitrogen dioxide (10) has been done. Hence, ozone (O_3) will be used to illustrate the methodologies needed to develop dosimetry models for reactive gases and to examine various aspects of delivered dose.

Ozone Dosimetry Models

Background

A brief overview of previous O_3 models and analyses will be given to provide the reader with a perspective of the development of research in this area. In 1972, McJilton et al. (1) proposed a model for predicting the uptake of O_3 in the human lung. However, since they did not consider chemical reactions of O_3 with constituents of the lining layer of the airways and gas exchange units, the model was more useful for studying the uptake of nonreactive gases. The model structure and illustrations of modeling results have been presented elsewhere (3,4). Miller

(2) incorporated an instantaneous reaction scheme (to account for chemical reactions in the liquid lining of the lung) into a mathematical model that described the transport and removal of O_3 in the lower respiratory tract of laboratory animals and man. Using this model, Miller et al. (5) demonstrated a general similarity in the tissue dose curves for guinea pigs, rabbits, and man, with the first generation of the pulmonary region predicted to receive the maximum O_3 dose. Mockros et al. (7) developed a mathematical model for the purpose of examining transport, absorption, and chemical reactions of gases in the lower respiratory tract. The model formulation and prediction of lower respiratory tract uptake of O_3 in man and rabbits are similar to the instantaneous reaction regime model developed by Miller (2) and to the dose predictions it yields (2,5).

Improved treatments of effective dispersion, radial mass transport, the use of pseudo-first-order chemical reactions, and the addition of distinct tissue and blood compartments were features of the modeling studies published in 1985 by Miller and colleagues (6). They showed that, for the human lung, model simulation results were more sensitive to mucous compartment thickness and reaction rate constant than to transport and blood parameters. In addition, for ventilation levels used in many human clinical studies (11), exercise showed a pronounced effect on pulmonary tissue uptake but little effect on tracheobronchial tissue uptake. Recently, modeling studies by Overton et al. (8) focused on the sensitivity of O_3 uptake in laboratory animal lungs to anatomical and ventilatory parameters. Since airway dimensions change during the breathing cycle, an advancement by Overton et al. (8) was to modify the dosimetry model (6) so that anatomical dimensions vary during the cycle. The anatomical models for rats and guinea pigs that were used showed a qualitative similarity in the shape of the dose versus airway number curves but significant differences in predicted percent total and percent pulmonary uptake. Tissue dose in the centriacinar region was found to decrease with increasing distance from the trachea when lobar specific anatomical models were used.

Concepts and Model Formulation

With the above as a brief overview of modeling results available for O_3, this section will describe relevant aspects of respiratory tract morphology and the formulation of the mathematical dosimetry model. The major features of the structure of the lower respiratory tract (LRT) and their relation to model compartments are illustrated in Fig. 9.1. Fig. 9.1a is a diagram of the tracheobronchial (TB) and pulmonary regions of the human lung. For mathematical modeling purposes, the complex branching pattern of the LRT is often summarized by anatomical models as a sequence of sets of cylinders, as symbolized just below the TB region in Fig. 9.1a. The cylinders correspond to airways; each set of cylinders corresponds to a generation. Anatomical models exist for man (12,13) and animals (14–16) that give the number of airways (cylinders) in each generation and the length and diameter of the model airway in each generation. To complete the definition of the air paths in the LRT, the dimensions of

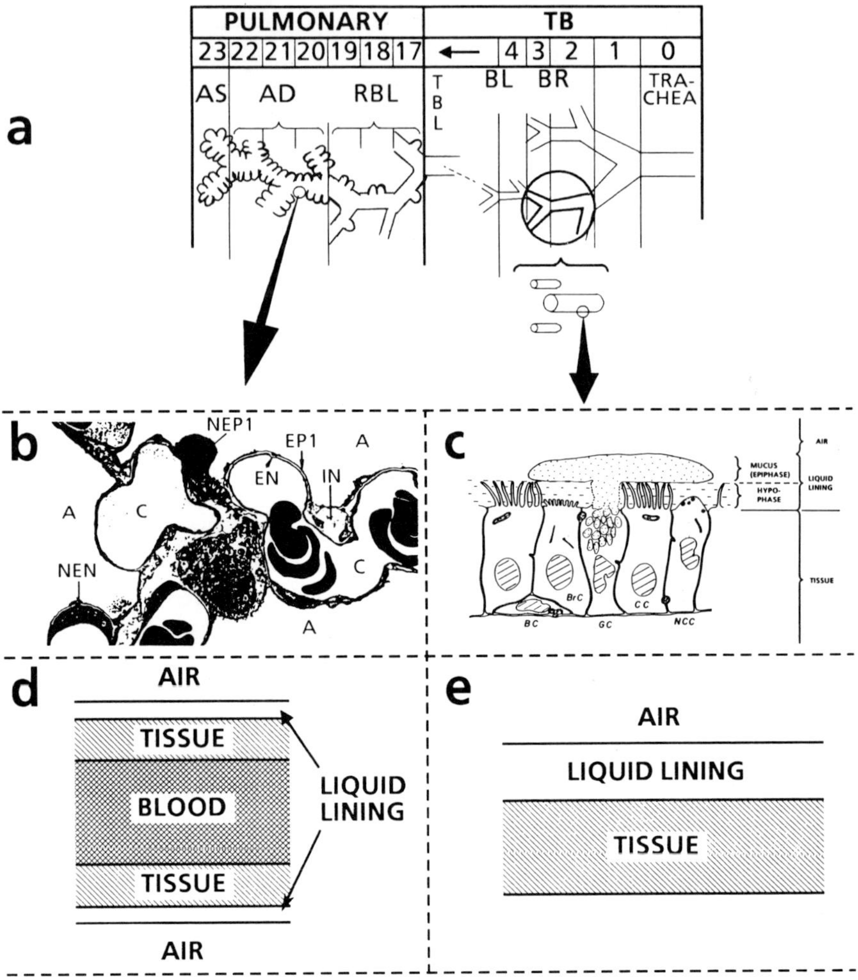

Fig. 9.1a-e. The relationships between morphologies and their model representations. **a**: Schematic of the branching airways of the TB and pulmonary region of man. The generations are labeled from the right, beginning with the trachea. BR, BL, and TBL indicate bronchi, brochioles and terminal bronchioles, respectively; the respiratory bronchioles, alveolar ducts, and alveolar sacs are indicated by RBL, AD, and AS, respectively. Below the TB portion of the lung schematic are three cylindrical figures that indicate the model representation of the airways. **c**: Diagram of the structure of the liquid lining and tissue of the TB region. The different cells represented are basal (BC), ciliated (CC), brush (BrC), goblet (GC), and nonciliated serous (NCC). **e**: Model representation of TB liquid lining and tissue compartments. On the left side of the figure: **b**: electron micrograph of the interalveolar septa. The air spaces (A), capillaries (C), type I cells and their nuclei (EP1 and NEP1), endothelial cells and their nuclei (En and NEN), and interstitial space (IN) are indicated. **d**: Model representation of the liquid lining, tissue, and capillaries of the pulmonary region. (Reprinted from Miller et al., ref. 35.)

pulmonary ducts and sacs, their number in each pulmonary generation, the number of alveoli, their volumes and surface areas must be available or estimated.

In Fig. 9.1b is a micrograph of the interalveolar septum, illustrating the physical structure of the tissue and capillary features of the pulmonary region that should be considered when developing a dosimetry model. At least 95% of the alveolar epithelial tissue is composed of type I cells which are very thin, allowing efficient gas exchange. The surface of the epithelial layer is covered with a liquid lining, the average thickness of which is less than 5% of the air-blood barrier (17). Beneath the epithelial layer is the interstitium followed by the endothelial cells that make up the wall of the capillaries. As illustrated in Fig. 9.1b, capillary blood is sandwiched between the air-blood barrier that consists mainly of a liquid lining, type I cells, interstitium, and endothelial cells. Fig. 9.1d is the model formulation of Miller et al. (6) for this arrangement in which the epithelium, interstitium, and endothelium have been combined into a single tissue compartment.

A diagram of the structure of the liquid lining and tissue of the TB region considered relevant for modeling O_3 uptake is shown in Fig. 9.1c. The liquid lining is made up of two layers, the epiphase and the hypophase. The former is composed of highly viscous mucus of varying thickness; as is illustrated, the layer may not completely cover the hypophase. The hypophase is a watery-like fluid in which cilia move back and forth in such a way as to propel the overlying mucus towards the trachea. The epithelial layer is made up of many cell types, the major types being illustrated in the figure. In the Miller et al. (6) dosimetry model formulation for the TB region, the liquid lining layers have been combined into one compartment and the cells into one tissue compartment (see Fig. 9.1e). A blood compartment in the TB region is not needed for O_3 since chemical reactions prevent any significant amount of O_3 from penetrating that deep (6).

In the dosimetry model of Miller et al. (6) and Overton et al. (8), the processes of transport and chemical reactions are described in terms of differential equations. Transport in the lumen of the airways and in the airspaces is described by a time-dependent partial differential equation that accounts for axial convection, axial dispersion, molecular diffusion, the loss of O_3 to the liquid lining, and lung expansion and contraction due to breathing.

$$\frac{\partial C}{\partial t} + U\frac{\partial C}{\partial x} = \mathrm{D}\frac{\partial^2 C}{\partial x^2} - \frac{S}{V}J_{\mathrm{w}} \qquad (1)$$

In Eq. 1, C is the average cross-sectional concentration at position x along a path in the lumen of the airways or airspaces at time t. U is the average air velocity along the x direction; D is the dispersion coefficient; S and V are the surface area and volume, respectively, of the air compartment of the relevant generation. J_{w} is the flux of O_3 to the liquid lining interface and is defined as

$$J_{\mathrm{w}} = k_{\mathrm{g}}\,(C - H\,C_{\mathrm{li}}). \qquad (2)$$

Henry's law constant, the gas phase mass transfer coefficient, and the liquid lining interfacial concentration of O_3 are, respectively, H, k_{g}, and C_{li}.

The processes considered for the liquid, tissue, and capillary blood compartments are molecular diffusion and chemical reactions. Chemical reactions are assumed to be first order, O_3 reacting only with the unsaturated fatty acids that are assumed to have a constant concentration that depends on the compartment. Because the rates of chemical reactions are much faster than changes in O_3 concentrations due to other processes, the steady state approximation is used (6). Thus, the equation used to describe the transport and loss of O_3 due to chemical reactions is

$$D_j \frac{\partial^2 C_j}{\partial y^2} = k_{lj} C_j . \tag{3}$$

The subscript, j, indicates the liquid lining, tissue or blood compartment; y is the distance perpendicular to the interface between compartments; C_j is the O_3 concentration at y; D_j is the molecular diffusion coefficient; k_{lj} is the first order rate constant. The value of this constant is equal to the product of the second order rate constant of the reaction of O_3 with unsaturated fatty acids and the concentration of the unsaturated fatty acids.

Analytical solutions are obtained from Eq. 3 for each compartment; solutions are matched at the compartment boundaries by using partition coefficients to relate interfacial concentrations and by requiring the flux of O_3 across boundaries to be continuous; the flux is assumed zero midway between the boundaries of the blood compartment. From the solutions, a mass transfer coefficient is obtained for the combined effect of the compartments. Given the compartmental mass transfer coefficient, Eq. 2, and the boundary and initial conditions, then Eq. 1 is solved numerically to obtain the quantity of O_3 absorbed and the dose of absorbed O_3 in each compartment and generation of the LRT. In the model formulation described above, the processes are linear. Hence, the LRT dose will be proportional to the concentration of O_3 entering the trachea.

Intra- and Interspecies Dosimetry of O_3

For discussion of comparative dosimetry, three types of illustrations are presented in this section. (1) An interspecies comparison of tissue dose curves is made, consisting of a plot of the tissue and net dose curves of man, rat, guinea pig, and rabbit versus lung generation. (2) Experimental LRT uptake data is compared to predicted uptake data. Plots are shown for LRT O_3 dose per breath versus tidal volume and versus minute volume. (3) O_3 dose-response curves are constructed using data on forced expiratory volume in 1 s (FEV_1) from a controlled human exposure study and using lavage fluid protein (LFP) data from animal studies. For the former, plots of FEV_1 versus estimated pulmonary tissue dose are presented; for the latter, a graph of LFP versus estimated pulmonary tissue dose for three animals are shown, allowing a comparison of results for all three animals species.

In order to use the dosimetry model to estimate the dose of O_3 that an exposed animal or man received, information that is needed includes the O_3 concentration, the length of time exposed, as well as the tidal volume (V_T) and breathing frequency (f) during exposure. Usually, all of this information is not reported, and the missing data must be estimated. For example, the ventilatory parameters for laboratory animals are often not measured; however, if the weight of the animals is reported, allometric equations can be used to estimate the absent parameters. Once all of the necessary data have been obtained, either as reported or estimated, then estimated doses can be computed using the mathematical dosimetry model. Using the parameters that characterize the particular animal and the conditions of exposure, the model is used to compute the dose for single or multiple breaths for the length of time necessary. If, during the time of exposure, conditions change (e.g., concentration, ventilatory parameters), then dose for these time periods is estimated using the model. Using the estimated doses and the times of exposure, the total estimated dose is computed. The dosimetry model yields dose per breath in several forms, including the quantity of O_3 absorbed per unit airway surface area in a given generation, quantity absorbed by region, quantity absorbed by region and compartment (tissue, liquid lining, blood). Given the experimental effects data, a plot of the effects versus the time integrated dose (e.g., TB tissue dose, pulmonary tissue dose, total LRT dose, etc.) can than be constructed.

Interspecies LRT Dosimetry Patterns

An example of LRT dose curves is illustrated in Fig. 9.2a and b, in which are plotted net and tissue O_3 dosimetry simulation data versus generation for rat and man, order for guinea pig, and zone for rabbit. (The particular segmentation of airways and ducts into generation, order and zone depends on the anatomical model.) Dose is expressed as micrograms of O_3 per square centimeter of segment (generation, order or zone) surface area per minute, standardized to a tracheal O_3 value of 1 $\mu g/m^3$. Thus, for a tracheal concentration of one part per million, multiply the plotted values by 1960 ($\mu g/m^3$ per ppm).

Because the number of sequential segments are different for all the anatomical models, there is a set of segment indices for each animal along the horizontal axis in Fig. 9.2. Although the predicted doses for each segment are calculated only for each segment of an anatomical model, the data for each species has been joined by lines to help in interpreting the plots. Further, we have matched the tracheas, the last TB segment (terminal bronchioles in the human and rat anatomical models; not defined for the guinea pig and rabbit anatomical models), the last pulmonary segment (defined as sacs in the human, rat and rabbit anatomical models; guinea pig's last order contains sacs and ducts), and the first airway of respiratory bronchioles in man with the first alveolated airway in the animal lungs. This latter location is where the histopathological data show the first and the most pronounced lesions in O_3 studies using rats (18–22) and monkeys (23–27). The maximal tissue dose in man, rat, and guinea pig is predicted to

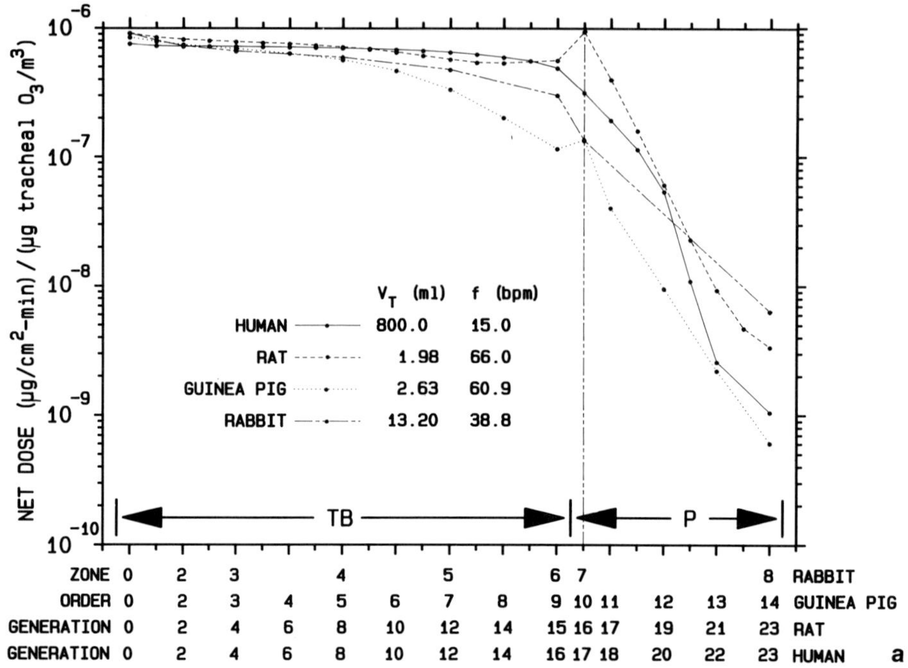

Fig. 9.2. Net dose (**a**) and tissue dose (**b**) versus sequential segments along anatomical model airway paths for man, rat, guinea pig, and rabbit. In general, each segment represents a group of airways or ducts with common features as defined by the designers of the anatomical model [man: generation (121); rat: generation (15); guinea pig: order (16); rabbit: zone (141)]. For a given species, the plotted "dots" represent a predicted dose that corresponds to a given segment. The dots have been joined by lines for ease of interpreting the plots; these lines do not represent predicted values except where they intercept the dots.

occur in this region (Fig. 9.2b). As can be seen from the figures, the shape of the dose curves of O_3 is very comparable in the lungs of these animal species and man. For the same unit tracheal O_3 value, almost a three fold increase in the absorption or removal of O_3 is predicted in the first nonciliated portion of the rat lung compared to man. However, the relative doses depend on the ventilatory parameters chosen.

To make more definitive interspecies dosimetric comparisons, upper respiratory tract removal of O_3 in man versus rat must be considered. Preliminary results of O'Neil et al. (28) indicate that upper respiratory tract removal of O_3 in man is about 40%–45%. In contrast, Wiester et al. (29) have shown that total respiratory tract removal of O_3 in the rat is only about 40%. Uptake studies are currently being conducted, and unconfirmed preliminary experiments (Drs. Jean Wiester and Gary Hatch, personal communication) indicate that the rat may remove only 10%–25% of the inhaled O_3 in the nasopharyngeal region. Further analyses

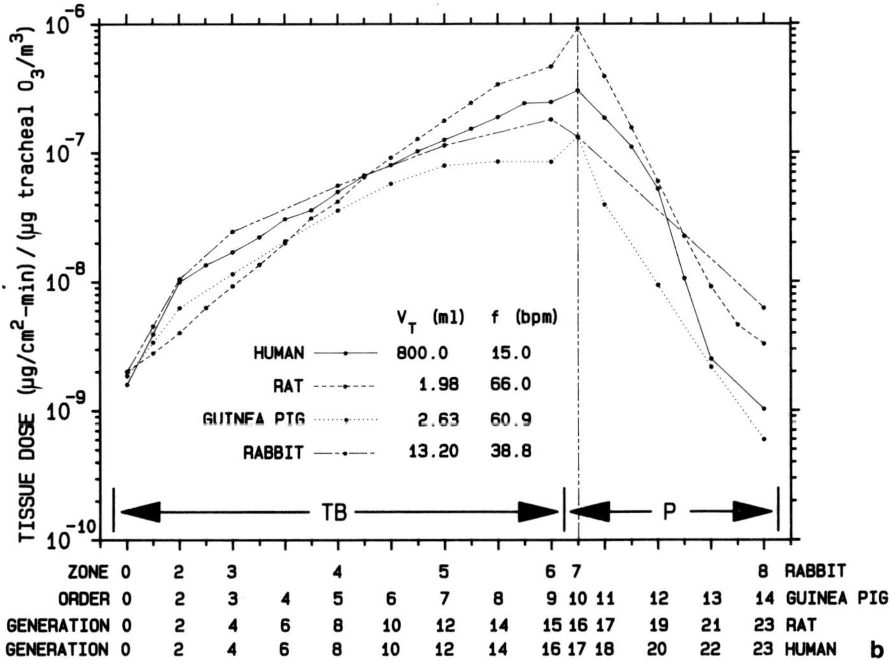

Fig. 9.2. (*Continued*)

presented in this chapter will assume upper respiratory tract removal values of 20% for rats, guinea pigs, and rabbits, and 40% for man.

Experimental LRT Data and Theoretical Predictions

The O_3 removal efficiency of the lower respiratory tract was measured in healthy nonsmoking male volunteers (28). A small polyethylene tube was inserted through a subject's nostril until the tip of the tube could be visualized orally 0.5 cm below the soft palate. While a subject was seated in an environmental O_3 exposure chamber, samples of air from the posterior pharynx were drawn through the tube and into an O_3 analyzer (Monitor Labs 8410) that had been modified so that it could respond rapidly to changing O_3 concentrations. Samples of air from the posterior pharynx were collected while the subject was exposed to either 0.1, 0.2, or 0.4 ppm. At each concentration a subject breathed at a breathing frequency of either 12 or 24 breaths per min (bpm), and either through his nose only, mouth only, or oronasally. Ventilation (f and V_T) was measured concurrently with pharyngeal O_3 concentration. Data were collected from each subject at all combinations of O_3 concentration, mode of breathing, and breathing frequency utilizing a randomized split-split-plot design. The O_3 removal efficiency F_X of that part of the respiratory tract distal to the posterior pharynx (ALRT; the LRT augmented by the segment of the respiratory tract from the

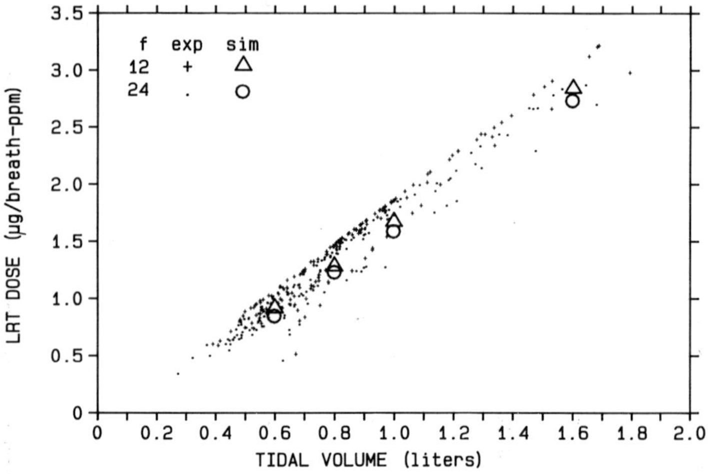

Fig. 9.3. Dose versus tidal volume. Plotted are the experimental data and the predicted values for the absorption of O_3 in human subjects in that part of the respiratory tract distal to the posterior pharynx. For the predicted values, V_T and f were chosen to encompass the range of experimental ventilatory parameters.

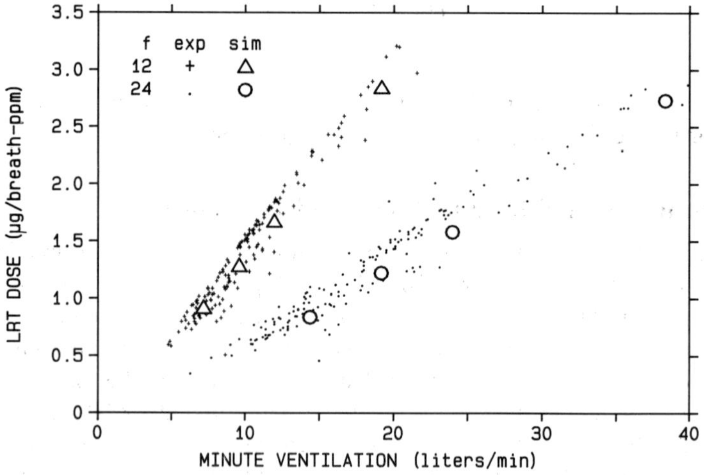

Fig. 9.4. Dose versus minute ventilation. Plotted are the experimental data and the predicted values for the absorption of O_3 in human subjects in that part of the respiratory tract distal to the posterior pharynx. For the predicted values, V_T and f were chosen to encompass the range of experimental ventilatory parameters.

posterior pharynx to the trachea) was calculated by dividing the O_3 concentration in the posterior pharynx during expiration by the O_3 concentration during inspiration and subtracting this from unity.

The mean O_3 removal efficiency of the ALRT over all subjects, O_3 concentrations, modes of breathing, and breathing frequency, and compared with the dosimetry model predictions for ALRT total dose. Figure 9.3 shows the dose of O_3 per breath defined as the product of *F*, tidal volume (reduced by the upper respiratory tract volume proximal to the posterior pharynx), and mass concentration equivalent to one ppm plotted against V_T. Figure 9.4 shows the dose of O_3 per breath per ppm plotted against minute volume ($\dot{V}_T$).

the predicted values are also shown in Figs. 9.3 and 9.4, indicating good agreement between the dosimetry model predictions and the values based on the measurements. To obtain the predicted values, the Weibel anatomical model (12) was used but adjusted to a functional residual capacity (FRC) of 3.32 liters. According to Morris et al. (30), this is the value that corresponds to the subjects' average age and height of 29 years and 117 cm. The tidal volume and breathing frequencies used for the simulations were chosen to represent the range of experimental values. All other parameters have the values as given in Miller et al. (6). The agreement was obtained without adjusting the values of any parameters (such as chemical rate constants, compartment thicknesses, partition coefficients, etc.) except of course, V_T, *f*, and FRC.

When plotted against V_T, the doses per breath fall within a straight band regardless of *f*; however, when plotted against $\dot{V}_E$, the data split according to whether *f* was 12 or 24 bpm. The slope of the line at 12 bpm is approximately half that at 24 bpm. These results indicate that V_T is a more important determinant of net dose per breath than is *f*. In addition, since the dosimetry model predictions of net dose agree well with experimental measurements of total ALRT uptake, it is reasonable to speculate that the LRT dose pattern for man given in Fig. 9.2 may be reflective of that occurring in vivo.

Decrements in FEV_1 Versus Pulmonary Tissue Dose in Man

Human clinical studies routinely employ exercise as a part of the experimental regimen in O_3 exposure studies (11). Probably FEV_1 is the pulmonary function parameter studied most often since this variable reflects a summation of changes in both volume and resistance. However, for O_3 exposures to 0.3 ppm or less, decrements in FEV_1 mainly reflect forced vital capacity changes of similar magnitude, with little to no contribution from resistive changes (11).

A detailed consideration of the numerous clinical studies in which FEV_1 changes have been studied with O_3 levels ranging from 0.11 to 0.75 ppm for $\dot{V}_E$ from 20 to 70 liter/min is beyond the scope of this paper [EPA (11) cites 25 such studies involving a total of more than 300 subjects]. Rather, this section focuses on one such concentration-response study (31) to illustrate an approach to intraspecies dose-response comparisons. McDonnell and coworkers (31) divided 135 healthy subjects into six groups, each group exposed to a different concentration of O_3 [(ppm, number of subjects): (0, 20), (0.12, 22), (0.18, 20), (0.24, 21), (0.3, 21), (0.4, 29)]. During the first 120 min of the 2.5-h exposure regimen, alternating 15-min periods of rest and exercise ($\dot{V}_E$ ranging from 64 to 68 liter/min) were employed. While still being exposed, forced expiratory spirometry was measured 5 min after the final exercise.

The average age and average height of all subjects were used to obtain a common FRC estimated from (30) to be used for simulating the dose of each exposure group. This was reasonable since the averages were not significantly different from one group to the next. Tidal volumes and breathing frequencies were dependent on the particular 15-min period and exposure groups. Values of these parameters were reported for two exercise periods, as well as were minute volume averaged over the four exercise periods for each group. Using this data, estimated one hour average V_T and f were made for the total time of exercise for each group (estimated average V_T and f ranged from 1820 ml and 35.5 bpm to 2251 ml and 30.2 bpm; $\dot{V}_E$ ranged from 65 to 68 liter/min). No measurements of ventilatory parameters for the rest periods were reported. For the first rest period, we assumed $V_T = 800$ ml and $f = 15$ bpm; for the rest periods after the exercise periods, including the 5-min rest period prior to measurement, we chose $V_T = 800$ ml and $f = 20$ bpm.

In Fig. 9.5 are plotted the changes in FEV_1 observed by McDonnell et al. (31) against the pulmonary tissue doses predicted by the mathematical dosimetry model after adjusting for upper respiratory tract removal (28). The dose-response curve is sigmoid in shape and similar to the concentration-response curve of (31). Differences in the shape of the two curves are due primarily to the number of additional factors, in addition to concentration, for which the dose is dependent and were accounted for in the dosimetry model estimates: upper respiratory tract removal efficiency, V_T and f changes over the exposure period, estimating the amount of O_3 delivered to the portion of the lung to which the FEV_1 changes relate, etc.

Interspecies Effects of O_3 on Lavage Fluid Protein (LFP)

Concentration response studies were conducted by Hatch et al. (32) in which groups of rabbits, guinea pigs, rats, hamsters, and mice were exposed for 4 h to either 0, 0.2, 0.5, 1.0, or 2.0 ppm of O_3. LFP accumulation 18–20 h after cessation of exposure was used as an indicator of O_3-induced pulmonary edema. Although the air-exposed animals for all species had similar basal levels of LFP, guinea pigs showed significant effects at 0.2 ppm O_3, mice, hamsters, and rats at 1.0 ppm O_3, and rabbits at 2.0 ppm O_3. There were also species differences in the percent of lavage fluid that could be recovered. The various concentration-response results did not appear to Hatch et al. (32) to be related to species difference in body weight.

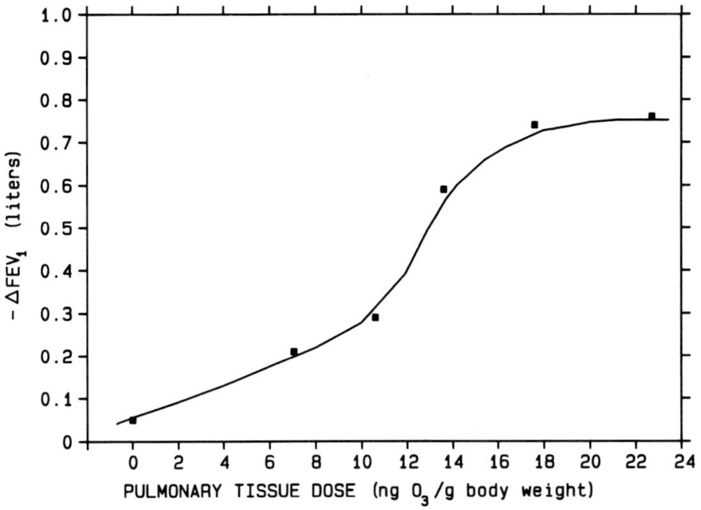

Fig. 9.5. Changes in FEV_1 versus pulmonary tissue dose. Plotted are decrements in FEV_1 (liters) for human subjects against predicted pulmonary tissue dose normalized to body weight. In order, from left to right, the dose values correspond to 0, 0.12, 0.18, 0.24, 0.30–, and 0.40 ppm O_3 exposure concentration. The continuous curve was "eye fit."

The values of the ventilatory parameters and the FRCs were not reported for the animals investigated; however, weight ranges were reported, and we chose the mean of the range as an animal's weight to be used with allometric equations to estimate ventilatory parameters and FRCs. FRC was defined as one-half of the TLC value of each animal, as predicted by the formulae of Takezawa et al. (33). The equations of Gunther (34) were used to estimate V_T and f.

The LFP concentration-response data reported by Hatch et al. (32) for the guinea pig, rat, and rabbit are depicted as dose-response data in Fig. 9.6. Anatomical models were not available for the hamster and mouse, so dose-response curves were not constructed for these two species. The mathematical dosimetry model estimates of the amount of O_3 delivered to pulmonary tissue over the 4-h exposure period have been divided by body weight to facilitate interspecies comparisons of possible differences in sensitivity to O_3 exposure. The partial horizontal line at LFP $\sim$ 470 μg/ml divides the data so that those values below the line are not (statistically) significantly ($p > 0.05$) different from the control values (zero dose). The LFP values above the line, including the second guinea pig but not the fourth rabbit data point, are all significantly different ($p < 0.05$) than the control values of LFP. The rats and rabbits respond similarly with the first significantly elevated level of protein corresponding to a pulmonary tissue dose of about 80 ng O_3/g body weight. On the other hand, the first significantly elevated level of protein for the guinea pig occurs at

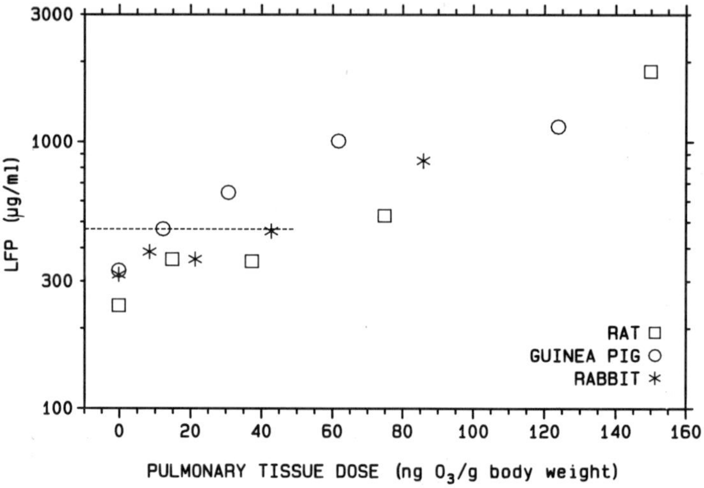

Fig. 9.6. LFP versus pulmonary tissue dose. Plotted for rat, guinea pig, and rabbit is lavage fluid protein (LFP, µm/ml) against predicted pulmonary tissue dose normalized to animal body weight. For each species, in order from left to right, the dose values correspond to 0.0, 0.2, 0.5, 1.0, and 2.0 ppm O_3 exposure concentration.

~12–13 ng O_3/g body weight. These results suggest, that for equivalent pulmonary tissue ozone doses, the guinea pig is more sensitive initially to O_3 than the rat and rabbit. Because of the predicted differences in species sensitivity, speculation as to the effect of equivalent doses in man is not feasible or at best ambiguous. For example, note that the maximal dose to the pulmonary region in the human studies associated with FEV_1 changes in Fig. 9.5 is about 22 ng O_3/g body weight. If man is as sensitive as the guinea pig then we would conclude that there was probably edema formation in the human study. However, if man is more like the rat and rabbit, we would predict no edema formation in any of the exposed human subjects. A third possibility, of course, is that man's sensitivity to O_3 is not similar to any of the three laboratory animals.

Summary

We have demonstrated the feasibility of using physiologically based dosimetry models to enable interspecies comparisons of responses following exposure to reactive gases. Although the specifics of the process and examples of lower respiratory tract dose patterns were presented for the reactive gas, O_3, the intent was to illustrate the type of biological, physical, and chemical information that must be synthesized for the development of dosimetry models that facilitate interspecies comparisons of dose delivered to comparable target sites. The critical information areas include respiratory tract morphology, route, rate, and depth of breathing, physicochemical properties of the gas, the physical processes governing gas transport, and the physical and chemical properties of the liquid lining and tissue of the airways and gas exchange units. Application of an O_3 dosimetry model to obtain intra- and interspecies dose-response curves highlights the potential impact of dosimetry models for collective assessments of toxicological data, thereby improving the overall risk assessment process, especially its quantitative aspects. Since the full array of potential effects from exposure to inhaled compounds can only be accomplished by integrating information from epidemiological, human clinical, and animal toxicological studies, improvements in our ability to make more quantitative comparisons among species are inextricably linked to an improved understanding of interspecies dosimetry.

Acknowledgment. The authors would like to express their appreciation to Mr. Andrew Barnett for his excellent technical assistance and to Ms. Carolyn Wheeler for her typing of the manuscript.

References

1. McJilton C, Thielke J, Frank R (1972) Ozone uptake model for the respiratory system. In: Abstracts of technical papers, American Industrial Hygiene Conference, 14–19 May 1972, paper no 45
2. Miller FJ (1977) A mathematical model of transport and removal of ozone in mammalian lung. Thesis, North Carolina State University, Raleigh
3. National Research Council (1977) Committee on medical and biological effects of environmental pollutants, subcommittee on ozone and other photochemical oxidants. Toxicology, ozone and other photochemical oxidants. National Academy of Sciences, Washington, DC, pp 323–387
4. Morgan MS, Frank R (1977) Uptake of pollutant gases by the respiratory system. In: Brain JD, Proctor DF (eds) Respiratory defense mechanisms, part I. Marcel Dekker, New York, pp 157–189
5. Miller FJ, Menzel DB, Coffin DL (1978) Similarity between man and laboratory animals in regional pulmonary deposition of ozone. Environ Res 17:84–101
6. Miller FJ, Overton JH Jr, Jaskot RH, Menzel DB (1985) A model of the regional uptake of gaseous pollutants in the lung. I. The sensitivity of the uptake of ozone in the human lung to lower respiratory tract secretions and exercise. Toxicol Appl Pharmacol 79:11–27
7. Mockros LF, Grotberg JB, Sheth BV (1985) Absorption of noxious gases in pulmonary airways. Abstract from 38th ACEMB meeting, 30 September to 2 October, Chicago
8. Overton JH, Graham RC, Miller FJ (1987) A model of the regional uptake of gaseous pollutants in the lung. II. The sensitivity of ozone uptake in laboratory animal lungs to anatomical and ventilatory parameters. Toxicol Appl Pharmacol 88: 418–432
9. Chang JCF, Gross EA, Swenberg JA, Barrow CS (1983) Nasal cavity deposition, histopathology, and cell proliferation after single or repeated formaldehyde exposure in B6C3F1 mice and F-344 rats. Toxicol Appl Pharmacol 68:161–176

10. Miller FJ, Overton JH, Meyers ET, Graham JA (1982) Pulmonary dosimetry of nitrogen dioxide in animals and man. In: Schneider T, Grant L (eds) Air pollution by nitrogen dioxide. Proceedings of US-Dutch international symposium on NO_x, Maastricht, Netherlands, Elsevier, Amsterdam, pp 377–386
11. U.S. Environmental Protection Agency (1986) Air quality criteria for ozone and other photochemical oxidants, vol V. EPA/600/8-84/020eF August 1986
12. Weibel ER (1963) Morphometry of the human lung. Academic, New York
13. Yeh HC, Schum GM (1980) Models of human lung airways and their application to inhaled particle deposition. Bull Math Biol 42:461–480
14. Kliment V (1973) Similarity and dimensional analysis, evaluation of aerosol deposition in the lungs of laboratory animals and man. Folia Morphol 21:59–64
15. Yeh HC, Schum GM, Duggan MT (1979) Anatomic models of the tracheobronchial and pulmonary region of the rat. Anat Rec 195:483–492
16. Schreider JP, Hutchens JO (1980) Morphology of the guinea pig respiratory tract. Anat Rec 196:313–321
17. Weibel ER (1973) Morphological basis of alveolar-capillary gas exchange. Physiol Rev 53(2):419–495
18. Stephens RJ, Sloan MF, Evans MJ, Freeman G (1973) Early response of lung to low levels of ozone. Am J Pathol 74:31–58
19. Stephens RJ, Sloan MF, Evans MJ, Freeman G (1974) Alveolar type 1 cell response to exposure to 0.5 ppm O_3 for short periods. Exp Mol Pathol 20:11–23
20. Plopper CG, Chow CK, Dungworth DL, Tyler WS (1979) Pulmonary alterations in rats exposed to 0.2 and 0.1 ppm ozone: a correlated morphological and biochemical study. Arch Environ Health 34:390–395
21. Boorman GA, Schwartz LW, Dungworth DL (1980) Pulmonary effects of prolonged ozone insult in rats. Lab Invest 43(2):108–115
22. Barry BE, Miller FJ, Crapo JD (1985) Effects of inhalation of 0.12 and 0.25 ppm ozone on the proximal alveolar region of juvenile and adult rats. Lab Invest 53:692–704
23. Dungworth DL, Castleman WL, Chow CK, Mellick PW, Mustafa MG, Tarkington B, Tyler WS (1975) Effect of ambient levels of ozone on monkeys. Fed Proc Fed Am Soc Exp Biol 34:1670–1674
24. Castleman WL, Tyler WS, Dungworth DL (1977) Lesions in respiratory bronchioles and conducting airways of monkeys exposed to ambient levels of ozone. Exp Mol Pathol 26:384–400
25. Eustis SL, Schwartz LW, Kosch PC, Dungworth DL (1981) Chronic bronchiolitis in nonhuman primates after prolonged ozone exposure. Am J Pathol 105:121–137
26. Mellick PW, Mustafa MG, Tyler WS, Dungworth DL (1975) Morphologic and biochemical changes in primate lung due to low-level ozone exposure. In: Proceedings of 23rd international tuberculosis conference, September, Mexico. Bull Int Union Tubercul 51:565–567
27. Mellick PW, Dungworth DL, Schwartz LW, Tyler WS (1977) Short term morphologic effects of high ambient levels of ozone on lungs of rhesus monkeys. Lab Invest 36:82–90
28. O'Neil JJ, Gerrity TA, Weaver RA, Berntsen JH, Overton JH, Miller FJ (1987) Ozone removal in the nasopharynx and lungs of normal man during tidal breathing. Abstract from international symposium on inhalation toxicology, 23–27 March, Hannover, FRG

29. Wiester MJ, Williams TB, King ME, Ménache MG, Miller FJ (1987) Ozone uptake in awake Sprague Dawley rats. Toxicol Appl Pharmacol 89:429–437
30. Morris AH, Kanner RE, Crapo RO, Gardner RM (1984) Clinical pulmonary function testing, 2nd edn. International Thoracic Society, Salt Lake City
31. McDonnell WF, Horstman DH, Hazucha MJ, Seal E Jr, Haak ED, Salaam S, House DE (1983) Pulmonary effects of ozone exposure during exercise: dose-response characteristics. J Appl Physiol: Respir Environ Exercise Physiol 54:1345–1352
32. Hatch GE, Slade R, Stead AG, Graham JA (1986) Species comparison of acute inhalation toxicity of ozone and phosgene. J Toxicol Environ Health 19:43–53
33. Takezawa J, Miller FJ, O'Neil JJ (1980) Single-breath diffusing capacity and lung volumes in small laboratory animals. J Appl Physiol: Respirat Environ Exercise Physiol 48(6):1052–1059
34. Gunther B (1975) Dimensional analysis and theory of biological similarity. Physiol Rev 55:659–699
35. Miller FJ, Overton JH, Smolko ED, Graham RC, Menzel DB (1987) Hazard assessment using an integrated physiologically-based dosimetry modeling approach: ozone. In: Pharmacokinetics in risk assessment/drinking water and health, vol. 8. National Academy Press, Washington, pp 353–368

CHAPTER 10

Behavior of Inspired Aerosol Boli in Humans

J. Heyder[1]

Introduction

The respiratory system is the initial target for inhaled pollutants. An assessment of the effects of air pollutants on the lungs is often based on measurements of lung volumes, maximum expiratory flow rates, and lung compliance during breathing of inert gases (8).

Inert monodisperse aerosols can also be used to characterize the respiratory system (6). Many investigators have measured the total deposition of particles during steady tidal breathing or during breath-holding. Others have studied the short-term clearance of particles from the lungs. However, little use has been made of the aerosol bolus technique. This approach utilizes monodisperse particles which are not distributed throughout the entire tidal air; rather, they are confined to a small volume within the tidal air, and the distribution of particles in the inspired and expired air is monitored (3).

Aerosol boli can be made to behave as a "nondiffusing" gas which is only slightly absorbed and which penetrates to different volumetric depths into the respiratory system. At each lung depth the following information can be obtained:

- Convective gas transport
- Particle deposition
- Particle clearance
- Airway dimensions
- Relative humidity

The purpose of this paper is to describe the aerosol bolus technique and to explain how it can be applied to the above topics.

---

[1]Gesellschaft für Strahlen- und Umweltforschung m.b.H., Projekt Inhalation, Ingolstädter Landstrasse 1, 8042 Neuherberg, FRG.

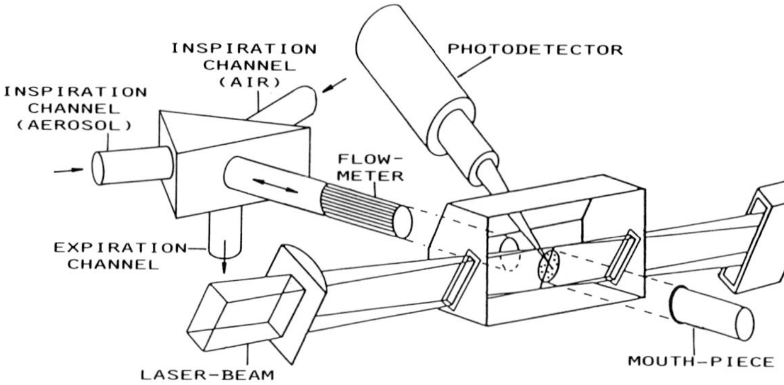

Fig. 10.1. The inhalation apparatus.

Description of the Aerosol Bolus Technique

A monodisperse aerosol with particles about 1 µm in diameter is continuously generated and is available when desired during inspiration. The intrinsic motion of these particles is almost entirely due to the action of gravity; particle transport by diffusion is negligible.

To study gas transport, particle deposition, and airway caliber, hydrophobic droplets generated by heterogeneous nucleation are usually used. Radioactively labelled hydrophobic particles generated by dispersion of solutions or suspensions are suitable to the study of particle clearance. Hydrophilic particles are required to study the relative humidity at various sites of the respiratory tree. These aerosols are usually generated by dispersion of aqueous solutions.

During the experiment a subject breathes air orally through a pneumotachograph which monitors instantaneous flow rate and, after time integration, respired volume. The inspired and expired air also passes through a laser aerosol photometer (Fig. 10.1). This device monitors either instantaneous particle number concentration (photometric mode of operation) or particle size (count mode of operation). After volume integration, the number of inspired and expired particles and thus particle losses in the lungs can be calculated. Poppet valves serve to separate expired from inspired air. To condition the inspired air and to avoid water vapor condensation during expiration, the pneumotachograph, photometer, and valves are kept above body temperature.

Assisted by a volume signal, visible on an oscilloscope screen, and an audible time signal, the subject is trained to breathe air with a 1000 cm^3 tidal volume and a 250 cm^3s^{-1} flow rate from functional residual capacity.

An aerosol bolus is introduced at a preselected volume in the inspired air by a computer which closes the solenoid valve of the air inlet and simultaneously opens the valve of the aerosol inlet. After about 50 cm^3 aerosol has entered the

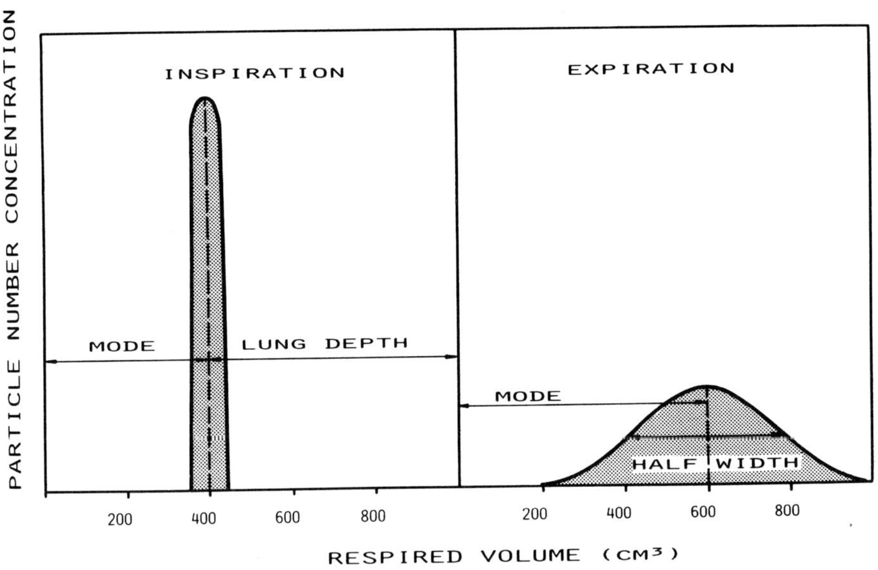

Fig. 10.2. Illustration of some measured and controlled variables in the aerosol bolus technique in a plot of particle number concentration in inspired and expired air as a function of the respired volume; the shadowed areas represent inspired and expired aerosol bolus.

inspired air, the valves reverse. After inspiration of 1000 cm^3 the computer closes both solenoid valves and the subject immediately (or after breath-holding) expires to residual volume at a flow rate of 250 cm^3s^{-1}. Thus, the subject inspires an aerosol bolus into the respiratory system to a preselected volumetric depth, and particle number concentration is plotted as a function of the respired volume (Fig. 10.2).

Controlled and Measured Variables

The controlled variable in this technique is the mode of the inspired bolus and thus the volumetric depth to which the bolus penetrates into the respiratory system. To achieve shallow penetration, the bolus is introduced late in the breath, to achieve deep penetration, it is introduced early. The mode of the bolus is the inspired air volume at which maximum particle number concentration occurs. Volumetric lung depth is the difference between the 1000 cm^3 tidal volume and the mode of the inspired bolus or, in other words, is the air volume which pushes the peak of the bolus into the respiratory system. Fig. 10.2 illustrates the case when an aerosol bolus is penetrating 600 cm^3 into the respiratory tract.

Table 10.1. Information obtained by the aerosol bolus technique

Measured variable	Information
Mode of expired bolus	Bulk gas transport (ventilation)
Half-width of expired bolus	Convective gas mixing
Particle losses in the lungs during breathing	Regional deposition
Particle losses in the lungs during breath holding	Airway caliber
Disappearance of deposited particles from the lungs	Regional clearance
Change of particle size within the lungs	Relative humidity

In the expired air, particles are no longer confined to the small air volume in which they were initially inspired. Rather, they are spread over much larger air volumes, so that an axially dispersed bolus is recovered from the lungs.

The measured variables are the mode and half-width of the expired bolus (Fig. 10.2) as well as particle losses and particle size in the respiratory system. The mode of the expired bolus is the expired air volume at which maximum particle number concentration occurs. The half-width is the air volume in which the particle number concentration exceeds half the maximum concentration. In the case illustrated in Fig. 10.2, the expired bolus is characterized by a mode of 600 cm³ and a half-width of 400 cm³.

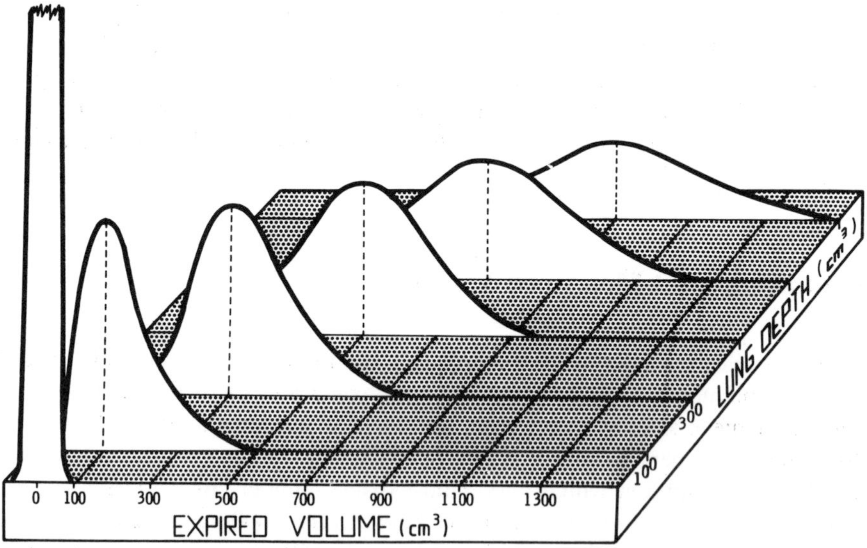

Fig. 10.3. Aerosol bolus dispersion (particle number concentration in expired air) as a function of the volumetric depth to which the bolus penetrates into the respiratory tract.

Information Obtained by the Aerosol Bolus Technique

Table 10.1 summarizes the information obtained by this technique from various measured variables.

Convective Gas Transport

The typical behavior of an aerosol bolus within the respiratory system is illustrated in Fig. 10.3. The mode of the expired bolus is identical with the volumetric depth to which the bolus penetrates into the lungs. In other words, the location of the bolus within the tidal air is usually unaffected by its passage through the respiratory system. However, a bolus undergoes progressively more axial dispersion the deeper it descends into the lungs. Consequently, the lungs fill and empty in a symmetric manner (*bulk gas transport*), but with superimposed asymmetric

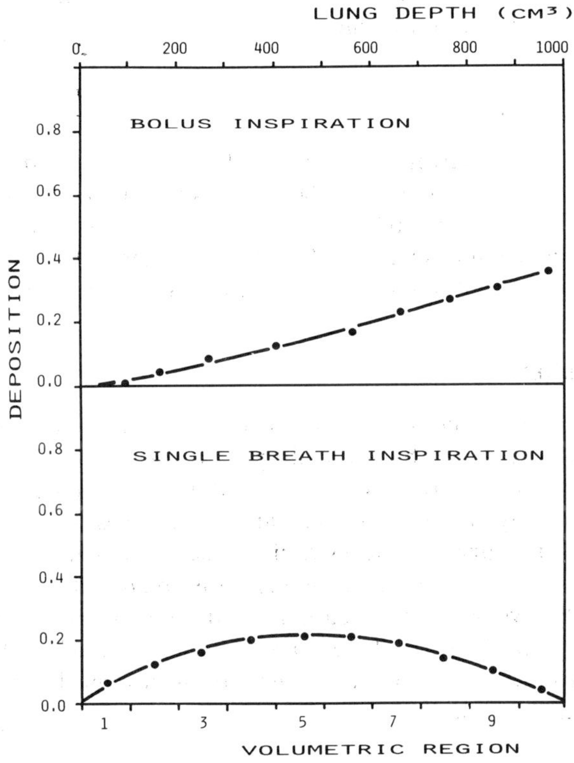

Fig. 10.4. Deposition of particles from aerosol boli inspired to various volumetric depths into the respiratory tract (upper panel); deposition of particles in volumetric regions of the respiratory tract from a single inspiration of 1000 cm^3 tidal volume at a flow rate of 250 cm^3s^{-1} (lower panel).

processes that cause the bolus to disperse (*convective gas mixing*). Usually, the dispersion function (half-width of expired bolus as a function of volumetric lung depth) is a linear function (5).

Particle Deposition

The aerosol bolus technique can also be used to study where particles deposit in the lungs. When the entire tidal air contains particles, dispersion can be neglected for this estimate. That portion of the lungs which is ventilated by the tidal air can be considered as a series of volumetric regions which collect particles. The disappearance of particles from the inspired bolus can then be used to calculate the particle collection efficiencies of these regions and, for a single aerosol inspiration, deposition in these regions (4).

Figure 10.4 shows experimental deposition data for aerosol boli inspired to different depths (upper panel) and calculated deposition data for ten volumetric regions (*regional deposition*) ventilated during a single aerosol inspiration of 1000 cm^3 tidal volume (lower panel).

Particle Clearance

The delivery of radioactively labelled particles by the aerosol bolus technique to a certain volumetric lung region can be used to study particle clearance from this region (*regional clearance*). It has been shown that clearance of nonsoluble particles delivered to the first 100 cm^3 of the respiratory tract exhibits a short-term and a long-term component, both, surprisingly, of about equal magnitude (7).

Airway Caliber

The estimation of airway caliber is based upon the measurement of gravitational losses of particles during breath-holding from aerosol boli in the respiratory tract. Provided that (a) an aerosol bolus is uniformly distributed over a system of identical, randomly oriented cylinders, and (b) particles settle from a monodisperse aerosol onto airway surfaces during breath-holding, then the number of particles expired decreases exponentially with breath-holding time. From the terminal settling velocity of the particles and the exponential loss rate during breath-holding, the diameter of the cylinders (airways) can be calculated. These diameters are in reasonable agreement with those described in current morphometric lung models (3).

Relative Humidity in Airways

Dry, hygroscopic particles delivered by the aerosol bolus technique to the lungs grow in size due to water vapor adsorption while passing through the respiratory system. These changes in particle size can be characterized with the laser

Table 10.2. Means and standard deviations of personal and predicted pulmonary function values

Group	Number of subjects	Age of subjects (years)	Lung function parameter			
			TLC (%)	VC (%)	FEV_1 (%)	R_{aw} $\left[\frac{kPa}{1/s}\right]$
Unexposed asymptomatic subjects	19	42.8±10.3	105±10	117±10	110±10	0.18±0.05
Exposed asymptomatic subjects	15	43.2±12.0	103±11	110±12	100±12	0.24±0.08
Exposed symptomatic subjects	8	48.3± 7.7	100±12	104±11	94± 7	0.25±0.06

TLC, total lung capacity; VC, vital capacity; FEV_1, volume forcefully expired in one second; R_{aw}, airway resistance

aerosol photometer by measuring particle size distribution in inspired and expired air (1).

Particles penetrating to a certain lung depth grow until the water vapor pressure at the particle surface is in equilibrium with that in the surrounding airways. Therefore, at each lung depth particles grow to a certain size which is related to the water vapor pressure or the relative humidity at this site. If particle growth as a function of relative humidity is known, either from model experiments or from theoretical calculations, the particle growth in the lungs can be used to study *relative humidity* in the lungs as a function of volumetric lung depth.

Application of the Aerosol Bolus Technique

As just described, aerosol boli can be used to study convective gas transport, regional particle deposition and clearance, airway dimensions, and relative humidity in the human respiratory tract. All these parameters can also be measured after acute or chronic exposure to air pollutants. The extent to which these parameters are altered by these exposures can then be used as indices in inhalation toxicology.

In a previous study, convective gas transport and airway dimensions have been evaluated in three groups of subjects (2):

Group 1 (normals): 19 subjects without occupational dust exposure and no respiratory symptoms

Group 2 (exposed asymptomatic subjects): 15 subjects with occupational dust exposure but no respiratory symptoms

Group 3 (exposed symptomatic subjects): 8 subjects with occupational dust exposure and respiratory symptoms (cough, wheeze, or phlegm)

Table 10.3. Aerosol-derived parameters of lung structure and lung function

Group	Number of subjects	Airway diameter (mm) at lung depth of 120 cm³	200 cm³	600 cm³	Dispersion function intercept (cm³)	slope
Unexposed asymptomatic subjects	19	1.36±0.32	0.85±0.16	0.40±0.07	139±73	0.42±0.20
Exposed asymptomatic subjects	15	1.20±0.40	0.76±0.14	0.35±0.06	153±86	0.46±0.21
Exposed symptomatic subjects	8	1.09±0.31	0.71±0.19	0.38±0.11	91±92	0.66±0.20

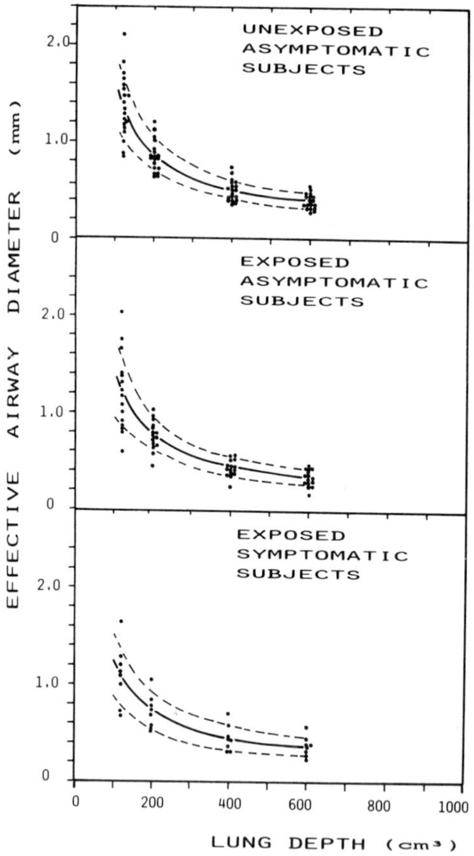

Fig. 10.5. Aerosol-derived airway dimensions as a function of volumetric lung depth in three groups of subjects.

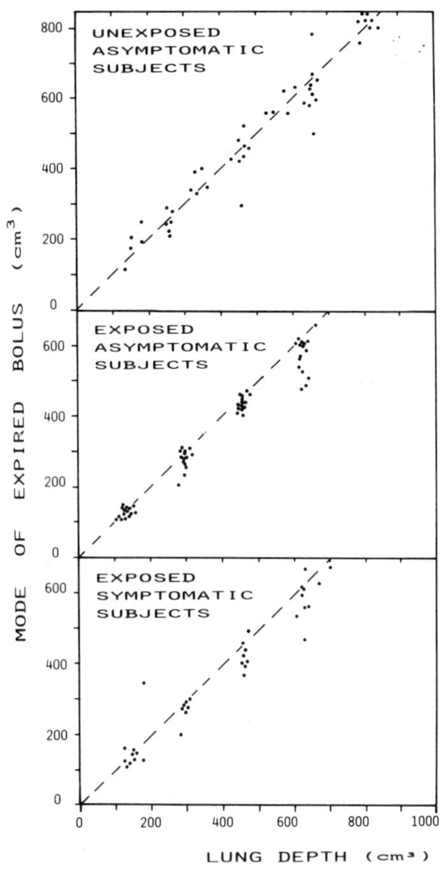

Fig. 10.6. Mode of expired bolus as a function of volumetric lung depth in three groups of subjects.

The exposed subjects were dental technicians exposed to various types of dusts while molding artificial teeth. The means of some personal data and pulmonary function values are listed in Table 10.2.

As a result of a reduced caliber of small airways in exposed symptomatic subjects (Table 10.3, Fig. 10.5), the forced expiratory volume in one second is reduced and airway resistance is increased (Table 10.2). The mode of the expired bolus is little affected by dust exposure (Fig. 10.6). In another (unpublished) study with patients with chronic obstructive pulmonary disease, however, the mode was often dramatically altered, so that inspiration and expiration could no longer be considered as symmetric processes. The first-in-last-out principle was disturbed.

The most significant finding is expressed in Table 10.3 and Fig. 10.7. Although the dispersion function was found to be linear in all subjects, its slope was significantly higher in the group of exposed symptomatic subjects than in the group of normal subjects.

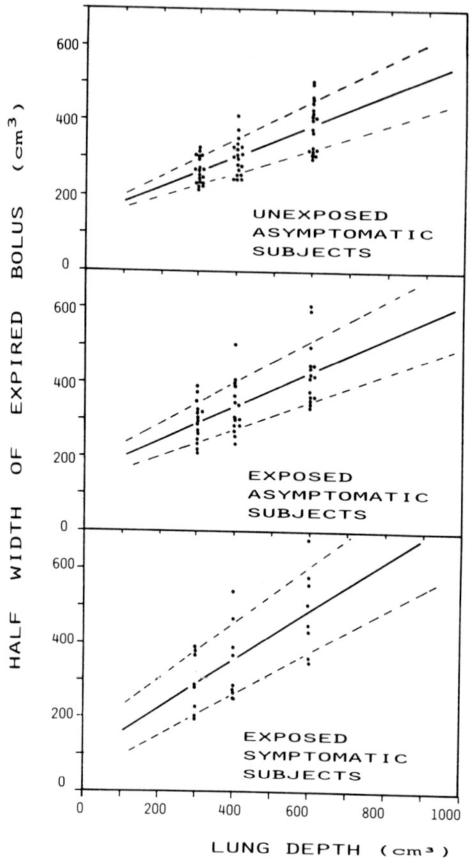

Fig. 10.7. Aerosol dispersion function (half-width of expired aerosol bolus as a function of lung depth) in three groups of subjects.

From the observations on normal subjects, occupational exposed subjects, and patients with chronic obstructive pulmonary disease, the following hypothesis may be put forward: *Progressive alterations in lung function are first expressed as altered convective gas mixing. Later on, altered bulk gas transport is also seen.*

Summary

The aerosol bolus technique is a useful way of relating lung structure to lung function. It is also a promising tool for human air pollution inhalation studies.

References

1. Anselm A, Gebhart J, Heyder J, Ferron G (1986) Human inhalation studies of growth of hygroscopic particles in the respiratory tract. In: Aerosols: Proc. 2nd Int. Aerosol Conf., Berlin. Pergamon, Oxford, p 252

2. Gebhart J, Heyder J, Scheuch G (1983) Nachweis von Funktionsstörungen der Lunge mit Hilfe der Aerosol-Pulstechnik. In: Schütz J (ed) Medizinische Physik. Hüthig, Heidelberg, p 265
3. Heyder J (1983) Charting human thoracic airways by aerosols. Clin Phys Physiol Meas 4:29–37
4. Heyder J, Blanchard JD, Brain JD (1988) Particle deposition in volumetric regions of the human respiratory tract. Ann Occup Hyg (in press)
5. Heyder J, Blanchard JD, Brain JD (1986) Examining convective gas mixing by aerosols. Prog Resp Res 21:111–113
6. Lippmann M (1985) Use of aerosols for measuring airway and airspace size and tracheobronchial mucociliary clearance rate. In: Frank R et al. (eds) Inhalation toxicology of air pollutants: Clinical research considerations, ASTM STP 872. American Society for Testing and Materials, Philadelphia, p 48
7. Stahlhofen W, Gebhart J, Rudolf G, Scheuch G (1986) Clearance from the human airways of particles of different sizes deposited from inhaled aerosol boli. In: Aerosols: Proc. 2nd Int. Aerosol Conf., Berlin. Pergamon, Oxford
8. Utell MJ (1985) Measurements of central and peripheral pulmonary function to assess response to air pollutants: An overview. In: Frank R et al. (eds) Inhalation toxicology of air pollutants: Clinical research considerations, ASTM STP 872. American Society for Testing and Materials, Philadelphia, p 48

CHAPTER 11

Respiratory Tract Clearance of Particles and Substances Dissociated from Particles

R.G. Cuddihy[1] and H.C. Yeh[1]

5719 272

Introduction

This report describes the clearance of particles and substances associated with particles deposited in the respiratory tract. It complements the report by Heyder (this volume) on inhaled particle deposition and the reports by Miller (this volume) and Andersen (1) on the deposition of inhaled reactive and nonreactive gases. Most of the information reported here was derived from studies using human subjects. Results of studies using laboratory animals are also described because some measurements cannot be made using human subjects and because it is necessary to compare respiratory tract clearance in people and animals for the purposes of toxicology and human health risk assessment.

The majority of studies on respiratory tract clearance have been done using inhaled particles containing radionuclides and the reported measurements of retained radioactivity reflect the clearance of both particles and radionuclides that may dissociate from the particles. Such measurements can be used to determine radiation dose to nearby tissues without great concern for chemical interactions between the radionuclides and components of the tissues; only the presence of the radionuclides is important. This type of information is the focus of the 1966 report by the Task Group on Lung Dynamics which was chaired by Morrow (2). Their work has guided much of our current thinking on the mechanisms, pathways, and rates of clearance in different regions of the respiratory tract. Information given in this report builds on the original Task Group work and is derived from the continuing efforts of new Task Groups of the National Council on Radiation Protection and Measurements and the International Commission on Radiological Protection that are updating the current radiation dosimetry models. However, this does not imply that the following material has been reviewed or accepted by the NCRP or ICRP.

---

[1]Inhalation Toxicology Research Institute, Lovelace Biomedical and Environmental Research Institute, P.O. Box 5890, Albuquerque, NM 87185, USA.

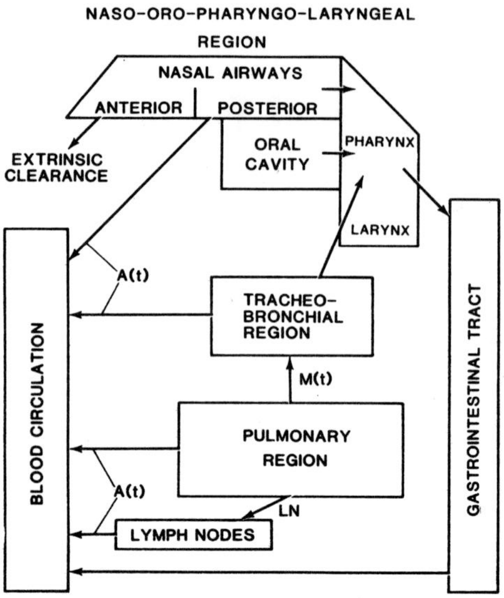

Fig. 11.1. Respiratory tract clearance model. *M(t)*, mucociliary transport; *A(t)*, absorption into the blood circulation; *LN*, clearance to lymph nodes.

A brief discussion of respiratory tract clearance of particles composed of organic compounds and organic compounds associated with inert vector particles is included. These studies also used radioactive labels to trace the organic compounds and the extent to which metabolism influenced clearance of the organic compounds or portions of the compounds is not fully understood. Nonetheless, when chemically toxic substances are inhaled, it should be remembered that the effective dose leading to injury of surrounding tissues may result from not only the inhaled compounds but also metabolic products of the inhaled compounds. Thus, measurements of the clearance of radioactivity from the respiratory tract may not provide all of the pertinent information needed for dosimetry.

Concepts of Respiratory Tract Clearance

The rates and pathways by which deposited substances are cleared from the respiratory tract mainly depend upon their sites of deposition and chemical interactions between the substances and components of the surrounding tissues. As discussed in another report (Heyder, this volume), the sites of deposition are influenced by: (a) aerosol particle size, shape and density, (b) respiratory parameters including breathing frequency, tidal volume, and residual air volume, (c) airway morphology, and (d) breathing mode, whether nasal or oral. Chemical factors that influence the rates of clearance of specific substances include: (a) their physical-chemical form and that of the total particle matrix, (b) their rates of elution from the particle surfaces, (c) particle dissolution, (d) reactions with constituents of lung fluids, especially those influencing dissolution, (e) chemical binding to cellular and extracellular tissue components, and (f) the chemical nature of the toxicant entering the lung fluids, lymph, or plasma. The interactions of these factors are complex, so that predicting inhaled particle deposition and clearance for toxicity evaluations requires extensive information on the specific inhaled material along with model calculations. A biomathematical model of respiratory tract clearance is described here, and some comparisons are made between model predictions and clearance measurements in human subjects.

The respiratory tract clearance model is subdivided into the naso-oro-pharyngo-laryngeal airways, tracheobronchial airways, pulmonary region, and lymph nodes (Fig. 11.1). In all regions, clearance is described in terms of competing mechanical and absorptive processes. Mechanical clearance processes move deposited substances to the oropharynx, where they are swallowed, or to the pulmonary lymph nodes. Absorptive processes transfer substances from the respiratory tract and lymph nodes to the blood circulation. Absorption mainly occurs for substances that dissolve or elute from particle surfaces; however, these substances may still react with tissue constituents and remain in the respiratory tract for a long time. Conversely, a small fraction of the deposited particles may pass into the blood circulation and translocate to other organs or be excreted (3,4). This rarely occurs for particles larger than 0.1 μm in diameter, but may be more common for smaller particles. Thus, absorptive processes represent

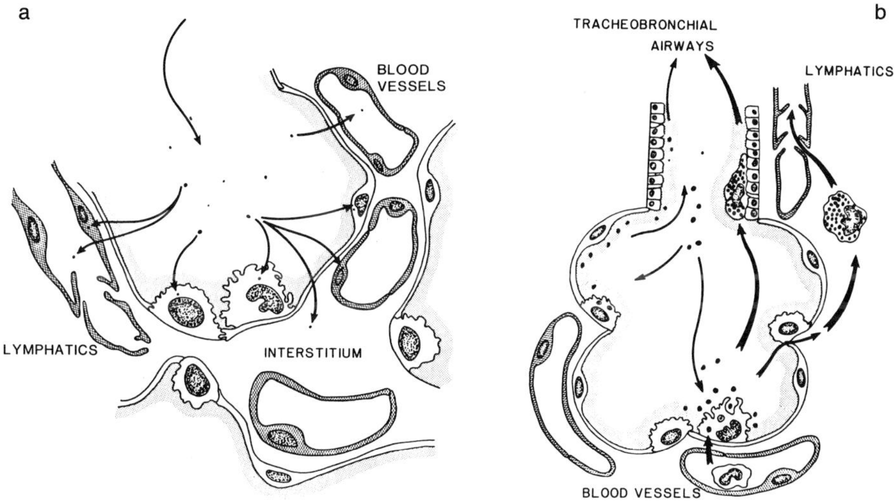

Fig. 11.2. Clearance pathways for particles in the pulmonary region. Particles smaller than one micrometer in diameter are found in virtually all types of cells and may pass into the interstitium and the endothelial cells of vessels without the aid of macrophages (**a**). Larger particles are mainly cleared to the tracheobronchial airways and lymphatics by pulmonary macrophages (**b**).

the net transfer of material from the respiratory tract to blood regardless of the mechanism.

Most of the conducting airway surfaces from the nasal passages through the terminal bronchioles are lined with ciliated epithelium and covered by mucus. Except for the most anterior area in the nose, substances depositing in these airways are effectively moved by mucociliary action toward the oropharynx. The velocity of mucus movement is more rapid in the larger airways and becomes progressively slower in the smaller distal airways. Mucus flow patterns are probably complicated, especially in convoluted airways and near bifurcations; however, simple linear flow in tubes of regular shape is assumed in the following discussions.

In some studies using laboratory animals, a small fraction of the inhaled particles has been shown to be retained in the nasal and tracheobronchial epithelium for several weeks after exposure (5–7). The mechanisms by which particles penetrate into the epithelium are unknown, but they may include pinocytosis by epithelial cells, phagocytosis by macrophages with subsequent translocation into epithelial tissues, passive movement along normal fluid clearance pathways, trapping in areas where clearance mechanisms have been damaged, and others. The importance of such focal accumulations of potentially toxic material in relation to the high average doses to tissues in other areas of the respiratory tract is uncertain. However, tumors of the nasal airways have been observed in some studies of laboratory animals and people who inhaled specific carcinogenic substances (8), and tumors of the central bronchial airways are the most common sites for lung cancer in cigarette smokers (9).

Clearance of particles from the pulmonary region appears to depend on their size, shape, and composition. Deposited particles smaller than one micrometer and down to molecular sizes are found in almost all types of cells (10). They can be taken into cells by phagocytosis, pinocytosis, and endocytosis, and cleared to the lymphatic vessels, tracheobronchial airways, or blood circulation (Fig. 11.2a). Larger particles are mainly taken up by phagocytic cells and cleared to the tracheobronchial airways or lymph vessels (Fig. 11.2b), although soluble material leaving the surfaces of the particles can pass directly into the blood circulation. Most likely, cells phagocytize the particles in the alveolar lumen and move to the tracheobronchial airways or through the epithelium and interstitial spaces to lymphatic vessels (11). Fibers greater than a few micrometers in length that deposit in the pulmonary region are cleared very slowly (12–14). Because they may be too large for cells to ingest and move along the pathways described above, dissolution with absorption into the blood circulation and mechanical penetration of whole fibers toward the lung pleura appear to be the main factors affecting clearance.

Because the state of particles in the pulmonary region changes with time after deposition, their availability for clearance through different pathways also changes. The manner in which these changes occur is difficult to predict and probably depends upon many of the particle characteristics. The fractional clearance rate of deposited material generally decreases with time, making it difficult to use simple first-order kinetic relationships for predicting the lung burdens and doses to tissues at risk for inhaled toxic substances. Thus, the mathematical model discussed below makes use of variable clearance rates that are expressed in terms of the fractions of the remaining tissue burdens cleared per day.

Particle Clearance in the Naso-oro-pharyngo-laryngeal Airways

To describe the clearance of deposited substances, the nasal airways may be divided into the anterior and posterior areas (Fig. 11.3). In the anterior area, clearance is toward the nostrils, and the cleared material may remain in the nasal vestibule for many hours because it is only removed by extrinsic means (15). Substances that deposit in the posterior area of the nasal airways are cleared to the oropharynx where they are rapidly swallowed. Direct absorption of dissolved substances in the anterior area is probably negligible because most of this area is lined with squamous epithelium similar to skin (16). However, absorption from the posterior region to blood can be significant, probably due to its rich vascular perfusion (17,18).

Quantitative measurements of the clearance of inhaled particles in the nasal airways of human subjects were reported by Lippmann (19) and Fry and Black (20). The particles had an aerodynamic diameter of 0.8–10 μm and the subjects breathed normally under resting conditions. In both studies, most of the deposited particles were in the forward portion of the nasal passages. About 40% of the total nasal deposits cleared within 3 h, and thus would be assigned to the posterior area; 60% showed the prolonged retention which is assumed to be associated with the anterior area. Model studies reported by Itoh et al. (21) indicate a shift in deposition toward the posterior nasal area for particles less than 0.5

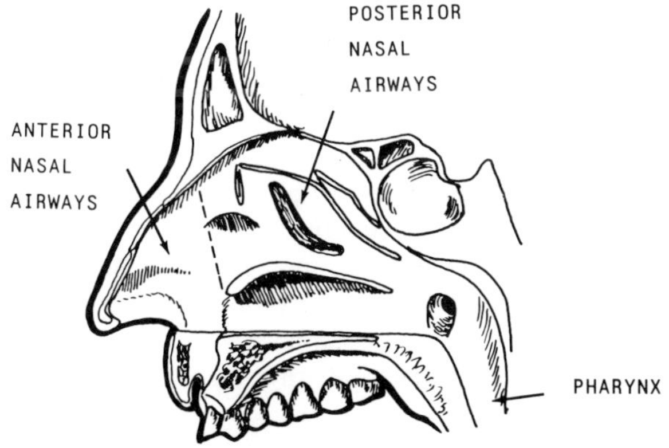

Fig. 11.3. Nasal airways showing the anterior area in which particles are cleared toward the nostrils and the posterior area in which particles are cleared toward the pharynx.

Table 11.1. Measurements of particle clearance velocities in the posterior nasal airways of human subjects

Measurement technique	Particle clearance velocity (mm/min)		Reference
	Mean	Range	
Inert powder	5.0	3–8	22
Inert powder	4.2	1–12	23
^{131}I-labeled albumin	6.0	1–20	15
^{99m}Tc-labeled resin beads	7.0	0–15	24
^{99m}Tc-labeled resin beads	8.4	2–24	25
^{99m}Tc-labeled polystyrene particles	6.8	2–18	26

μm in diameter. For such particles, it is reasonable to assume 50% deposition in each of the anterior and posterior areas.

Mucus flow velocity in the nasal airways has been studied after instilling or inhaling insoluble beads or powders (Table 11.1). Most of these measurements focused on the posterior area beginning just forward of the nasal turbinates. Particle clearance velocities were reported between 0 and 24 mm/min; an average value is 6 mm/min. Because the posterior nasal area is about 6 cm long, the effective retention time for inhaled particles in this area is about 10 min (20).

Particle Clearance in Tracheobronchial Airways

Clearance of insoluble particles deposited in the tracheobronchial region has been studied using fiberoptic bronchoscopy with visible particles, fluoroscopy with radiopaque particles, and external counting with radioactive particles. Fiberoptic bronchoscopes have been used to instill small teflon discs into the lower trachea and to observe their rates of movement along with mucus clearing toward the oropharynx (27,28). A similar technique has been used to instill radiopaque teflon discs into the trachea, but their movement was measured using a fluoroscopic image intensifier (29). The most common technique is to instill or have the subjects inhale radioactive particles and follow the clearance of boli moving up the trachea by external counting using a gamma camera (30,31). All of these studies measured particle clearance velocities in the trachea, but only one study measured velocities in the major bronchi (Table 11.2). Transport rates in medium-size human bronchi have been calculated to be 0.2–1.3 mm/min (32), and those in the most distal ciliated airways were calculated to be 0.001–0.6 mm/min (33–35).

Since direct measurements of mucus flow rates in the distal airways of humans are very difficult to make, the time pattern for clearance of material deposited in the thorax is generally used as an index of clearance function. Measurements of

Table 11.2. Measured clearance velocities for insoluble particles in the trachea and main bronchi of normal humans

Technique	Location	Particle velocity (mm/min)	Reference
Fiberoptic bronchoscopy with teflon discs (both 0.68 mm diam., 0.13 mm thick)	Midtrachea Midtrachea	20.1 21.5	27 28
Fluoroscopy of instilled radiopaque teflon discs (1 mm diam., 0.8 mm thick)	Trachea	5.8–10.1[a]	29
Gamma camera imaging of instilled albumin microspheres (3–7 μm diam.)	Trachea	15.5	30
Gamma camera imaging of inhaled albumin microspheres (1.4 μm diam., 0.5 μm count median diam.)	Trachea	3.6	31
Gamma camera imaging of inhaled ferric oxide (4.13–5.34 μm, aerodynamic diam.)	Trachea Main bronchi	5.5 2.4	32

[a]Higher value for individuals less than 30 years of age; lower value for individuals over 55 years of age.

thoracic clearance of insoluble radioactive particles beginning immediately after inhalation show a rapid clearance phase during the first 20–40 h followed by a prolonged clearance phase lasting hundreds of days (Fig. 11-4). The rapid phase has been attributed to clearance of particles deposited in the tracheobronchial region and the prolonged phase to clearance from the pulmonary region (36–38). In healthy nonsmoking humans, material has been reported to clear from the tracheobronchial region within 24 h (39,40), but the presence of disease or exposure to irritants may depress mucociliary function and extend the time for clearance well beyond 24 h. Other investigators have suggested that bronchial clearance in peripheral airways extends beyond 24 h, even in healthy individuals (41). Svartengren et al. (42) reported a slow phase of clearance for 6-μm teflon particles instilled into the trachea and at the first bifurcation of rabbits; the clearance half-time at the latter site was 39 h.

Effective particle clearance velocities can be estimated for individual bronchial airway generations using information on respiratory tract airway dimensions, inhaled particle deposition fractions for individual airways, and thoracic clearance measurements. The first detailed attempt to estimate effective particle clearance velocities for individual airways was reported by Altshuler et al. (43); this was later extended by Harley and Pasternack (44). These analyses were based upon particle clearance studies reported by Albert and Arnett (45) and on considerations of mucus thickness in the tracheobronchial airways. Using new clear-

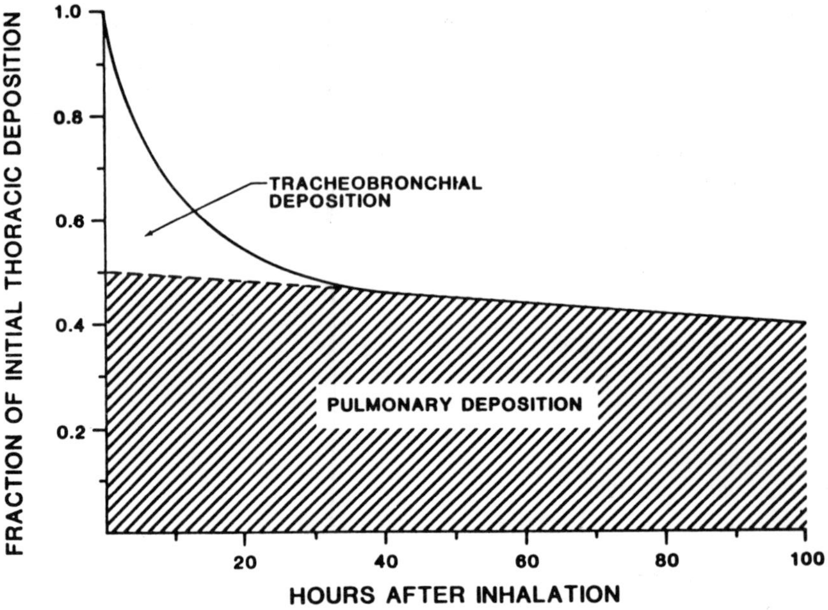

Fig. 11.4. Early thoracic clearance pattern for inhaled insoluble particles and assignment of deposited fractions to the tracheobronchial airways and pulmonary region.

Table 11.3. Effective particle clearance velocities calculated for tracheobronchial airways of the human lung

	Effective clearance velocities (mm/min)		
Airway generation	Harley and Pasternack [44]	Lee et al. [46]	Cuddihy and Yeh (this report)
1 (trachea)	15.0	5.5	5.5
2	8.0	4.1	3.5
3	2.5	3.0	2.0
4	2.5	2.2	1.1
5	0.9	1.4	0.9
6	0.9	0.88	0.9
7	0.9	0.55	0.7
8	0.25	0.34	0.6
9	0.25	0.21	0.4
10	0.25	0.13	0.3
11	0.01	0.074	0.2
12	0.01	0.044	0.1
13	0.01	0.025	0.05
14	0.01	0.015	0.02
15	0.01	0.0082	0.007
16 (terminal bronchioles)	0.01	0.0046	0.001

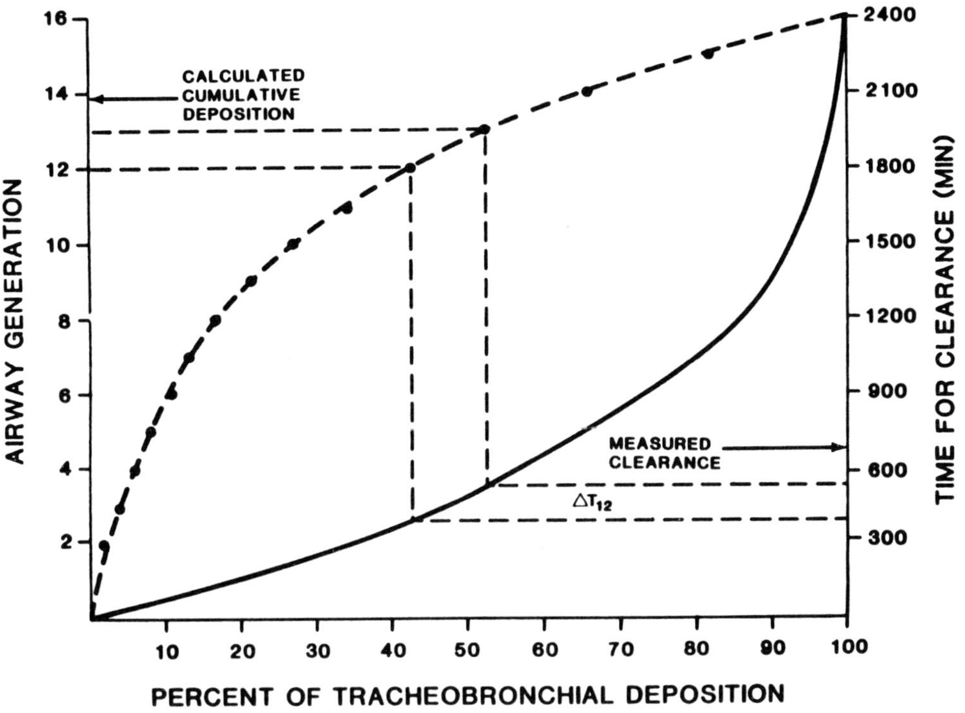

Fig. 11.5. Relationship between the calculated cumulative deposition of inhaled particles in tracheobronchial airway generations (*upper curve*) and time for clearance of the deposited particles (*lower curve*). The method of estimating the time for clearance of each airway generation (ΔT_i) is indicated by the *dashed lines* (generation 12 used as an example).

ance studies with monodisperse aerosols (7.9 μm aerodynamic diameter) and the Weibel A anatomic model, Lee et al. (46) also calculated effective airway particle clearance velocities. The results of these model calculations are summarized in Table 11.3, together with a third set obtained by ourselves from analyses of particle deposition and clearance studies reported by Stahlhofen et al. (47). They used monodisperse aerosols of 1.1–9.5 μm aerodynamic diameter, two different breathing patterns, and three subjects. In these analyses, we first calculated particle deposition for each airway generation using the model of Yeh and Schum (48). The particle size and breathing pattern corresponding to an individual human clearance study was used for these calculations (Fig. 11.5, upper curve). Next, measured clearance in the exposed individual was represented (Fig. 11.5, lower curve). The time for clearance of each airway generation was then calculated (Fig. 11.5, dashed lines). These values were divided by the typical airway lengths reported by Yeh and Schum to obtain effective particle clearance velocities for each airway generation (Fig. 11.6; see also Table 11.3).

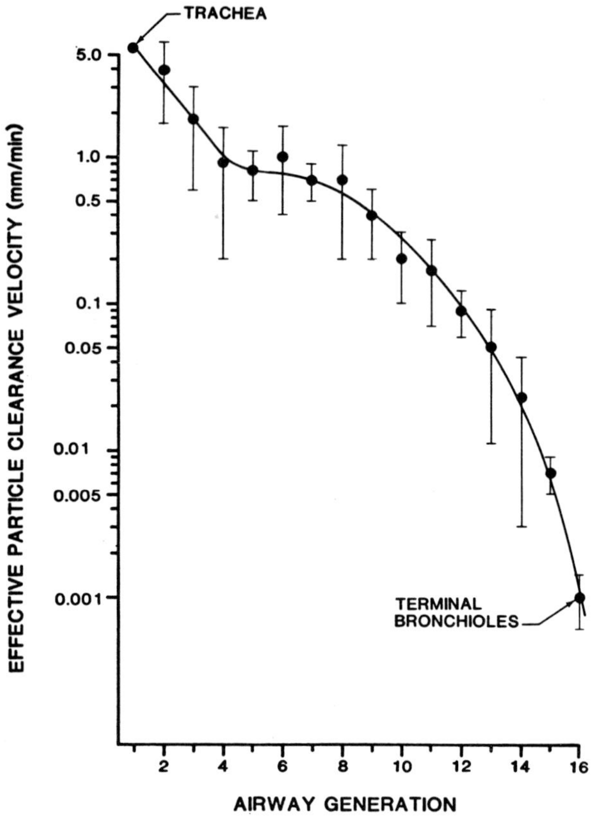

Fig. 11.6. Relationship between effective particle clearance velocity and tracheobronchial airway generation, beginning with the trachea (measured value) and ending with the terminal bronchioles.

Particle Clearance in the Pulmonary Region

Due to the absence of efficient clearance mechanisms, inhaled and deposited particles may remain in the pulmonary region for several hundred days. Thus, the rates at which these particles are cleared to the tracheobronchial airways and gastrointestinal tract must be determined from studies of people who inhaled very insoluble aerosols. To be most useful, the studies should also furnish information on the slow dissolution or absorption of material from the pulmonary region to blood over very long periods of time. This is necessary because the fractional long-term clearance rate for particles in the pulmonary region is only about 1×10^{-3} per day. Thus, dissolution and absorption of respirable-size particles, which generally occur at comparable rates, would introduce considerable uncertainty

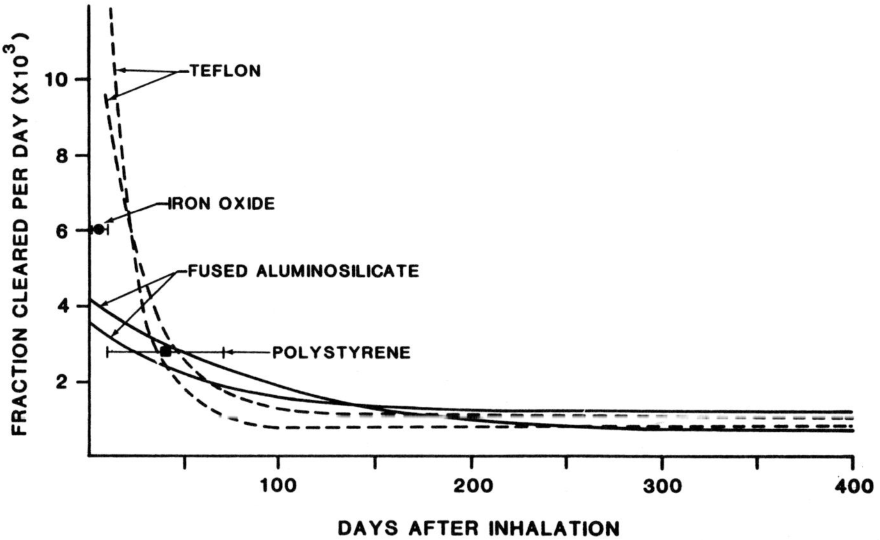

Fig. 11.7. Calculated fractional daily clearance rate, *M(t)*, for the pulmonary region based on experimental measurements using inhaled Teflon (50), iron oxide (47), fused aluminosilicate (51), and polystyrene (52) particles.

in the estimates of particle clearance rates unless information is provided to correct for this effect. Only two studies meet this requirement; Bailey et al. (49) measured the retention of ^{85}Sr- and ^{88}Y-labeled fused aluminosilicate particles in 12 adult men for 372–533 days, and Philipson et al. (50) measured the retention of ^{51}Cr-labeled teflon particles in six adult men for 300 days. In both studies, the long-term rate of dissolution of the radioactive label was similar to the rate of particle clearance; however, measurements of in vitro solubility and urinary excretion were provided so that appropriate corrections could be made in calculating the rates of particle clearance. Other clearance studies in humans can also be used for the early time periods (e.g., less than 100 days), during which particle clearance rates are much higher than rates of absorption of the radioactive label into the blood circulation (47,51,52).

A summary of information on particle clearance rates from the pulmonary region of humans is shown in Fig. 11.7. At early times, the fractional clearance rate is approximately 6×10^{-3}, corresponding to a half-time of 115 days. By 200 days after inhalation exposure, this decreases to a value of about 1×10^{-3}, corresponding to a half-time of 700 days. A mathematical function representing the daily fractional clearance rate for particles in the pulmonary region of people is:

$$M(t) = 0.005\, e^{-0.02t} + 0.001$$

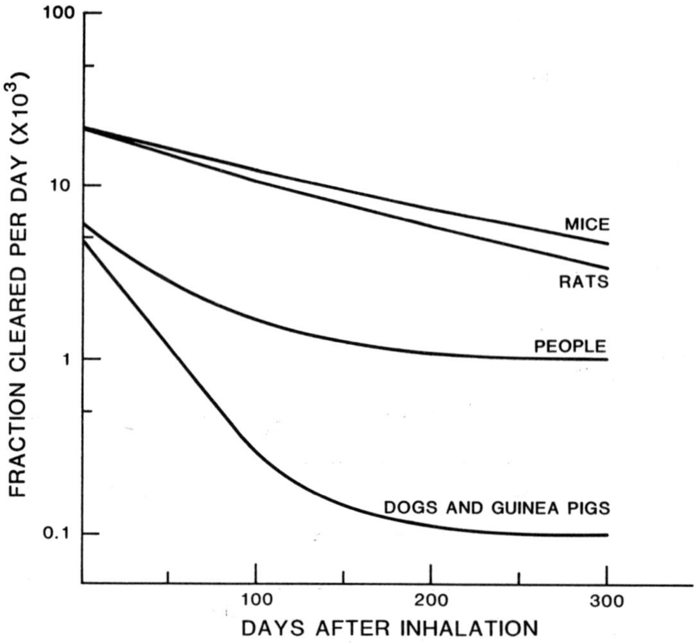

Fig. 11.8. Daily fractional clearance rate, *M(t)*, from the pulmonary region to the tracheobronchial region estimated from laboratory studies using inhaled insoluble particles.

The rates at which insoluble particles are cleared from the pulmonary region varies markedly among different species (53,54). Mathematical functions representing particle clearance to the tracheobronchial airways are compared in Fig. 11.8. Similar aerosols (radiolabeled fused aluminosilicate particles) were used in the studies from which these functions were derived. Clearance in mice and rats is notably faster than that in people, and clearance in guinea pigs and dogs is slower than in people for more than 300 days. The reasons for these differences in particle clearance are not certain, but they may result from species differences in the structures of airways between the terminal bronchioles and alveoli.

The rate of transport of insoluble particles from the pulmonary region to lymph nodes has not been studied quantitatively in people. Thomas suggested that this rate is relatively independent of animal species and derived a value of 1×10^{-4} for the daily fractional transfer rate constant (53). This value is similar to those derived for inhaled niobium oxide in dogs (55) and inhaled fused aluminosilicate particles in dogs and guinea pigs (54). Therefore, 1×10^{-4} may be used to represent a constant daily transfer of particles from the pulmonary region to pulmonary lymph nodes in people.

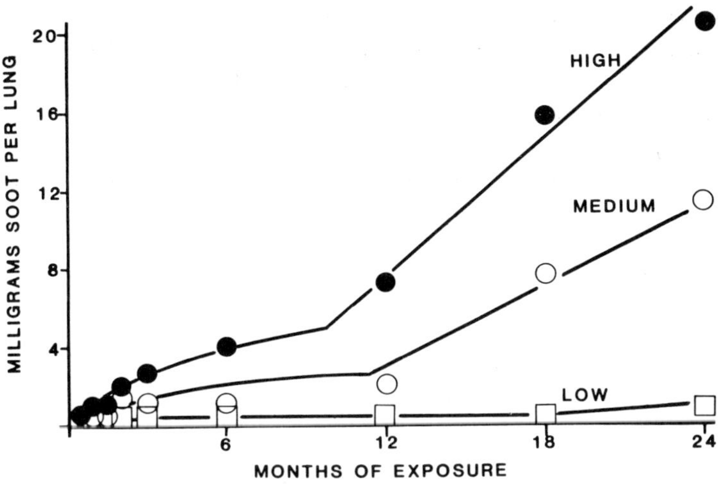

Fig. 11.9. Accumulated lung burdens of diesel engine exhaust particle in the lungs of rats exposed daily to air concentrations of 0.35 (low), 3.5 (medium), and 7 (high) mg/m³. Pulmonary clearance of particles appeared to cease after 12 or 18 months of inhalation exposure.

The clearance studies described above involved total pulmonary depositions of tens to hundreds of micrograms of particles. Other studies oriented toward assessing the toxicity of substances have used much higher aerosol concentrations and resulted in pulmonary burdens exceeding 1 mg/g lung tissue (56–58). In these studies, long-term clearance of particles from the respiratory tract was impaired or nearly ceased after about 12 months of chronic inhalation exposure. This pattern of clearance is illustrated in Fig. 11.9. These measurements were made using rats exposed to whole diesel engine exhaust at particle concentrations of 0.35, 3.5, and 7 mg/m³ for 7 h/day and 5 days/week. Thus, impaired clearance of particles from the respiratory tracts of industrial workers who are exposed to high air concentrations of insoluble dusts is likely to be an important health concern. It is interesting to note that long-term clearance in most cigarette smokers is not impaired to the extent observed in rats exposed to diesel engine exhaust even though smokers may inhale more than 1 g of tar each day (51).

Absorption to the Blood Circulation

Inorganic Cations

The rate at which material deposited in the respiratory tract is absorbed into the blood circulation depends upon many factors, even for particles of similar chemical form. These include particle surface area, chemical structure, previous temperature history, radionuclide specific activity, and probably other unknown factors that are difficult to predict. Mercer suggested that particle dissolution is the major determinant controlling the rate of absorption for material retained in the respiratory tract, and that dissolution rate is proportional to particle surface area (59). This concept would provide an excellent basis for mathematical modeling of lung clearance if (a) all factors controlling particle dissolution were known, (b) sufficient data were available to project dissolution rates for different substances in biological fluids, and (c) dissolution was the only factor controlling absorption of substances from the respiratory tract. To date, scientific information is not available to adequately model these factors. Thus, a more pragmatic approach to predicting absorption is described here that uses experimental observations of clearance rates for specific substances that were inhaled by people or laboratory animals.

For this approach to be successful, it is necessary that systemic absorption rates for material deposited in the respiratory tract be similar among different species, including humans. If different rates exist among species, they are not likely to be detected for highly soluble or insoluble particles. Likewise, the related errors in dosimetry model calculations are not apt to be significant when laboratory-derived absorption rates are used for people. The greatest difficulties arise with inhaled particles that have intermediate rates of dissolution and when projecting absorption of substances incorporated into particles having a mixed chemical composition.

Experimental measurements of cerium absorption from the lungs of dogs, mice, rats, and hamsters that inhaled either aerosols of cerium chloride or cerium oxalate have been reported to be similar (60). Also, absorption rates for cesium incorporated into fused aluminosilicate particles and deposited in the lungs of dogs, guinea pigs, rats, and mice were reported to be independent of species (61). The most extensive interspecies comparison to test this hypothesis is currently under way and is using cobalt oxide aerosols inhaled by rats, mice, dogs, baboons, and people (62). The early results indicate that absorption rates for cobalt are similar in rats and mice, about twice as fast in dogs, and one-half as fast in baboons. It will be possible to determine how humans compare with other species when these studies are complete.

At present, several hundred radionuclide inhalation studies are available in the scientific literature and they deal with a large portion of the most important or probable types of worker exposures. Absorption rate functions can be derived from these studies in the manner discussed below. Ideal studies for this purpose provide information on radionuclide contents of the head airways, lungs (including the trachea and bronchi), gastrointestinal tract, internal organs, and excreta as a function of time after inhalation exposure. Measurements should also be provided for absorption in the gastrointestinal tract and endogenous fecal excretion of material after absorption into the blood circulation. Because few studies report such complete kinetic information for inhaled aerosols, values for some model parameters must be assumed or estimated from separate studies using the

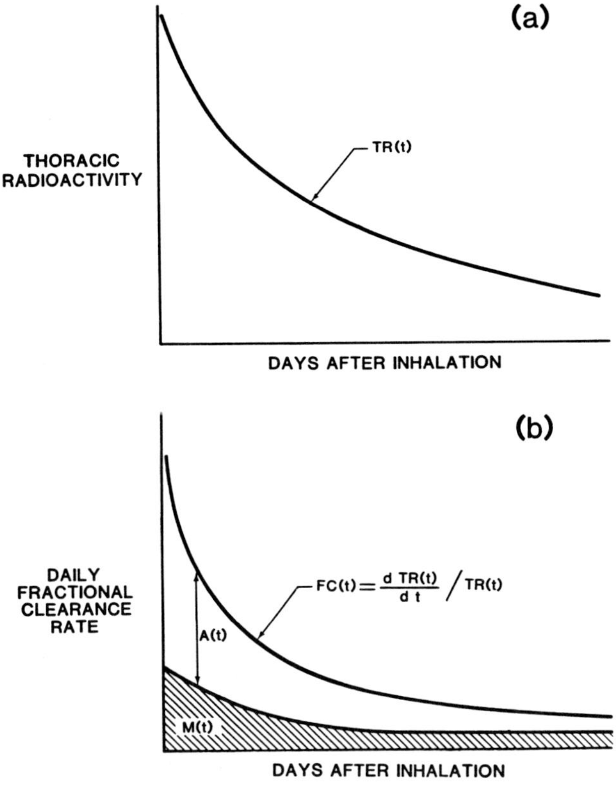

Fig. 11.10a,b. Method for estimating the absorption rate function, *A(t)*, using **a** measurements of thoracic radioactivity, *TR(t)*, over long periods of time, and **b** the derivative of *TR(t)* expressed as a fraction of the remaining radioactivity.

same or similar radionuclides and chemical forms. This problem is likely never to be completely resolved.

For radioactive particles, the most important measurements used in respiratory tract dosimetry modeling are of thoracic radioactivity as a function of time after inhalation exposure, *TR(t)*. This generally includes radioactivity in the tracheobronchial airways, pulmonary region, and lymph nodes. The decrease in thoracic radioactivity results from (a) clearance of material up the conducting airways to the oropharynx, (b) absorption into the blood circulation, and (c) radioactive decay. After correcting for radioactive decay, mathematical functions are fit to the measurements of thoracic radioactivity and the derivatives of the functions are obtained. The overall daily fractional clearance rate, *FC(t)*, can then be calculated:

$$FC(t) = \frac{d\,TR(t)}{dt} \quad TR(t)$$

This process is illustrated in Fig. 11.10.

For modeling purposes, the total daily fractional clearance rate for the thorax is composed of clearance rates to the gastrointestinal tract, $M(t)$ as given above, and to the blood circulation, $A(t)$:

$$FC(t) = A(t) + M(t)$$

In using this relationship to calculate $A(t)$, it is assumed that (a) the rate of absorption or clearance to the blood circulation is similar for all material retained in the thorax (including that in the pulmonary region, tracheobronchial region, and lymph nodes), and *(b)* $A(t)$ is independent of species, so that absorption rates calculated from studies in laboratory animals can be directly applied to model calculations for people.

To ascertain whether the derived function for absorption of radioactivity into the blood circulation is reasonable, further evaluation using information on radionuclide uptake by internal body organs and excreta is useful. The amount of radionuclide absorbed from the respiratory tract into the blood circulation, $(\mathrm{ABS}_{RT})_t$, between the exposure and time, t, is calculated from the expression:

$$(\mathrm{ABS}_{RT})_t = \Sigma \text{ (internal organ burdens)}_t + \Sigma_t \text{ (urine + endo. feces)} - \text{gastrointestinal absorption}$$

Here, radioactivity is summed for all internal organs (except the respiratory tract and gastrointestinal tract) at time, t, and for urinary and endogenous fecal excretion from exposure to time, t. The amount of radioactivity absorbed from the gastrointestinal tract is deducted from the sums. The amount of radioactivity absorbed from the respiratory tract should also be equal to the integrated product of the fractional absorption rate and amount of radioactivity remaining in the respiratory tract;

$$(\mathrm{ABS}_{RT})_t = \int_0^t A(t)\,[TR(t) + HR(t)]dt$$

where $HR(t)$ is the amount of radioactivity retained in the head airways. This application of radionuclide kinetic information is illustrated in Fig. 11.11.

Organic Compounds

Compared to the abundance of quantitative information available on absorption of inorganic cations from the respiratory tract to blood, much less is known about absorption of organic compounds. This imbalance is probably due to the relative ease with which radioactive elements can be measured in biological samples compared to the more difficult chemical analysis that may be necessary to quantify the kinetic behavior of inhaled organic compounds and their metabolic products. Also, most of the available information on organic compounds relates to individual gases or vapors encountered in work environments; less information is available for complex mixtures of chemicals inhaled as droplets or particles. However, the chemical forms of the deposited organic compounds and the sites of deposition probably determine their rates of absorption and the fractions

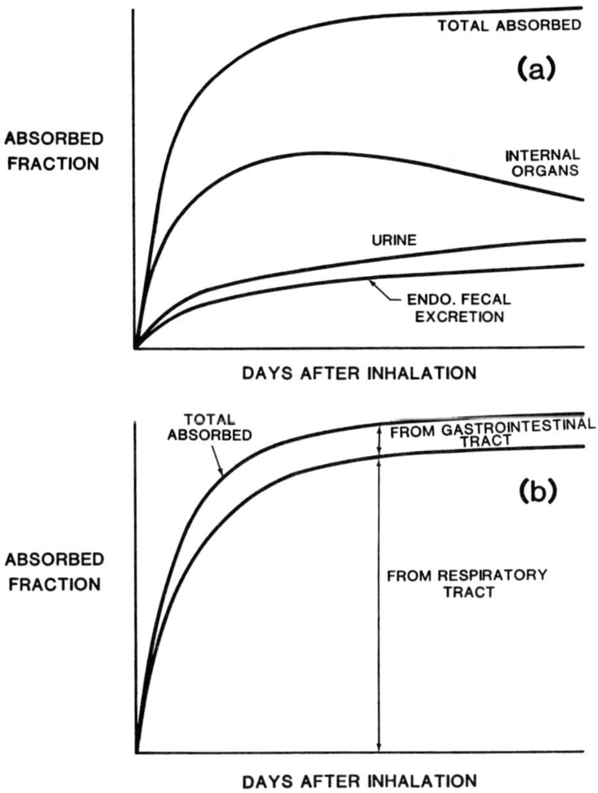

Fig. 11.11a,b. Method for estimating the amount of an inhaled substance absorbed from the respiratory tract using (**a**) measurements of the cumulative urine and endogenous fecal excretion and internal organ contents, and (**b**) calculated absorption of the substance in the gastrointestinal tract.

absorbed into the blood circulation in a similar manner as discussed above for inorganic cations.

Bond et al. compared the rates at which several different organic compounds were cleared from the lungs of rats after being inhaled in different chemical forms (63). A summary of measurements for benzo[*a*]pyrene (BaP) is shown in Fig. 11.12. The aerosols were composed of pure BaP and BaP associated carbonaceous diesel exhaust particles, organic coal tar particles, and inorganic gallium oxide particles. Although it is not possible to determine what fractions of the BaP were absorbed directly into the blood circulation in all cases, most likely its association with diesel particles markedly reduced the rate of absorption. Similar results were reported for inhaled nitropyrene.

One additional factor that has been related to the rate at which organic compounds are cleared from the lung is their lipophilicity (64–66). This has been measured using the octanol/water partition coefficient and related to the half-

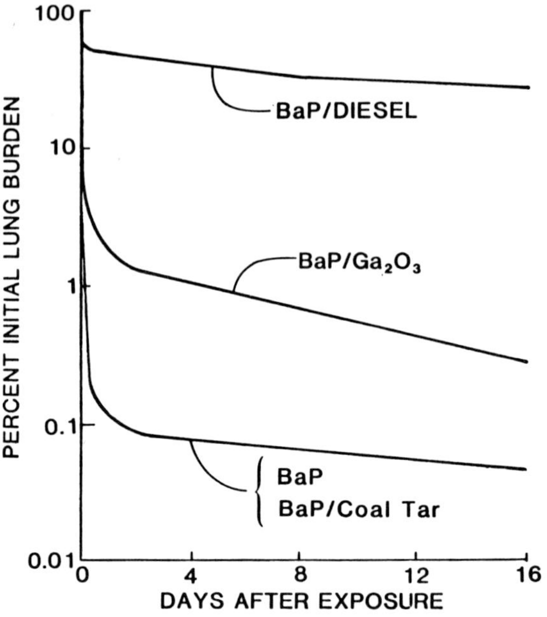

Fig. 11.12. Clearance of radiolabeled BaP from the lungs of rats that received a single inhalation exposure to BaP alone and BaP associated with particles of diesel engine exhaust, gallium oxide, and coal tar. Reprinted with permission from ref 63.

time of the long-term component of the lung retention function. Results of studies reported to date indicate that more lipophilic compounds are more slowly absorbed from the pulmonary region to blood.

Much additional work is needed before quantitative models can be developed to predict respiratory tract clearance of inhaled organic compounds. The experience developed in performing kinetic studies with radioactive inorganic cations can provide a useful framework for designing the necessary quantitative studies. These studies should attempt to measure the rates of absorption of the inhaled compounds from all regions of the respiratory tract and gastrointestinal tract, organ uptake and metabolism, and all pathways for excretion.

Comparison of Clearance Model Projections with Experimental Measurements

The mathematical model of respiratory tract deposition and clearance (see Fig. 11.1) was formulated by combining particle deposition calculations described by Yeh and Schum (48) with tracheobronchial clearance as represented by a series of 16 airway generations (effective particle clearance velocities summarized in Table 11.2), and pulmonary clearance as represented by the daily fractional rate

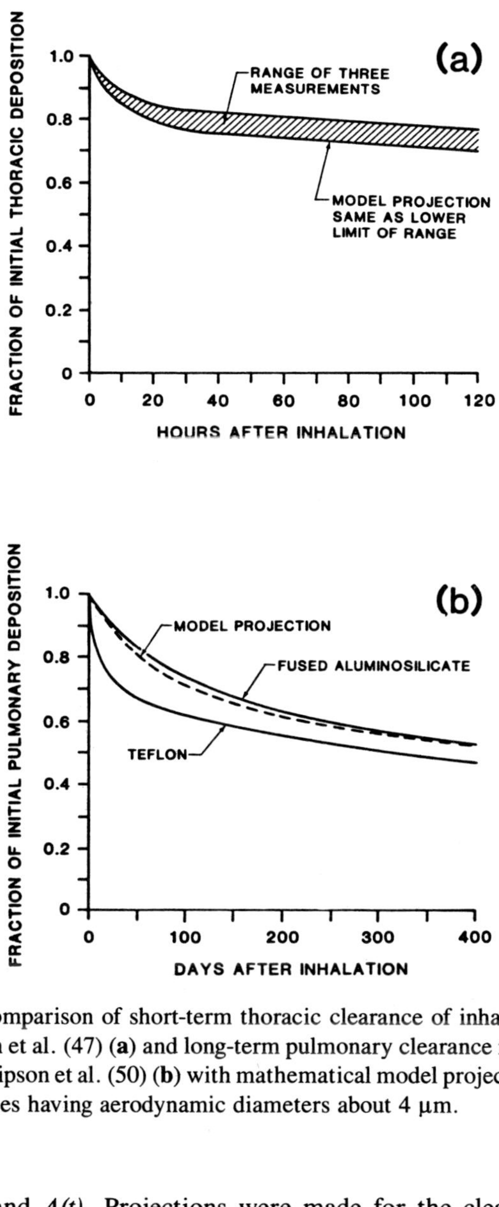

Fig. 11.13a,b. Comparison of short-term thoracic clearance of inhaled particles measured by Stahlhofen et al. (47) (**a**) and long-term pulmonary clearance measured by Bailey et al. (49) and Philipson et al. (50) (**b**) with mathematical model projections. All measurements used particles having aerodynamic diameters about 4 μm.

functions *M(t)* and *A(t)*. Projections were made for the clearance of inhaled insoluble particles having an aerodynamic diameter of 4 μm, and inhaled with a tidal volume of 1000 cm^3 and frequency of 7.5 per minute. The results are compared with short-term clearance measurements in three subjects reported by Stahlhofen et al. (47) and long-term clearance measurements reported by Bailey et al. (49) and Philipson et al. (50). These are shown in Figure 11.13.

In general, there is a good agreement between the model projections and experimental measurements. However, this is not surprising since these and

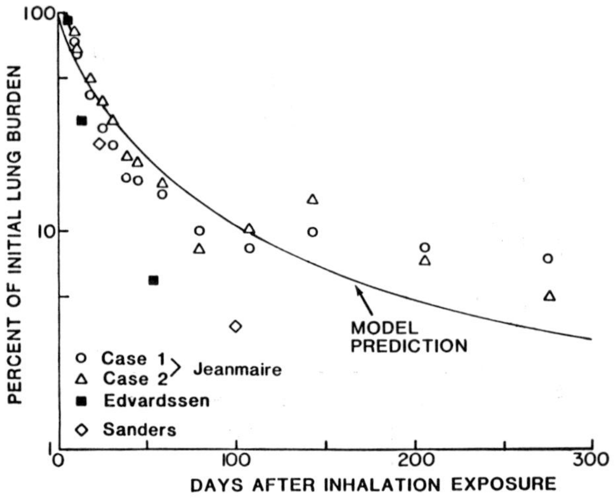

Fig. 11.14. Measured thoracic clearance of americium oxide in people compared with clearance model prediction. Reprinted with permission from ref 67. Copyright 1982, Pergamon Journals, Ltd.

other similar measurements formed the basis for the model formulation. The composite deposition and clearance model tended to produce an overestimation of the amount of early clearance of inhaled particles having less than 7 μm aerodynamic diameter and an underestimation of the amount of early clearance for larger particle sizes. Long-term clearance projected by the model was corrected for dissolution and absorption of the radioactive label, which accounted for 20%–30% of the daily fractional clearance beyond 200 days after inhalation.

Finally, model projections were made for respiratory tract clearance of AmO_2 inhaled by people. When inhaled in the oxide form, americium is slowly absorbed into the blood circulation and mainly transfers to bone and liver or is excreted in urine. Several sets of data obtained from studies of accidental human exposures were summarized by Mewhinney and Griffith (67) and are shown in Fig. 11.14. Thoracic retention is expressed as a percentage of the measured or calculated burden at 4 days after inhalation. The model projection used a fractional daily absorption rate expressed by the function:

$$A(t) = 0.03e^{-0.016t} + 0.0014$$

This was derived from the results of inhalation studies using dogs. All other parameters used in the model projection are described above. The good agreement between model calculations and measurements of clearance in humans supports the use of absorption rate information derived from studies with laboratory animals.

Although the model described above was mainly based upon studies using radioactive cations, many of its features apply equally well to projecting clearance of a variety of inhaled chemical substances. Unless chemical toxicity or mass loading alters the clearance mechanisms, virtually all respirable-size particles should be cleared in a similar manner. Dissociation of more complex chemical compounds from particles will likewise control their absorption into the blood circulation and this may be determined from studies using laboratory animals. However, the chemical changes induced by metabolism and the importance of these changes in estimating dose to target tissues are unique to each type of inhaled substance. These factors are beyond the scope of the model calculations described here, but they must be taken into account when estimating chemical dose.

Summary

Relationships between exposure air concentrations of toxic substances and the probability of inducing biological effects can vary greatly depending upon the physical-chemical characteristics of the inhaled aerosols, the species of laboratory animal studied, and the mode of exposure. Thus, further information is needed when using the results of laboratory toxicology studies in human health risk assessments. By modeling the kinetics of deposition and retention of inhaled toxic substances, a unique understanding of dose to tissues at risk is developed, and this is a necessary step in the risk assessment process. Modeling also provides a basis for designing experiments and hypothesis testing by toxicologists. In addition, kinetic models are now being used as a basis for developing standards for controlling exposures to radioactive aerosols (68). However, much more effort is needed before regulations to control exposures to chemically toxic substances can be placed on a similar quantitative basis.

For radioactive particles, dose is proportional to the product of time and concentration in the tissues at risk; for chemically toxic particles, the appropriate expression of dose is more difficult to define. The effective chemical dose may be proportional to the time averaged or integrated concentration of the substance, metabolic products of the substance, or chemically bound moieties such as DNA adducts. It may also be crucial to know dose rate over short periods of time. However, in all of these cases, kinetic models are an asset, if not a necessity, to the dosimetry process.

Acknowledgments. This work was supported by the US Department of Energy, Office of Health and Environmental Research, under contract no. DE-AC04-76EV01013. The authors gratefully acknowledge the suggestions of many members of the National Council on Radiation Protection and Measurement Task Group on Respiratory Tract Dosimetry Modeling, including Drs. Robert Phalen, Owen Moss, Gerald Fisher, David Swift, and Richard Schlesinger, and members of the staff of the Inhalation Toxicology Research Institute, including Drs. Patrick Haley, Michele Medinsky, James Bond, Roger McClellan, and Bruce Boecker.

References

1. Andersen ME (1987) Toxicokinetics of non-reactive gases. Paper delivered at an international symposium on inhalation toxicology, the design and interpretation of inhalation studies and their use in risk assessment, held in Hanover, Federal Republic of Germany, March 1987
2. Task Group on Lung Dynamics (1966) Deposition and retention models for internal dosimetry of the human respiratory tract. Health Phys 12:173–207
3. Stradling GN, Ham GJ, Smith H, Cooper J, Breadmore SE (1978) Factors affecting the mobility of plutonium-238 dioxide in the rat. Int J Radiat Biol 34:37–47
4. Gearhart JM, Diel JH, McClellan RO (1980) Intrahepatic distribution of plutonium in beagles. Radiat Res 84:343–352
5. Gore DM, Patrick G (1978) The distribution and clearance of inhaled UO_2 particles on the first bifurcation and trachea of rats. Phys Med Biol 23:730–737
6. Watson MS, Brain SD (1979) Uptake of iron oxide aerosols by mouse airway epithelium. Lab Invest 40:450–459
7. Benjamin SA, Boecker BB, Cuddihy RG, McClellan RO (1979) Nasal carcinomas in beagles after inhalation of relatively soluble forms of beta-emitting radionuclides. J Nat Cancer Inst 63:133–139
8. Boecker BB, Hahn FF, Cuddihy RG, Snipes MB, McClellan RO (1986) Is the human nasal cavity at risk from inhaled radionuclides? In: Thompson RC, Mahaffey JA (eds) Life-span radiation effects studies in animals: What can they tell us? pp 564–577 Published by; Office of Scientific and Technical Information; United States Department of Energy
9. Schlesinger RB, Lippmann M (1978) Selective particle deposition and bronchogenic carcinoma. Environ Res 15:424–431
10. Lauweryns JM, Baert JH (1977) Alveolar clearance and the role of the pulmonary lymphatics. Am Rev Respir Dis 115:625–683
11. Harmsen AG, Muggenburg BA, Snipes MB, Bice DE (1985) The role of macrophages in particle translocation from lungs to lymph nodes. Science 230:1277–1280
12. Vincent JH, Johnston AM, Jones AD, Balton RE, Addison J (1985) Kinetics of deposition and clearance of inhaled mineral dusts during chronic exposure. Br J Ind Med 42:707–715
13. Morgan A, Holmes A, Davison W (1982) Clearance of sized glass fibres from the rat lung and their solubility in vivo. Ann Occup Hyg 25:317–331
14. Roggli VL, George MH, Brody AR (1987) Clearance and dimensional changes of crocidolite asbestos fibers isolated from the lungs of rats following short-term exposure. Environ Res 42:94–105
15. Proctor DF, Andersen I, Lundquist G (1977) Nasal mucociliary function in humans. In: Brain JD, Proctor DF, Reid LM (eds) Respiratory defense mechanisms, part 1. Dekker, New York, pp 427–452
16. Swift DL, Proctor DF (1977) Access of air to the respiratory tract. In: Brain JD, Proctor DF, Reid LM (eds) Respiratory defense mechanisms, part 1. Dekker, New York, pp. 63–93
17. Cuddihy RG, Ozog JA (1973) Nasal absorption of CsCl, $SrCl_2$, $BaCl_2$ and $CeCl_3$ in Syrian hamsters. Health Phys 29:219–224
18. Stather JW, Howden S (1975) The effect of chemical form on the clearance of 239-plutonium from the respiratory system of the rat. Health Phys 28:29–39

19. Lippmann M (1970) Deposition and clearance of inhaled particles in the human nose. Ann Otol Rhinol Larygnol 76:519–528
20. Fry FA, Black A (1973) Regional deposition and clearance of particles in the human nose. J Aerosol Sci 4:113–124
21. Itoh H, Smaldone GC, Swift DL, Wagner HN (1985) Mechanisms of aerosol deposition in a nasal model. J Aerosol Sci 16:529–534
22. van Ree JHL, van Dishoeck HAE (1962) Some investigations on nasal ciliary activity. Pract Ororhinolaryngol 24:383–390
23. Ewert G (1965) On the mucus flow rate in the human nose. Acta Otolaryngol [Suppl] (Stockh) 200:1–62
24. Quinlan MF, Salmon SD, Swift DL, Wagner HN, Proctor DF (1969) Measurement of mucociliary function in man. Am Rev Respir Dis 99:13–23
25. Andersen I, Lundqvist GR, Proctor DF (1971) Human nasal mucosal function in a controlled climate. Arch Environ Health 23:408–420
26. Black A, Evans JC, Hadfield EH, Macbeth RG, Morgan A, Walsh M (1974) Impairment of nasal mucociliary clearance in woodworkers in the furniture industry. Br J Ind Med 31:10–17
27. Wood RE, Wanner A, Hirsch J, Farrell PM (1975) Tracheal mucociliary transport in patients with cystic fibrosis and its stimulation by terbutaline. Am Rev Respir Dis 111:733–738
28. Santa Cruz R, Landa J, Hirsch J, Sackner MA (1974) Tracheal mucus velocity in normal man and patients with obstructive lung disease; effects of terbutaline. Am Rev Respir Dis 109:458–463
29. Goodman RM, Yergin BM, Landa JF, Golinvaux MH, Sachner MA (1978) Relationship of smoking history and pulmonary function tests to tracheal mucus velocity in nonsmokers, young smokers, ex-smokers and patients with chronic bronchitis. Am Rev Respir Dis 117:205–214
30. Chopra SK, Taplin GV, Elam D, Carson SA, Golde D (1979) Measurement of tracheal mucociliary transport velocity in humans – smokers versus nonsmokers (preliminary findings). Am Rev Respir Dis 119:205
31. Yeates DB, Aspin M, Levison H, Jones MT, Bryan AC (1975) Mucociliary tracheal transport rates in man. J Appl Physiol 39:487–495
32. Foster WM, Langenback EG, Bergofsky EH (1982) Lung mucociliary function in man: Interdependence of bronchial and tracheal mucus transport velocities with lung clearance in bronchial asthma and healthy subjects. Ann Occup Hyg 26:227–244
33. Yeates DB, Aspin M (1978) A mathematical description of the airways of the human lungs. Respir Physiol 32:92–104
34. Morrow PE, Gibb FR, Gazioglu KM (1967) A study of particulate clearance from the human lungs. Am Rev Respir Dis 96:1209–1221
35. Yeates DB (1974) The clearance of soluble and particulate aerosols deposited in the human lung. Doctoral thesis, University of Toronto
36. Bair WJ, Willard H (1963) Plutonium inhalation studies. III. Effect of particle size and total dose on deposition, retention and translocation. Health Phys 9:253–266
37. Hatch TF, Gross P (1964) Pulmonary deposition and retention of inhaled aerosols. Academic, New York
38. Lippmann M, Albert R (1969) The effect of particle size on the regional deposition of inhaled aerosols in the human respiratory tract. Am Ind Hyg Assoc J 30:257–275
39. Albert RE, Lippmann M, Briscoe W (1969) The characteristics of bronchial clearance in humans and the effect of cigarette smoking. Arch Environ Health 18:738–755

40. Camner P, Philipson K (1978) Human alveolar deposition of 4 μm teflon particles. Arch Environ Health 36:181–185
41. Clarke SW, Parvia D (1980) Lung mucus production and mucociliary clearance: Methods of assessment. Br J Clin Pharmacol 9:537–546
42. Svartengren M, Widtskiold-Olsson K, Philipson K, Camner P (1981) Retention of particles on the first bifurcation and the trachea of rabbits. Bull Eur Physiopathol Respir 17:87–91
43. Altshuler B, Nelson N, Kuschner M (1964) Estimation of lung tissue dose from the inhalation of radon and daughters. Health Phys 10:1137–1161
44. Harley NH, Pasternack BS (1972) Experimental absorption measurements applied to lung dose from radon daughters. Health Phys 23:771–782
45. Albert RE, Arnett LC (1955) Clearance of radioactive dust from the human lung. AMA Arch Ind Health 12:99–106
46. Lee PS, Gerrity TR, Hass FJ, Lourenco RV (1979) A model for tracheobronchial clearance of inhaled particles in man and a comparison with data. IEEE Trans Biomed Eng BME-26, 11:624–630
47. Stahlhofen W, Gebhart J, Heyder J (1980) Experimental determination of the regional deposition of aerosol particles in the human respiratory tract. Am Ind Hyg Assoc J 41:385–398
48. Yeh HC, Schum GM (1980) Models of human lung airways and their application to inhaled particle deposition. Bull Math Biol 42:461–480
49. Bailey MR, Fry FA, James AC (1985) Long-term retention of particles in the human respiratory tract. J Aerosol Sci 16:295–305
50. Philipson K, Falk R, Camner P (1985) Long-term lung clearance in humans studied with teflon particles labeled with chromium-51. Exp Lung Res 9:31–42
51. Bohning DE, Atkins HL, Cohn SH (1982) Long-term particle clearance in man: Normal and impaired. Ann Occup Hyg 26:259–271
52. Newton D, Fry FA, Taylor BT, Eagle MC, Sharma RC (1978) Interlaboratory comparison of techniques for measuring lung burdens of low-energy photon-emitters. Health Phys 35:751–771
53. Thomas RG (1972) An interspecies model for retention of inhaled particles. In: Mercer TT, Morrow PE, Stöber W (eds) Assessment of airborne particulates. Thomas, Springfield, pp 405–419
54. Snipes MB, Boecker BB, McClellan RO (1984) Respiratory tract clearance of inhaled particles in laboratory animals. In: Smith H, Gerber G (eds) Lung modeling for inhalation of radioactive materials, pp 63–71
55. Cuddihy RG (1978) Deposition and retention of inhaled niobium in beagle dogs. Health Phys 34:167–176
56. Strom KA, Chan TL, Johnson JT (1985) Pulmonary retention of inhaled submicron particles in rats: Diesel exhaust exposures and lung retention model. Inhaled Particles VI, proceedings of an international symposium organized by the British Occupational Hygiene Society held in Cambridge, England, September 1985
57. Vostal JJ, Schreck RM, Lee PS, Chan TL, Soderholm SC (1982) Deposition and clearance of diesel particles from the lung. In: Lewtas J (ed) Toxicology of diesel exhaust emissions. Elsevier Biomedical, New York, pp 143–159
58. Wolff RK, Henderson RF, Snipes MB, Griffith WC, Mauderly JL, Cuddihy RG, McClellan RO (1987) Alterations in particle accumulation and clearance in lungs of rats chronically exposed to diesel exhaust. Fundam Appl Toxicol 9:154–166

59. Mercer TT (1967) On the role of particle size in the dissolution of lung burdens. Health Phys 13:1211–1221
60. Cuddihy RG, Boecker BB, Griffith WC (1979) Modeling the deposition and clearance of inhaled radionuclides. In: Proceedings of an international symposium on biological implications of radionuclides released from nuclear industries, 26–30 March 1979, Vienna. International Atomic Energy Agency, pp 77–90
61. Snipes MB, Boecker BB, McClellan RO (1983) Retention of monodisperse or polydisperse aluminosilicate particles inhaled by dogs, rats and mice. Toxicol Appl Pharmacol 26:264–273
62. Bailey MR, Kreyling WG, Andre S, Batchelor A, Black A, Collier CG, Drosselmeyer E, Ferron GA, Foster P, Haider B, Hodgson A, Metivier H, Moores SR, Morgan A, Muller HL, Patrick G, Pearman I, Pickering S, Ramsden D, Stirling C, Talbot RG (1985) EULEP interspecies comparison of the lung clearance of inhaled cobalt oxide particles: interim summary of the results. Inhaled Particles VI, proceedings of an international symposium organized by the British Occupational Hygiene Society, Cambridge, England, September 1985
63. Bond JA, Sun JD, Mitchell CE, Dutcher JS, Wolff RK, McClellan RO (1986) Biological fate of inhaled organic compounds associated with particulate matter. In: Lee SD, Schneider T, Grant LD, Verkerk PJ (eds) Aerosols: Research, risk assessment and control strategies, Lewis, Chelsea, Michigan, pp 579–592
64. Bond JA, Baker SM, Bechtold WE (1985) Correlation of the octanol/water partition with clearance half-times of intratracheally instilled aromatic hydrocarbons in rats. Toxicology 36:285–295
65. Medinsky MA, Cheng YS, Kampcik SJ, Henderson RF, Dutcher JS (1986) Disposition and metabolism of ^{14}C-solvent yellow and solvent green aerosols after inhalation. Fundam Appl Toxicol 7:170–178
66. Bond JA (1986) Factors modifying the disposition of inhaled organic compounds. Paper presented at the 4th Inhalation Toxicology Workshop held in Albuquerque, NM, October 1986
67. Mewhinney JA, Griffith WC (1982) Models of Am metabolism in beagles and humans. Health Phys 42:629–644
68. International Commission on Radiological Protection: Report of Committee 2 (1979) Limits for intakes of radionuclides by workers. Pergamon, Oxford

Part IV
Interpretation of Results Using Laboratory Animals

CHAPTER 12

Interpretation of Early Lesions in the Mouse Lung: Fibrogenesis and Tumorigenesis

H.P. Witschi[1]

Up to the late 1960s, there was only a limited amount of information available on cytodynamics in the lung parenchyma. Morphometry provided insights on qualitative and quantitative changes in lung injury and repair, but was technically demanding and time-consuming. Nevertheless, the role of the alveolar type II epithelial cell in repairing damaged pulmonary epithelium became apparent (41). Autoradiography allows the study of cell renewal in airways and lung parenchyma. With the advent of plastic sections, the technique became a powerful tool. Embedding lung tissue in glycol methacrylate enabled one to cut sections thin enough (1 μm or less) to permit identification of individual cell types with much more precision than can be done with conventional paraffin sections. In addition, entire mouse lung lobes can be sectioned; this allows the examination and sampling of many more lung cells than can be done on Epon sections usually cut prior to electron microscopy. As a result of these developments there is now a considerable body of data available on cell injury and tissue repair in lungs damaged by toxic inhalants and by bloodborne agents (1,10,20).

Cell kinetic studies are done with pulse labeling or continuous labeling techniques. In pulse labeling experiments, animals receive a single injection of ^{3}H-labeled thymidine and are killed 1 hour later (3). Cells synthesizing DNA during this time become labeled. To obtain a profile of cell proliferation, animals have to be examined at selected intervals, usually daily, after initial lung injury (see Fig. 12.1 for an example). In continuous labeling studies, animals are given an implant with an osmotic minipump filled with the radiolabel (16). Minipumps release their content at a controlled rate over 10–20 days. The animals thus receive a constant infusion of radiolabeled thymidine and, as a result, all cells going through S phase during 1 or 2 weeks will become labeled. This technique allows one to determine the cumulative labeling index, as reflected by the area under the curve obtained with multiple pulse labelings (Fig. 12.2).

Analysis of autoradiographs involves counting cells (mostly 2000–3000 per mouse lung) and calculating the percentage of labeled cells, called the labeling

[1]Toxic Substances Research and Training Program, University of California, Davis, CA 95616, USA.

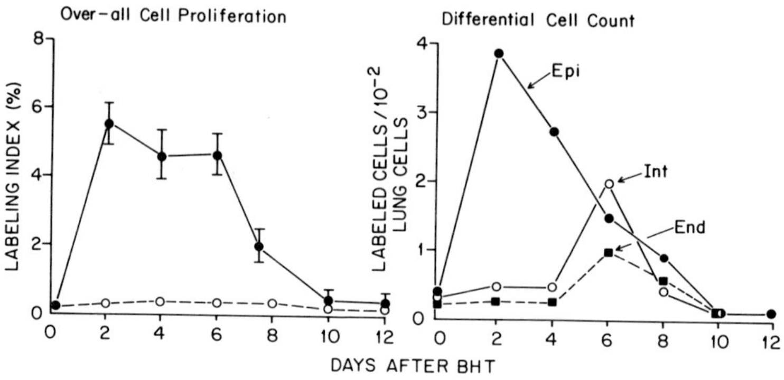

Fig. 12.1. Cell proliferation following acute lung injury as measured with pulse labeling. Animals were given 400 mg BHT/kg body wt. and on days indicated on abscissa received 50 μCi ^{3}H-labeled thymidine intraperitoneally. They were killed 1 h later. The lefthand panel shows labeling indices on the different days, the righthand one relative number of labeled cells, calculated from labeling index and differential cell count. Abbreviations: Epi, type II alveolar epithelial cells; Int, interstitial cells; End, capillary endothelial cells.

index (LI). The labeled cells can be classified according to morphologic criteria into type I and type II alveolar epithelial cells, alveolar macrophages, capillary endothelial cells and interstitial cells (30,48). By having both LI and percentage distribution of labeled cells it is possible to calculate the number of a certain labeled cell type per 10,000 lung cells, a calculation which often gives a better indication of shifts in the size of a proliferating cell population than would the differential percentage alone (16).

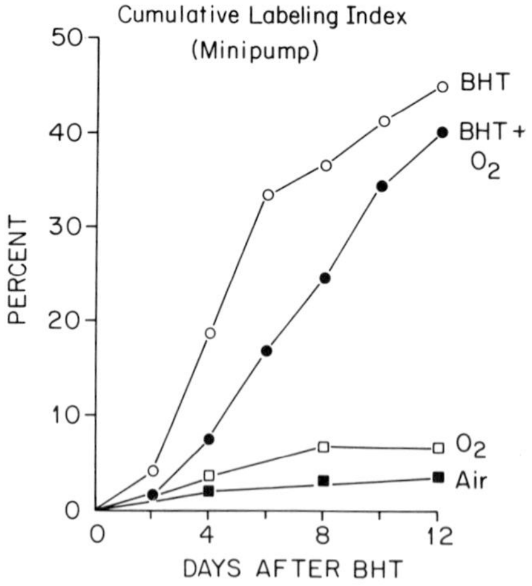

Fig. 12.2. Cumulative labeling index following acute lung injury. BHT-treated mice received ^{3}H-labeled thymidine-filled minipumps subcutaneously and were killed on days indicated. The single cumulative LI of the animals treated with BHT alone (open circles) at day 12 (45%) corresponds to the area under the curve (days 0 through 12) represented by the data on pulse-labeling in BHT-treated animals in Fig. 12.1 (closed circles in Fig. 12.1). Data from ref. 16 (with permission).

In the following section we will examine how a detailed knowledge of cell proliferation pattern may or may not help to predict long-term patterns of changes in pulmonary structure and function.

The Two-Injuries Model of Lung Fibrosis in the Mouse

In 1972 it was reported for the first time that the antioxidant butylated hydroxytoluene (BHT) would elicit diffuse alveolar damage in mouse lung (29). Initially, both epithelial and endothelial cells in the alveolar zone undergo widespread necrosis. Within a few days, however, the lesions become repaired through an extensive and diffuse proliferation of the surviving parenchymal cells (17,38). In a detailed study it was described how alveolar wall cell proliferation following administration of BHT would follow an orderly pattern. Type II alveolar epithelial cells would proliferate early, i.e., within 2–4 days after BHT-induced lung injury, whereas interstitial and capillary endothelial cells would undergo division only later, i.e., 5–7 days after BHT. Between 1 and 10 days after the initial insult, cell proliferation would return back to normal levels (3).

The BHT model of acute diffuse lung injury and repair offered the possibility to examine the effect of oxygen on dividing cells in the lung. Exposure of animals with damaged lungs to an atmosphere of 100% oxygen for up to 24 h resulted in a profound inhibition of thymidine incorporation into pulmonary DNA. It was observed however, that hyperoxia inhibited DNA synthesis only if applied early after BHT, e.g., on the 2nd day following lung injury. Exposure to hyperoxia 6 days after BHT no longer had an effect upon DNA synthesis in the lung (46).

One interpretation of these experiments was that, in the lung, dividing epithelial cells might be particularly vulnerable to oxygen toxicity. On the other hand, it appeared that cells proliferating late after BHT, e.g., interstitial cells, and perhaps capillary endothelial cells, would be somewhat more resistant. It was then speculated that inhibition of reepithelialization by oxygen (and perhaps by other agents) following diffuse alveolar damage might enhance the growth of fibroblasts in the lung. Eventually, such an event would lead to the development of fibrosis.

A series of experiments seemed to fulfill the prediction. Mice given BHT and exposed to hyperoxia (40–80% O_2 during the first 6 days after BHT) developed extensive pulmonary fibrosis (13). Increased levels of pulmonary hydroxyproline, a measurement used to quantitate the development of fibrosis, persisted up to 1 year later (15). If oxygen exposure was delayed and begun only 7 days after BHT, when epithelial cell proliferation following the BHT insult was completed, no fibrosis developed (Fig. 12.3).

Experiments done with irradiation of the thorax appeared to be even more conclusive (14). Only if animals were given 200 rad to the thorax on days 1 and 2 after BHT did extensive lung fibrosis develop. Delay of thorax irradiation was without any further effect. It therefore appeared that, in mouse lung, fibrosis was a result of diffuse alveolar injury and exposure to a second injurious agent during

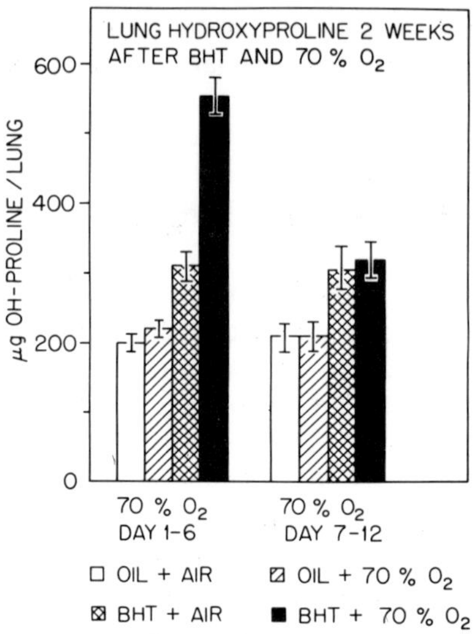

Fig. 12.3. Development of pulmonary fibrosis in animals treated with oxygen immediately following acute diffuse lung injury (*left*) or after allowing time for reepithelialization (*right*). Data from ref. 13 (with permission).

a particularly critical phase in the recovery. This critical phase appeared to be the time of epithelial cell regeneration. Interference with reepithelialization of the alveolar wall would lead to abnormal collagen accumulation. Some observations made in humans supported the hypothesis (6).

Further Testing of the Hypothesis

Diffuse lung injury in mice was produced with several other agents, such as methylcyclopentadienyl manganese tricarbonyl (MMT), oleic acid, $CdCl_2$ and the cytostatic drugs bleomycin and cyclophosphamide. All agents elicit diffuse lung damage in mice. We established that hyperoxia, induced early after drug exposure, potentiated fibrosis produced by all agents except oleic acid. It appeared that the two-injury model of lung fibrosis had some general validity (12).

There was one inconsistency. For the model to be universally applicable, it was required that fibrosis would not only develop if reepithelialization was interfered with by hyperoxia but also by X irradiation of the thoracic region. However, when we examined this possibility, we found that we could not potentiate lung damage produced by cyclophosphamide or by bleomycin with X rays, although it was perfectly possible to do so with hyperoxia (11). The difference between X rays and hyperoxia, of course, was that animals were exposed to elevated concentrations of oxygen for several days after lung injury. X irradiation, on the other hand, lasted only a few minutes. It seemed therefore possible that in the experiments with X rays we had missed the critical timepoint when epithelial cells would proliferate. This called for a reexamination of the cell kinetics in mouse lungs damaged by cytostatic drugs.

Pulmonary Cell Kinetics Following Administration of Cytostatic Drugs

A paper on bleomycin was the only information available on pulmonary cell kinetics following exposure to cytostatic drugs (2). An interesting finding was reported: following intravenous injection of bleomycin, alveolar wall cell proliferation, particularly proliferation of the type II epithelial cells, occurred somewhat late, i.e., more than 1 week after the drug was injected intravenously. This was at variance with all observations made on cell kinetics in lung damaged by a variety of agents (10,30). In almost all cases examined it appeared that a proliferation of the alveolar epithelial type II cell population was an early event following lung injury, destined to accomplish a quick restoration of a normal air-blood barrier (45).

It must be pointed out that at one time it was thought type II cell proliferation would only take place as a response to widespread damage to the alveolar type I cell population. Such a view is no longer tenable. It was recently shown that type II cell proliferation may also occur without any prior damage to the alveolar epithelium. Inflammatory cells, by the simple expedient of migrating across the alveolar wall, presumably break contact inhibition between epithelial cells. The net result is a round of type II and interstitial cell proliferation in an otherwise undamaged lung (35).

Nevertheless, the observation made with bleomycin called for a further investigation of the pulmonary cell kinetics following exposure to cytostatic drugs. We chose four agents, all known to produce pulmonary damage and eventually pulmonary fibrosis in man (4,8). The drugs were bleomycin, cyclophosphamide, busulfan and 1,2-*bis*(2 chloroethyl)-1-nitrosourea (BCNU; carmustine) (26,51). All drugs were given intraperitoneally once at doses which produced lung damage without excessive mortality. In addition, bleomycin was given intratracheally and busulfan, in one experiment, was also given orally.

Results obtained with all four cytostatic drugs had some striking similarities. Following intravenous administration of bleomycin, the peak labeling index was observed only about 2 weeks later, i.e., on day 15 after bleomycin injection. When the drug was given intratracheally, it produced an early peak of cell labeling 7 days later, followed by a second peak on days 9–11 (26). A delayed overall cell proliferation with a peak around days 7–9 was also observed following intraperitoneal injection of cyclophosphamide. With busulfan, alveolar cell proliferation occurred only as late as days 17–21 (intraperitoneal experiment) or even after 4 weeks (oral administration). BCNU produced a similarly delayed proliferation response (51).

A second striking feature was that the cytostatic drugs seemed to suppress rather than to stimulate the proliferation of the alveolar type II cell population.

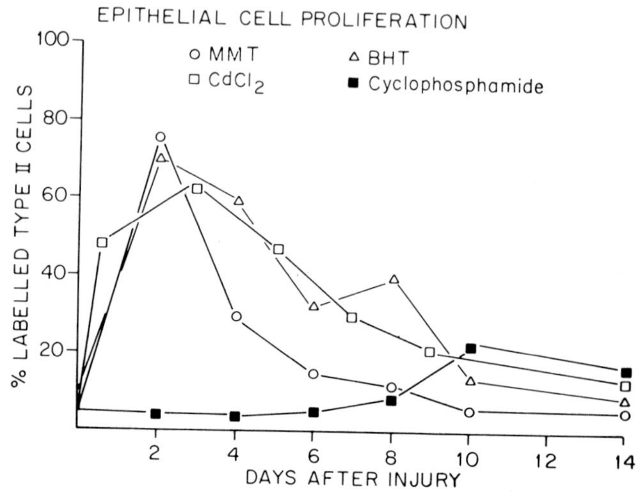

Fig. 12.4. Percentage of labeled type II alveolar cells on different days after lung injury caused by methylcyclopentadienyl manganese tricarbonyl (MMT), butylated hydroxytoluene (BHT), inhalation of $CdCl_2$ aerosol ($CdCl_2$) or cyclophosphamide. Note initial suppression of type II proliferation following administration of the cytostatic drug.

Following cyclophosphamide, the biggest percentage of labeled type II cells was found 10 days after injection of the drug and then only 22% of all labeled cells were type II epithelial cells. This finding is in stark contrast with observations made following administration of BHT, oleic acid or even $CdCl_2$, where early after injury up to 50–70% of all labeled cells have been identified as type II alveolar epithelial cells (Fig. 12.4).

Patterns of Cell Proliferation as a Predictive Tool for Fibrogenesis

Available data on cell proliferation in mouse lung following acute injury and on resulting long-term consequences may allow some cautious generalizations. An abnormal accumulation of collagen may occur if lung is acutely damaged and if the repair process is disturbed by a second toxic agent which interferes with proper repair of the epithelial layer in the alveolar zone. There is evidence that such a mechanism accounts for some forms of lung fibrosis in humans. In adult respiratory distress syndrome, the original lung damage is often of unknown etiology (34). Diffuse alveolar damage then may become amplified by secondary exposure to (therapeutically needed) oxygen (22). Fibrosis often develops as a consequence (52).

However, we now also have learned that not all chemicals apparently produce a similar sequence of events in acute lung damage. Proliferation of alveolar epithelial cells is not always an early hallmark of repair processes. It occurs following lung damage produced by such agents as oxidant air pollutants, BHT, oleic acid, MMT, and others. However, there appears also to exist a second class of agents, exemplified by cytostatic drugs. Following administration of these agents, cell proliferation in the lung is delayed 1–3 weeks, and epithelial cell proliferation appears to be impaired rather than stimulated. It is tempting to speculate that this is directly related to the well-established fibrogenic potential of these agents. In our own experiments we have observed that acute exposure to $CdCl_2$ aerosol produces a comparatively late (day 5) peak proliferation of type II epithelial cells. A one-time exposure is followed by a progressive accumulation of lung collagen (30). Cyclophosphamide produces an even more delayed cell proliferation. In a 1-year study we found that one single injection of 100 mg/kg of the drug is followed by progressive pulmonary fibrosis with accompanying decrease in pulmonary compliance (31).

Why cell proliferation is delayed after lung injury by cytostatic drugs remains at the present time open to speculation. It could be, of course, that a late migration of inflammatory cells across the alveolar epithelium was enough to trigger some cell division (35). In analyzing the slides in our study, we did not see abnormal accumulation of inflammatory cells in the alveolar parenchyma. Although we cannot rule out the possibility that inflammatory cells might ultimately have been involved, we favor at present a second possible mechanism to explain the delayed cell proliferation. Cytostatic drugs are designed to interfere with DNA synthesis. Available data show that small amounts of bleomycin or of cyclophosphamide remain in the lung for several days following administration of a single drug dose (2,51). The persistence of the drug might thus effectively prevent any proliferative response to injury produced by the same agent.

Tumor Promotion in Mouse Lung

A detailed knowledge of cell kinetics might also be of some use in assessing the likelihood of tumor development or of tumor promotion. For example, it has recently been claimed that differences in rate of alveolar cell renewal might be linked to the incidence and prevalence of spontaneous or chemically induced lung tumors in mice (39). Alveolar cell hyperplasia may also play a role in tumor promotion. In 1974, Boutwell reviewed the then existing information on mechanisms of two-stage carcinogenesis (5). Among several conclusions made was one of particular importance: that practically all agents known to have promoting activity in mouse skin were capable of producing skin epithelial hyperplasia (although it was also pointed out that not all agents capable of producing hyperplasia would be promoting agents in mouse skin). The second conclusion was that virtually no evidence existed that the elements of two-stage carcinogenesis would apply to internal organs.

Certain mouse strains have a high spontaneous incidence of pulmonary tumors. If mice from such a susceptible strain are treated with a carcinogen, they will within a few months develop an additional number of tumors (36). Many of these tumors are derived from alveolar type II cells; others are derived from the Clara cells in the small airways (21). Thus, knowing that many lung tumors in mice were type II cell tumors, having read that all agents active as skin tumor promoters were capable of producing a hyperplasia of the target cell population, and having shown that BHT would produce a proliferation of type II alveolar cells, we reasoned that BHT should promote tumor development in mouse lung.

This prediction was fully borne out in a series of experiments, the first one published in 1977 (49). In several mouse strains, BHT enhances the development of lung tumors, provided exposure to BHT is begun after exposure to the carcinogen. The effect of BHT is independent of route of administration, and intake of BHT may be for as little as 2 weeks at as low a concentration as 0.05% of the diet. Also, BHT enhances tumor development even if administered for the first time 5 months after the carcinogen (42). It must be pointed out, however, that it has not been possible to enhance lung tumor development with BHT in mice which are treated with a "subcarcinogenic" dose of a carcinogen. BHT does thus not meet all criteria developed for skin tumor promotion and, for the time being, it would appear more appropriate to refer to BHT not as a promoter but as a tumor-enhancing agent (42,43). Nevertheless, BHT is capable of enhancing tumor development not only in mouse lung but in other systems such as mouse and rat liver (28,32), bladder (18), thyroid and stomach (37), as well as in several in vitro systems (9,33,40).

Enhancement of Lung Tumor Development and Cell Hyperplasia in the Lung

After having shown that BHT could enhance lung tumor development, the prediction was made that any agent capable of producing alveolar cell hyperplasia in mouse lung would act as a tumor-enhancing agent. When the hypothesis was tested, no supporting evidence was found.

Cell hyperplasia quite similar to the one observed following BHT can be produced by exposing mice for 72 h to 100% oxygen, a treatment they survive well. When SWR mice were treated with urethan and exposed to 100% oxygen on 3 consecutive days a week for 6 weeks, tumor development was not influenced (47). The organometal compound MMT produces diffuse lung injury in mice, followed again by a substantial hyperplasia of the type II alveolar cell population. Treatment of A/J mice with repeated MMT injections after urethan was without any effect on lung tumor development (50).

Two additional experiments yielded even more surprising results. Instead of treating mice intermittently with 100% oxygen, we exposed them continuously to an atmosphere of 70% oxygen. This treatment produces an initial burst of type II cell proliferation in the lung; after 3–4 weeks proliferation abates somewhat, but remains significantly elevated over control animals kept in air for the entire duration (16 weeks) of oxygen exposure (Fig. 12.5). Under these conditions,

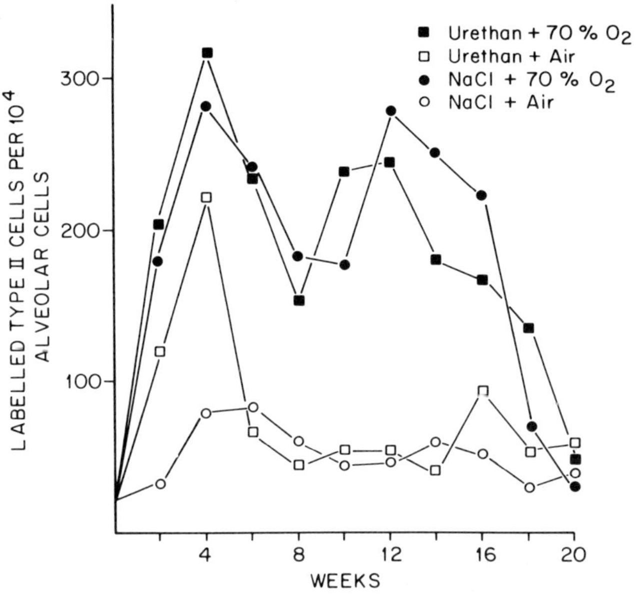

Fig. 12.5. Cumulative labeling indices (measured biweekly) over a 4½-month period. In animals kept continuously in 70% oxygen, there was a sustained increased in alveolar type II cell proliferation, although tumor development during the same time was severely curtailed. Data from ref. 27 (with permission).

however, substantially fewer (20% of controls) tumors develop in the lungs of oxygen-exposed mice compared to control animals kept in air (Fig. 12.6). Oxygen is cytotoxic for developing tumor cells and is an effective means for preventing lung tumor development in both mice and in rats (25,27). These observations are at variance with two widely accepted mechanisms of tumor promotion. Increased activity of ornithine decarboxylase (ODC) is usually taken to be a hallmark of tumor promotion. In the mouse lung tumor system, ODC activity is increased when tumor development is inhibited (27). It also can be assumed that exposure to hyperoxia may increase the production and flux of active oxygen species in the lung in vivo. In vitro evidence is available to suggest such a possibility. Oxygen free radicals are thought to be implicated in tumor promotion (7,23). However, in mouse lung oxygen severely curtails tumor development.

Chronic exposure to ozone also produces alveolar cell hyperplasia, and it might be expected that such a treatment would enhance the development of murine lung tumors. Again we found the opposite to be true. In both A/J and SWR mice, ozone exposure (0.8 ppm or 0.4 ppm) reduced the number of developing tumors (24).

A generalization made originally—that any agent capable of producing cell hyperplasia would enhance lung tumor development in mouse lung—could thus not be corroborated in experiments involving such diverse agents as MMT,

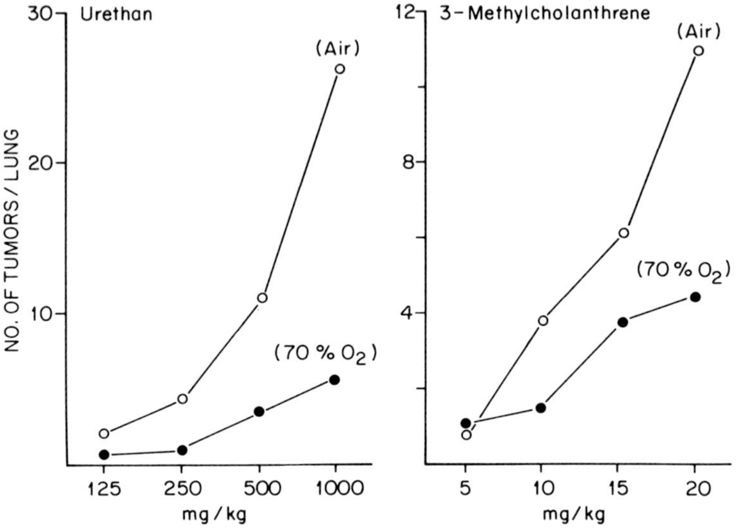

Fig. 12.6. Inhibition of lung tumor development by hyperoxia. Mice were treated with carcinogen at doses indicated and killed 4 months later. Oxygen severely suppressed tumor growth. Data from ref. 25 (with permission).

oxygen, or ozone. It has recently been reported that glycerol would enhance tumor development in mouse lung (19). The authors suggest that this occurs because, glycerol produces hyperplasia of the smooth endoplasmic reticulum, and development of peculiarly shaped mitochondria in the Clara cells of mouse lung, a precursor cell for lung tumors (53). So far in our studies, we have not found an effect of glycerol on tumor development in mouse lung (Witschi, unpublished observations).

Cell Proliferation as a Factor in Mouse Lung Tumor Promotion

It was discussed above that sustained or repeated hyperplasia does not always enhance tumor development in mouse lung and may even be accompanied by the opposite effect. There is also evidence now available to show that cell hyperplasia is not a prerequisite for tumor promotion in mouse lung. Originally it was assumed that after each BHT injection the alveolar cells would undergo a cycle of division. When this was actually measured, it was found that cell proliferation occurs only after the first two BHT injections; further injections no longer have any effect. Yet more than two BHT injections are required to enhance tumor development. We also found that tumor development was enhanced in animals given injections of SKF prior to BHT, a treatment which abolishes BHT-induced cell proliferation (47). Recently, we have documented that in animals made

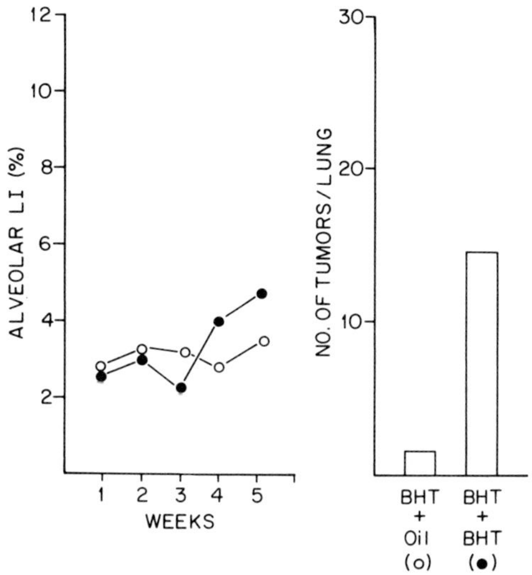

Fig. 12.7. Enhancement of tumor development in mouse lung in the absence of overall cell hyperplasia. The left panel shows that repeated injections of BHT in BHT-conditioned animals (closed circles) do not significantly increase cumulative labeling indices (measured weekly). The right panel shows that BHT treatment significantly enhances tumor development. Data from ref. 44 (with permission).

"tolerant" to BHT, enhanced tumor development can be found even in the absence of any detectable hyperplasia in the alveolar zone (Fig. 12.7). Available evidence thus suggests that cell hyperplasia is not a prerequisite for tumor promotion in mouse lung (44).

Conclusion

Detailed analysis of cell kinetics following acute lung injury has given us some insight into possible pathogenetic mechanisms underlying chronic lung disease. Possible correlations between defective reepithelialization and development of fibrotic changes need to be explored in future work. On the other hand, certain concepts generally thought to apply to tumor promotion have been found not be correct in mouse lung. It will be challenging to see whether other experimental model systems of two-stage carcinogenesis follow the mouse lung or the mouse skin paradigm.

Acknowledgment. Research sponsored by the Office of Health and Environmental Research, US Department of Energy under contract DE-AC05-840R21400 with the Martin Marietta Energy Systems, Inc.

References

1. Adamson IYR (1985) Cellular kinetics of the lung. In: Witschi HP, Brain JD (ed) Toxicology of inhaled materials. Springer, Berlin Heidelberg New York, pp 289–318
2. Adamson IYR, Bowden DH (1979)Bleomycin-induced injury and metaplasia of alveolar type 2 cells. Am J Pathol 96:531–544
3. Adamson IYR, Bowden DH, Côté MG, Witschi HP (1977) Lung injury induced by butylated hydroxytoluene. Cytodynamic and biochemical studies in mice. Lab Invest 36:28–32
4. Batist G, Andrews JL (1981) Pulmonary toxicity of antineoplastic drugs. JAMA 246:1449–1453
5. Boutwell RK (1974) The function and mechanism of promoters of carcinogenesis. CRC Crit Rev Toxicol 2:419–443
6. Brody AR, Soler P, Basset F, Haschek WM, Witschi HP (1981) Epithelial mesenchymal association of cells in human pulmonary fibrosis and in BHT-oxygen induced fibrosis in mice. Exp Lung Res 2:207–220
7. Cerutti PA (1985) Prooxidant states and tumor promotion. Science 227:375–381
8. Cooper JAD Jr, White DA, Mathey RA (1986) Drug-induced pulmonary disease. Part 1: Cytotoxic drugs. Am Rev Respir Dis 133:321–340
9. Djurhuus R, Lillehaug JR (1982) Butylated hydroxytoluene: Tumor promoting activity in an in vitro two-stage carcinogenesis assay. Bull Environ Contam Toxicol 29:115–120
10. Evans MJ (1982) Cell death and cell renewal in small airways and alveoli. In: Witschi HP, Nettesheim P (eds) Mechanisms in respiratory toxicology, vol 2, CRC Press, Boca Raton, pp 189–218
11. Hakkinen PJ, Whiteley JW, Witschi HP (1982) Hyperoxia but not thoracic X-irradiation potentiates bleomycin and cyclophosphamide-induced lung damage in mice. Am Rev Respir Dis 126:281–285
12. Hakkinen PJ, Morse CC, Martin FM, Dalbey WE, Haschek WM, Witschi HP (1983) Potentiating effects of oxygen in lungs damaged by methylcyclopentadienyl manganese tricarbonyl, cadmium chloride, oleic acid and antitumor drugs. Toxicol Appl Pharmacol 67:55–69
13. Haschek WM, Witschi HP (1979) Pulmonary fibrosis: A possible mechanism. Toxicol Appl Pharmacol 51:475–487
14. Haschek WM, Meyer KR, Ullrich RL, Witschi HP (1980) Potentiation of chemically induced lung fibrosis by thorax irradiation. Int J Radiat Oncol Biol Phys 6:449–455
15. Haschek WM, Klein-Szanto AJP, Last JA, Reiser KM, Witschi HP (1982) Long-term morphologic and biochemical features of experimentally induced lung fibrosis in the mouse. Lab Invest 46:438–449
16. Haschek WM, Reiser KM, Klein-Szanto AJ, Last JA, Witschi HP. (1983) Potentiation of butylated hydroxytoluene induced acute lung damage by oxygen: Cell kinetics and collagen metabolism. Am Rev Respir Dis 127:28–34
17. Hirai KI, Witschi HP, Côté MG (1978) Electron microscopy of butylated hydroxytoluene-induced lung damage. Exp Mol Pathol 27:295–308
18. Imaida K, Fukushima S, Shirai T, Ohtani M, Nakanishi K, Ito N (1983) Promoting activities of butylated hydroxyanisole and butylated hydroxytoluene on 2-stage urinary bladder carcinogenesis and inhibition of γ-glutamyl transpeptidase-positive foci development in the liver of rats. Carcinogenesis 4:895–899.

19. Inayama Y (1986) Promoting action of glycerol in pulmonary tumorigenesis model using a single administration of 4-nitroquinoline-1-oxide in mice. Gann 77:345–350
20. Kauffman SL (1980) Cell proliferation in the mammalian lung. Int Rev Exp Pathol 22:131–191
21. Kauffman SL, Alexander L, Sass L (1979) Histologic and ultrastructural features of the Clara cell adenoma of the mouse lung. Lab Invest 40:708–716
22. Katzenstein AA, Bloor CM, Liebow AA (1976) Diffuse alveolar damage—the role of oxygen, shock, and related factors. Am J Pathol 85:210–222
23. Kensler TW, Trush MA (1984) Role of oxygen radicals in tumor promotion. Environ Mutagen 6:593–616
24. Last JA, Warren DL, Pecquet-Goad E, Witschi HP (1987) Modification of lung tumor development in mice by ozone. JNCI 78:149–154
25. Lindenschmidt RC, Margaretten N, Griesemer RA, Witschi HP (1986) Modification of lung tumor growth by hyperoxia. Carcinogenesis 7:1581–1586
26. Lindenschmidt RC, Tryka AF, Godfrey GA, Frome EL, Witschi HP (1986) Intratracheal versus intravenous administration of bleomycin in mice: acute effects. Toxicol Appl Pharmacol 85:69–77
27. Lindenschmidt RC, Tryka AF, Witschi HP (1986) Inhibition of mouse lung tumor development in hyperoxia. Cancer Res 46:1994–2000
28. Maeura Y, Williams GM (1984) Enhancing effect of butylated hydroxytoluene on the development of liver altered foci and neoplasms induced by *N*-2-fluorenylacetamine in rats. Fd Chem Toxicol 22:191–198
29. Marino AA, Mitchell JT (1972) Lung damage in mice following intraperitoneal injection of butylated hydroxytoluene. Proc Soc Exp Biol Med 140:122–125
30. Martin FM, Witschi HP (1985) Cadmium-induced lung injury: cell kinetics and long-term effects. Toxicol Appl Pharmacol 80:215–227
31. Morse CC, Sigler C, Lock S, Hakkinen PJ, Haschek WM, Witschi HP (1985) Pulmonary toxicity of cyclophosphamide: a 1-year study. Exp Mol Pathol 42:251–260
32. Peraino C, Fry RJM, Staffeldt E, Christopher JP (1977) Enhancing effects of phenobarbital and butylated hydroxytoluene on 2-acetylaminofluorene-induced hepatic tumorigenesis in the rat. Food Cosmet Toxicol 15:93–96
33. Potenberg J, Kahl R, Hildebrandt AG, Schiffmann D, Henschler D (1985) Promotional effect of butylated hydroxytoluene and butylated hydroxyanisole on morphologic transformation of cultured hamster embryo cells by benzo(*a*)pyrene. Naunyn-Schmiedebergs Arch Pharmacol 330:R22
34. Rinaldo JE, Rogers RM (1982) Adult respiratory-distress syndrome. Changing concepts of lung injury and repair. N Engl J Med 306:900–909
35. Shami SG, Evans MG, Martinez LA (1986) Type II cell proliferation related to migration of inflammatory cells into the lung. Exp Mol Pathol 44:344–352
36. Shimkin MB, Stoner GD (1975) Lung tumors in mice: application to carcinogenesis bioassay. Adv Cancer Res 21:1–58
37. Shirai T, Fukushima S, Ohshima M, Masuda A, Ito N (1984) Effects of butylated hydroxyanisole, butylated hydroxytoluene and NaCl on gastric carcinogenesis initiated with *N*-methyl-*N'*-nitro-*N*-nitrosoguanidine in F344 rats. JNCI 72:1189–1198
38. Smith LJ (1984) Lung damage induced by butylated hydroxytoluene in mice: biochemical, cellular and morphologic characterization. Am Rev Respir Dis 130:895–904

39. Thaete LG, Beer DG, Malkinson AM (1986) Genetic variation in the proliferation of murine pulmonary type II cells: Basal rates and alterations following urethan treatment. Cancer Res 46:5335–5338
40. Trosko JE, Yotti LP, Warren S, Tushimoto G, Chang CC (1982) Inhibition of cell-cell communication by tumor promoters. In: Hecker E, Kunz W, Marx S, Fusenig NE, Phielman HW (eds) Carcinogenesis and biological effects of tumor promoters. Raven, New York, pp 565–585 (Carcinogenesis: A comprehensive survey, vol 7)
41. Witschi HP (1976) Proliferation of type II alveolar cells: A review of common responses in toxic lung injury. Toxicology 5:267–277
42. Witschi HP (1983) Enhancement of tumor formation in mouse lung. In: Slaga TJ (ed) Tumor promotion in internal organs, CRC Press, Boca Raton, pp 71–90 (Mechanisms of tumor promotion, vol 1)
43. Witschi HP (1985) Enhancement of lung tumor formation in mice. In: Mass MJ, Kaufman DG, Siegfried JM, Steele VE, Henson S (eds) Cancer of the respiratory tract: predisposing factors, Raven, New York, pp 147–158 (Carcinogenesis, vol 8)
44. Witschi HP (1986) Separation of early diffuse alveolar cell proliferation from enhanced tumor development in mouse lung. Cancer Res 46:2675–2679
45. Witschi HP, Côté MG (1977) Primary pulmonary responses to toxic agents. CRC Crit Rev Toxicol 5:23–66
46. Witschi HP, and Côté MG (1977) Inhibition of butylated hydroxytoluene induced mouse lung cell division by oxygen: time-effect and dose-effect relationships. Chem Biol Interact 19:279–289
47. Witschi HP, Kehrer JP (1982) Adenoma development in mouse lung following treatment with possible promoting agents. J Am Coll Toxicol 1:171–184
48. Witschi HP, Morse CC (1985) Cell kinetics in mouse lung following administration of carcinogens and butylated hydroxytoluene. Toxicol Appl Pharmacol 78:464–472
49. Witschi HP, Williamson D, Lock S (1977) Enhancement of urethan tumorigenesis in mouse lung by butylated hydroxytoluene. JNCI 58:301–305
50. Witschi HP, Hakkinen PJ, Kehrer JP (1981) Modification of lung tumor development in A/J mice. Toxicology 21:37–45
51. Witschi HP, Godfrey G, Frome E, Lindenschmidt RC (1987) Pulmonary toxicity of cytostatic drugs: Cell kinetics. Fundam Appl Toxicol 8:253–262
52. Zapol WM, Tretstad RL, Coffey JW, Tsai T, Solvador RA (1979) Pulmonary fibrosis in severe acute respiratory failure. Am Rev Respir Dis 119:547–554
53. Kitomura H, Iuayoma Y, Ito T, Yabana M, Piegorseh W and Kauisawa M (1987) Morphologic alteration of mouse Clara cells induced by glycerol: ultrastructural and morphometric studies. Exp Lung Res 12:281–302

CHAPTER 13

Relevance to Humans of Experimentally Induced Pulmonary Tumors in Rats and Hamsters

519273

U. Mohr[1] and D.L. Dungworth[2]

Introduction

Extrapolation of data from animal experiments to the human situation is a necessary part of risk assessment. Because both qualitative and quantitative results of carcinogenicity studies vary widely from one animal species to another, it is well recognized that there is a need to use data from several species in extrapolating to possible human effects. Accurate extrapolation requires an understanding of why there are large interspecies differences, and this understanding is beginning to be developed. Two important aspects, namely, interspecies differences in dosimetry of inhaled materials and in epithelial cell biology, are covered elsewhere in this book, and only a few specific examples will be considered here. This article concentrates on lesions observed in lungs of rats and hamsters during in vivo carcinogenicity trials (1) and on comparative information being derived from in vitro studies.

The discussion will be limited to tumors caused by inhalation and will exclude those caused by instillation and implantation. As background information we review briefly the tumor types inducible by various inhaled compounds in rats and hamsters and compare them with the epidemiological data in man. Recent findings on tumor markers, such as oncogene expression, will be mentioned briefly because the demonstration that the same oncogenes are expressed in both human and rodent tumors may confirm the relevance of rodent findings for man. Lastly, mention will be made of our attempt to make a direct experimental comparison of human and hamster cells using in vitro techniques. For such an attempt to be fruitful, however, the fundamental requirements are that the in vitro systems should mimic the in vivo circumstances as closely as possible and the findings obtained in vitro should be correlated closely to those obtained in vivo.

[1]Institut für Experimentelle Pathologie, Medizinische Hochschule Hannover, Konstanty-Gutschow-Str. 8, 3000 Hannover 61, FRG.

[2]Department of Veterinary Pathology, University of California, Davis, CA 95616, USA.

Factors Responsible for the Interspecies Differences in Incidence and Types of Pulmonary Tumors

One of the major factors responsible for the interspecies differences in incidence, localization, and types of pulmonary tumors is *species-dependent variation in the dosimetry of inhaled carcinogens or cocarcinogens.* In inhalation experiments using monodisperse ^{169}Yb-labelled aluminosilicate aerosols, bronchial deposition of particles with diameters smaller than 2.09 μm aerodynamic equivalent diameter was observed more constantly in hamsters than in rats, while the pulmonary deposition was variable between the two species, depending on the particle size (2). In the same study, tracheal deposition of particles larger than 1.04 μm aerodynamic equivalent diameter was greater in hamsters than in rats, whilst that of smaller particles showed a reversed relationship. Therefore, it is important to determine the deposition profile of test compounds in various bronchopulmonary regions when the carcinogenic sensitivity of each region is specifically to be addressed. In hamster tracheal tissues examined by fluorescence microscopy after intratracheal injection of benzo(*a*)pyrene-ferric oxide, penetration of the carcinogen into the epithelium was clearly indicated (3). In rats, however, this was not the case, despite significant amounts of the material being detected in the tracheal lumen. In the bronchioloalveolar region, deposition of the compounds was detected in the same amount in both species, although only rats developed squamous cell nodules. Clearance of compounds deposited in target areas will also affect the dosimetric profile, and macrophages are known to play a large part in this. The faster uptake of insoluble gold particles by pulmonary macrophages of hamsters compared to rats (4) is an example of a functional difference capable of influencing local dosimetry.

A second factor causing interspecies variations is the *sum of differences in susceptibility of cells at risk* in various species. Such differences are attributable to various aspects of cellular biology. For instance, rat tracheal epithelial cells may be more protected from carcinogen penetration than hamster tracheal epithelial cells, because of the more abundant mucus production in the rat trachea compared with the hamster trachea (3,5). Recently, a protective role of cellular glycoprotein synthesis against toxicity of xenobiotics has been suggested (6). Another example is the difference in capability for metabolizing indirect-acting carcinogens such as benzo(*a*)pyrene. Benzo(*a*)pyrene-directed monooxygenase levels were 2- to 3-fold greater in microsomes from lungs of methylcholanthrene-preinduced rats than in comparable preparations from hamster lungs (7). By contrast, organ-cultured tracheae of hamsters produced a larger amount of benzo(*a*)pyrene metabolites and more binding of them to DNA than those of rats (8). Differences between hamsters and rats in these studies correlate well with differences in incidence, types, and localization of the preneoplastic and neoplastic changes induced by benzo(*a*)pyrene in the two species (3,9). Later in this paper, human and hamster bronchioloalveologenic epithelial cells will also be compared.

A third set of factors responsible for interspecies differences is the *sequence of carcinogenetic events* from initiation to promotion and progression, which are influenced by species-related processes. Experimental evidence for multistage carcinogenesis in the respiratory tract has so far been provided mainly by combined in vivo–in vitro investigations on rat tracheal epithelial cells (10), but there is good reason to suspect that analogous processes occur in other species, including humans. Provided that initiation is closely associated with the binding of carcinogenic metabolites, cancer should be more easily initiated by benzo(*a*)pyrene in hamster tracheal epithelial cells than in rat tracheal epithelial cells, according to the information mentioned previously (8). If the human chromosomal apparatus is more stable than that of rodents (11,12), human cells should be more resistant than rodent cells to mutational events occurring during initiation as well as those leading to clonal selection during promotion and progression (13,14). The concept of relative genetic instability in rodent cells is also being used in the explanation of solid-state carcinogenesis (15).

Classification of Pulmonary Tumors in Rats

In a simplified system, tumors are classified into four types: bronchioloalveolar adenoma, bronchioloalveolar carcinoma, squamous cell tumor, and miscellaneous tumor (for example, sarcoma or hemangioendothelioma). Adenomas

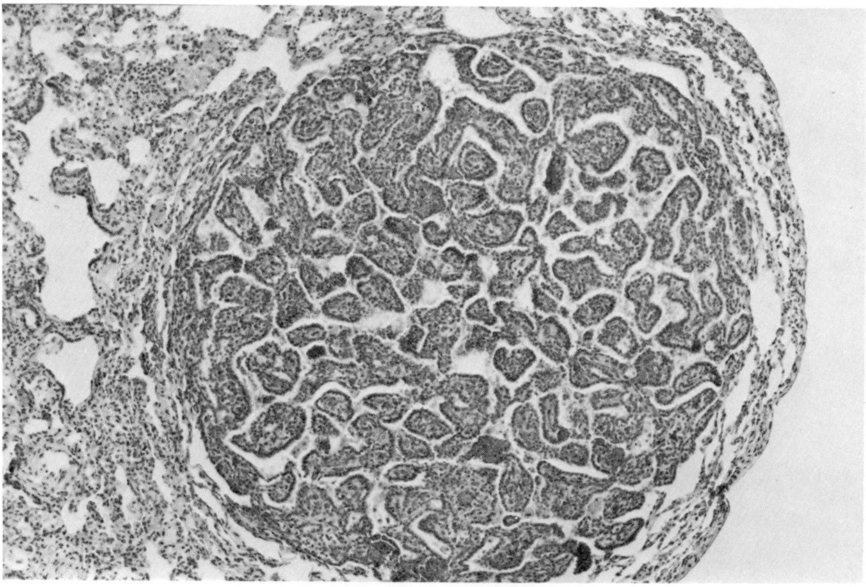

Fig. 13.1. Bronchioloalveolar adenoma in a rat receiving $CaCrO_4$. Regular papillary pattern and discrete border. H & E, ×90.

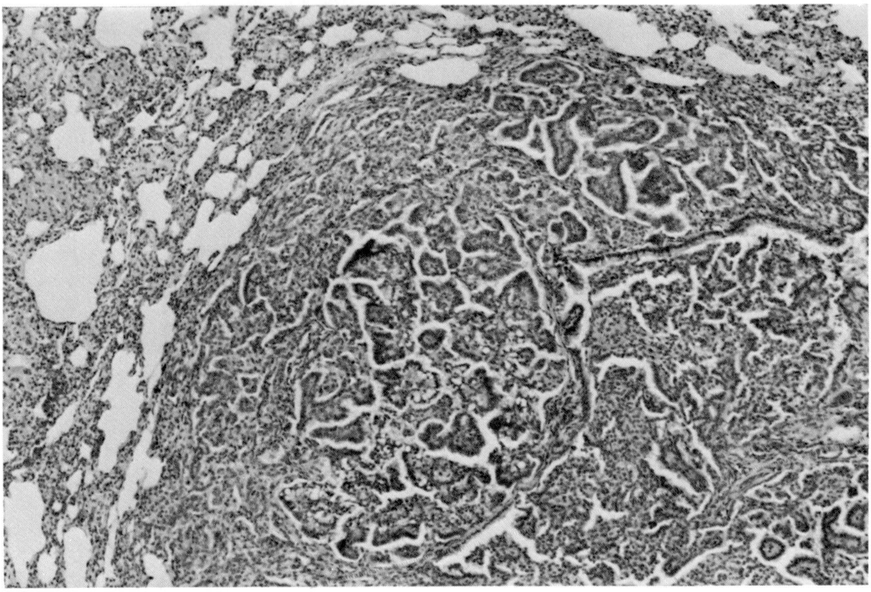

Fig. 13.2. Bronchioloalveolar adenoma with atypia in a rat receiving $CaCrO_4$. Distorted papillary and alveolar pattern with intrabronchiolar growth. H & E, ×90.

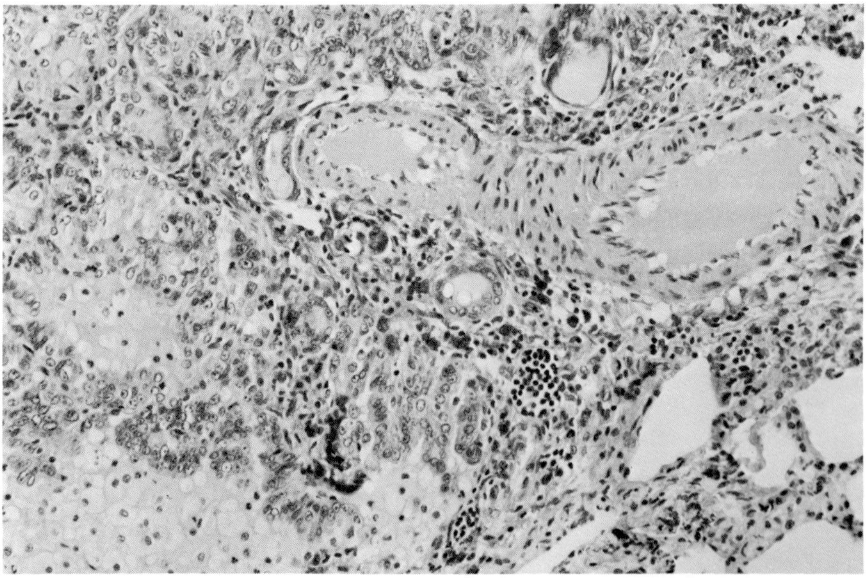

Fig. 13.3. Bronchioloalveolar carcinoma in a female rat receiving $Na_2Cr_2O_7$. Invasion of perivascular connective and lymphatic tissues by tumor cells. H & E, ×115.

Table 13.1. Keratinizing squamous cell tumors in rat lungs

Classification		Behavior	Cytology
	Cystic ↑		
1. Benign, keratinizing, cystic		Slow peripheral extension by air spaces	Regular, no atypia, rare to occasional mitoses
2. Grade I carcinoma		Slight evidence of stromal invasion (peribronchial/perivascular), possibly minimal scirrhous response	Borderline atypia, few to moderate mitoses
3. Grade II carcinoma		Definite stromal invasion, especially lymphatic or vascular, usually some scirrhous response	Mild atypia, moderate mitotic index
4. Grade III carcinoma		Invasive/destructive/scirrhous pleural/mediastinal spread	Moderate atypia, moderate to high mitotic index
	↓ Malignant		

Reprinted with permission from ref 1.

and adenocarcinomas are sometimes difficult to differentiate. However, it is even more difficult to classify squamous cell tumors according to their grade of malignancy.

The bronchioloalveolar adenoma is characterized by a regular alveolar, papillary, or mixed pattern, usually formed by a single layer of cuboidal or low columnar cells without cytologic features of atypia (Fig. 13.1). The tumor is usually demarcated from the surrounding tissues by compressed parenchyma.

An irregular, disorganized tumor with prominent papillary and/or cribriform pattern can be classified as a bronchioloalveolar adenoma with atypia (Fig. 13.2). This tumor often shows regional variations in architecture with associated variability of cell type from cuboidal to columnar.

The bronchioloalveolar carcinoma is similar but shows more exaggerated features than described for adenomas with atypia, and there is definite evidence of local invasion of interstitial tissues or of discontinuous spread of tumor cells to nearby alveoli (Fig. 13.3).

In an effort to define different types of squamous cell tumors, these have been classified according to the behavioral and histological criteria listed in Table 13.1. These specimens were obtained from a diesel exhaust experiment (1). Class 1 includes benign, keratinizing, cystic tumors which are characterized microscopically by a cystic cavity filled with keratin squames and squamous-cell "ghosts" and a thin wall of well-differentiated squamous epithelium (Fig. 13.4a). The tumor cells extend into alveolar spaces at the periphery of the tumor, but no clear evidence of stromal invasion is detected (Fig. 13.4b). Though there might be rare mitotic figures in some tumors, cellular atypia and dysplasia are not observed. Class 2 squamous cell tumors have a keratinizing cystic structure with a relatively thick wall of squamous epithelium which appears to have invaded the perivascular and peribronchiolar spaces (Fig. 13.5). Tumor cells show slight

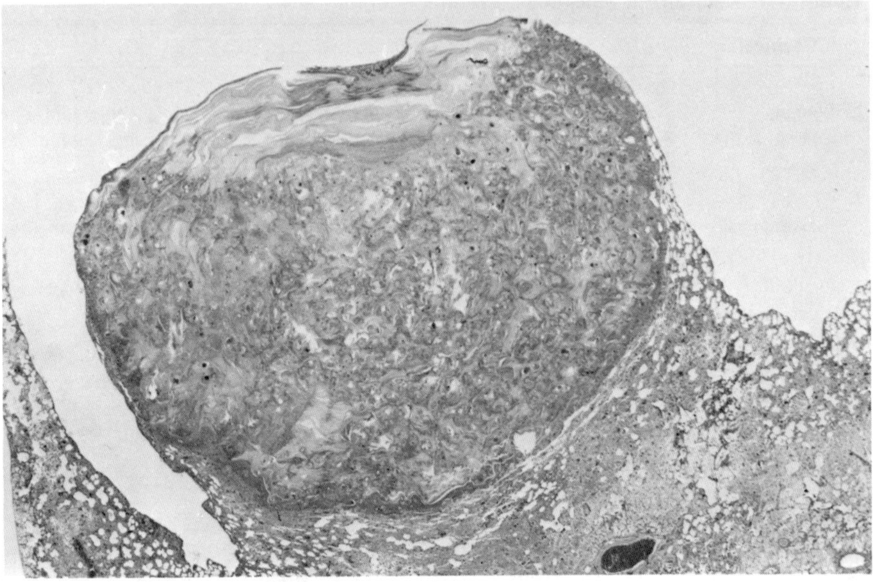

a

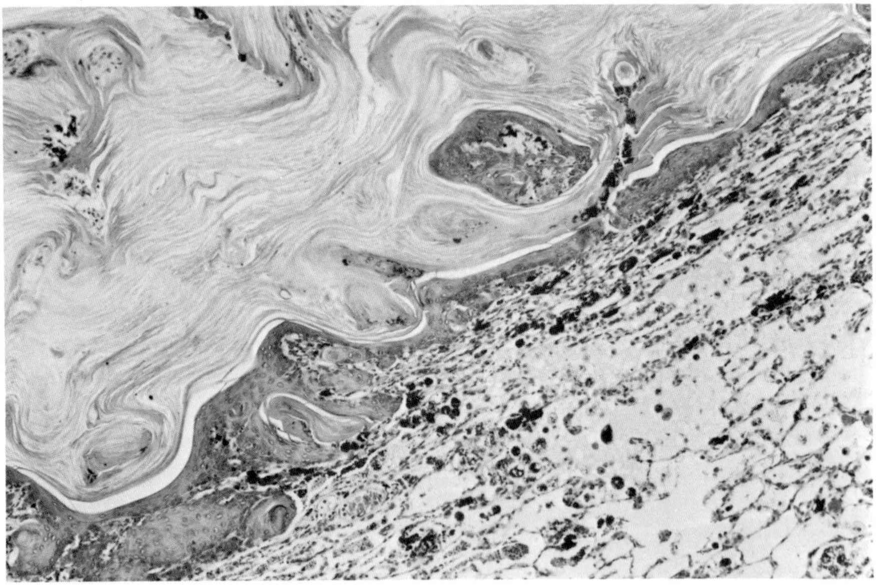

b

Fig. 13.4a,b. Lung of a rat exposed to unfiltered diesel exhaust. Benign, keratinizing, cystic squamous-cell tumor (class 1). H & E, ×9 (**a**) and 90 (**b**).

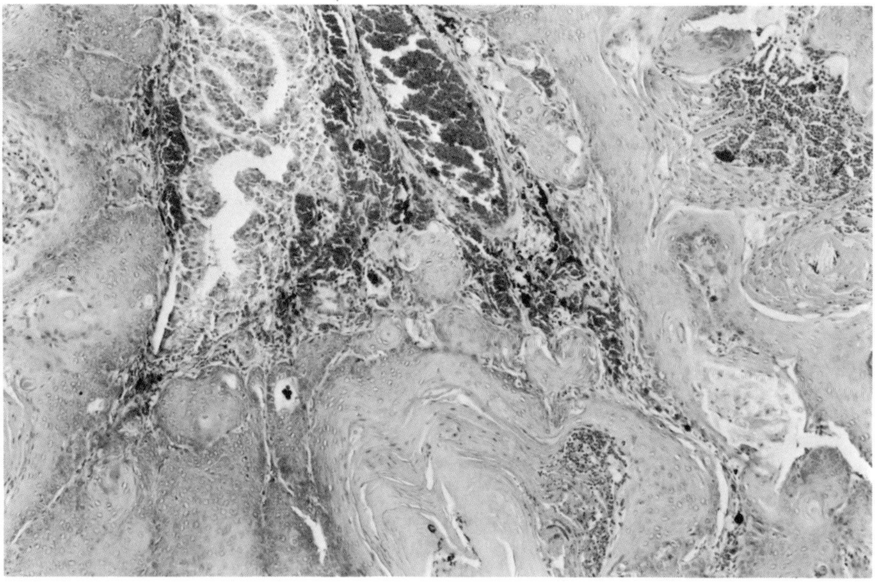

Fig. 13.5. Lung of a rat exposed to unfiltered diesel exhaust. Grade I squamous cell carcinoma (class 2). Tumor cells appear to be invading peribronchiolar/perivascular connective tissue. H & E, ×90.

atypia, moderate mitoses, and slight lack of polarity. In class 3 tumors (grade II carcinoma) definite stromal invasion occurs in lymphatic and blood vessels. Some scirrhous response is usually associated with these tumors. Class 4 tumors (grade III carcinoma) are composed of poorly differentiated cells, and mediastinal spread of tumor cells occurs.

Comparison of Pulmonary Tumors in Humans and Laboratory Rodents

Major epithelial tumors observed in humans and laboratory rodents are listed in Table 13.2. In laboratory rodents, especially in rats, pulmonary tumors usually occur in the peripheral regions, whereas in humans tumors occur predominantly in hilar regions. Although, as the table indicates, there has not been a rodent model of small-cell carcinomas up to now, recent work by Schuller and Witschi (16) indicates that combined use of imbalanced pulmonary oxygen levels and diethylnitrosamine in Syrian golden hamsters will produce a high incidence of small-cell carcinomas of the lung within 8 weeks.

Table 13.3 presents the carcinogenic potential of various inhaled substances which were examined in humans, rats, and hamsters. For humans, the data were obtained by epidemiological studies. Some substances, such as radionuclides, are

Table 13.2. Major pulmonary carcinomas observed in humans and laboratory rodents

	Human	Rat and hamster
Squamous-cell carcinoma	+	+
Large-cell carcinoma	+	+ (seldom)
Adenocarcinoma (bronchogenic)	+	+ (seldom)
Small-cell carcinoma	+	−
Bronchioloalveolar carcinoma	+	+

carcinogenic to the lung in humans as well as in both rats and hamsters. On the other hand, polycyclic aromatic hydrocarbons (PAH) and cigarette smoke, which induce pulmonary tumors in humans and rats, induce only tumors of the upper respiratory tract in hamsters. The second group in the table shows substances which are carcinogenic in humans and rats but not in hamsters. Tumor induction by diesel exhaust has been observed in rats only. As for humans, the epidemiological data concerning the tumor risk constituted by diesel exhaust are equivocal. As was outlined in the introduction, reasons for these differences between species must be established before reliable extrapolations can be made from rodents to humans.

Table 13.3. Inhaled substances causing pulmonary tumors in humans, rats, and hamsters

	Human	Rat	Hamster
Radioactive substances (51)	+	+	+
PAH with SO_2 or coal oven flue gas (52)	+	+	− (positive in the upper respiratory tract)
Cigarette smoke (53)	+	+	− (positive in the upper respiratory tract)
Asbestos (53)	+	+	+
Beryllium and its compounds (53)	+	+	−
Cadmium and its compounds (53–56)[a]	+	+	−
Nickel and its compounds (53)	+	+	−
Silica (57)[a]	+	+	−
Diesel exhaust (58)	?	+	−

[a]Although from epidemiological investigations it is strongly suspected that this compound is carcinogenic for humans, direct evidence is still limited because workers are usually exposed to a mixture of various compounds including silica or cadmium.

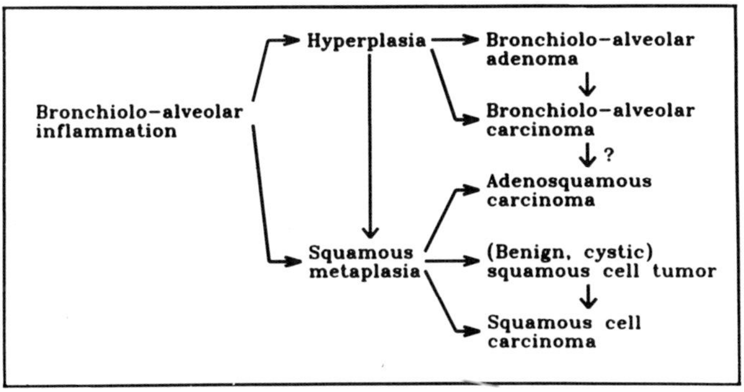

Fig. 13.6. Schematic outline of possible events occurring during pulmonary carcinogenesis.

Sequence of Carcinogenic Events

A schematic outline of possible events occurring during pulmonary carcinogenesis is shown in Fig. 13.6.

An important observation in rats is that the pattern of events leading to tumor development is different depending on whether a strong carcinogen or a weak carcinogen or cocarcinogen is involved. In studies with PAH-enriched coal oven flue gas (1) and of $^{239}PuO_2$ (17), pulmonary tumors developed in the absence of significant inflammatory responses. Figure 13.7 shows a benign squamous tumor without accompanying inflammation. By contrast, in lungs of rats exposed to diesel exhaust or some heavy metals, severe inflammation precedes the development of tumors (Fig. 13.8).

Slight to moderate squamous metaplasia was found mainly within the bronchioloalveolar inflammatory and hyperplastic lesions (Fig. 13.9). A more exaggerated type of squamous metaplasia characterized by nodular proliferation, with or without keratinization, was also observed (Fig. 13.10). There was confluent filling of alveolar spaces without appreciable disruption. The squamous cells were regular and lacked any evidence of dysplasia. In association with these changes, primary pulmonary tumors, i.e., bronchioloalveolar adenomas and squamous cell tumors, occurred in 16% of the rats exposed to diesel exhaust.

The constant association between severe inflammatory changes and development of squamous cell tumors in the lungs of rats exposed to diesel exhaust and absence of a correlation between inflammatory changes and tumors in rats exposed to PAH-enriched coal oven flue gas leads to the tentative conclusion that by causing severe persistent inflammation, particularly hyperplasia and metaplasia, diesel exhaust has a promotional effect rather than being a complete carcinogen. By contrast, PAH-enriched coal oven flue gas appears to be more of a complete carcinogen.

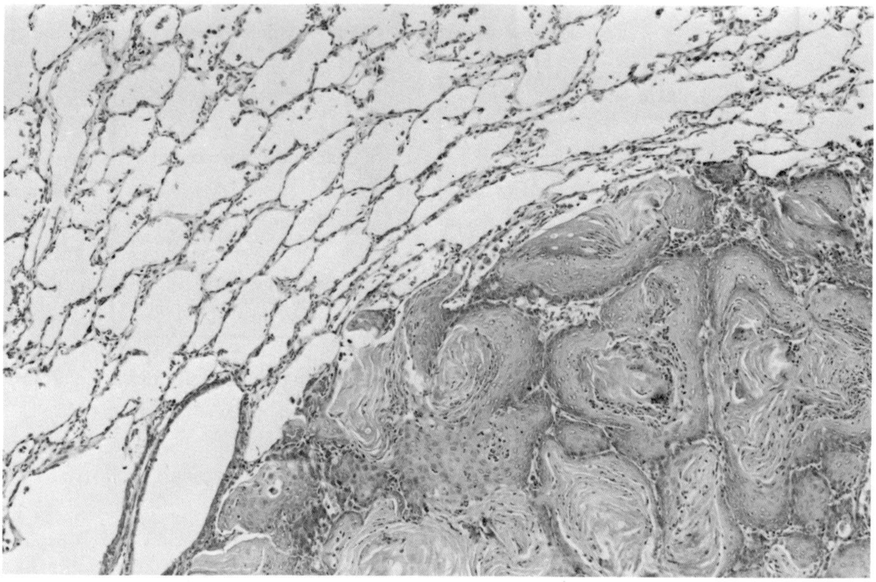

Fig. 13.7. Lung of a rat exposed to coal oven flue gas mixed with pyrolyzed pitch for 133 weeks. Benign, keratinizing, cystic squamous-cell tumor. Note relatively normal lung parenchyma except for compression adjacent to tumor: compare to Fig 8. H & E, ×90.

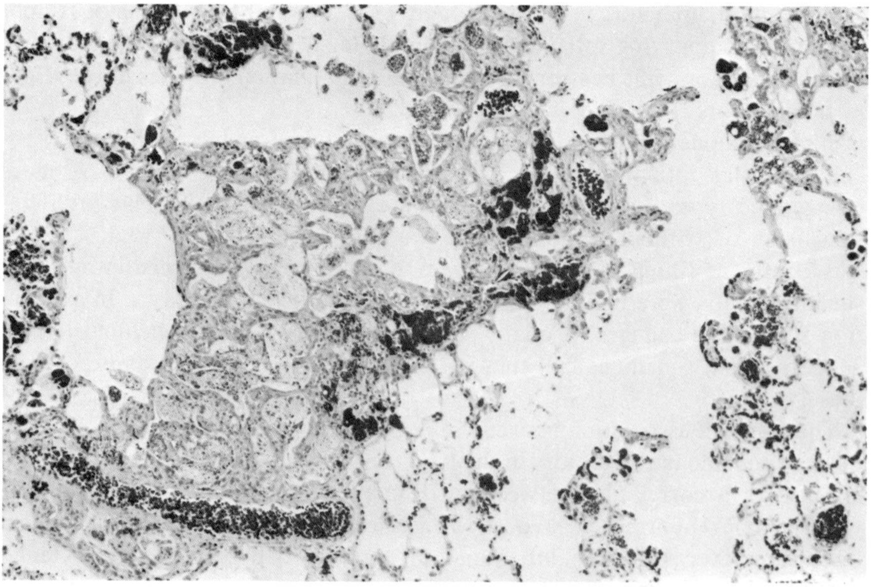

Fig. 13.8. Lung of a rat exposed to unfiltered diesel exhaust. Septal thickening by accumulation of large mononuclear cells and mild fibrosis. Masson-Goldner, ×180.

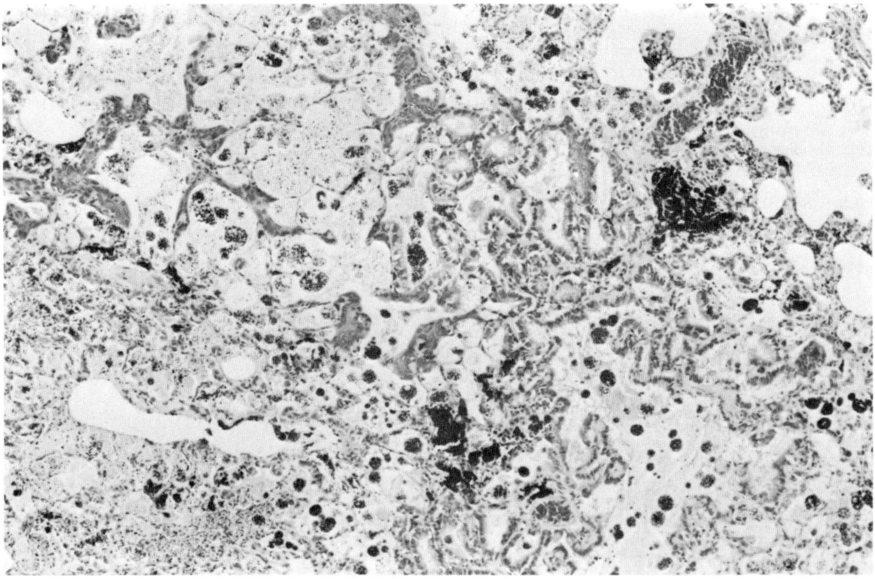

Fig. 13.9. Lung of a rat exposed to unfiltered diesel exhaust. Slight multifocal squamous metaplasia within the hyperplastic lesions. H & E, ×90.

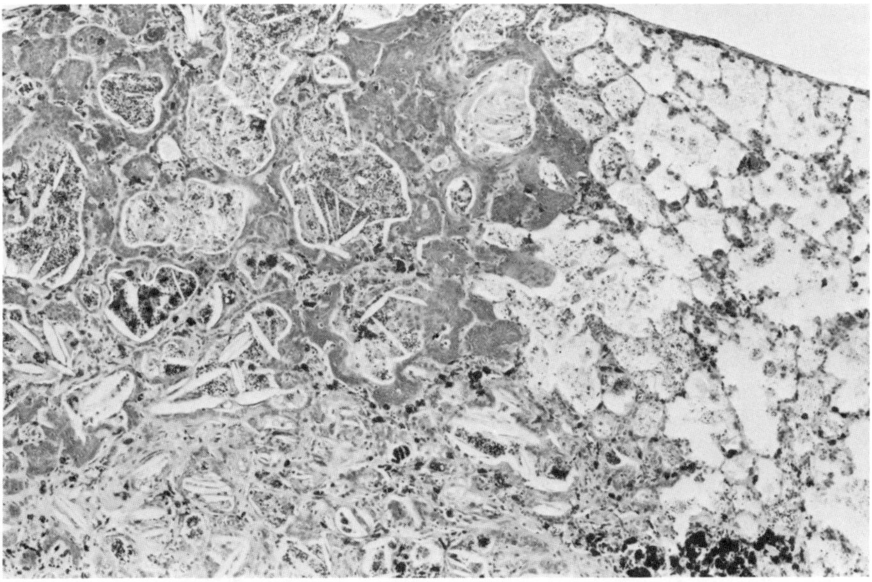

Fig. 13.10. Lung of a rat exposed to unfiltered diesel exhaust. Exaggerated squamous metaplasia with nodular proliferation and occasional keratinization. Cholesterol crystals are present at the periphery. H & E, ×90.

In lungs of hamsters exposed to diesel exhaust, marked deposition of carbonaceous pigments and slight bronchioloalveolar hyperplasia was observed. Unlike in lungs of rats exposed to diesel exhaust, there were neither severe inflammatory changes nor squamous metaplasia (Fig. 13.11). No primary pulmonary tumors occurred. Reasons for the differences between rat and hamster with respect to the amount of inflammation caused by inhaled particles such as those of diesel exhaust are unknown. A fruitful area for exploration would be differences between the two species in generation and release of inflammatory mediators by alveolar macrophages and epithelial cells.

Tumor Markers

Tumor markers are used for three main related purposes: providing clues for histogenetic classification; serving as criteria to aid in selection of therapeutic regimens; and for exploration of carcinogenetic mechanisms.

Major examples of functional markers which have been used in pulmonary carcinomas are cytokeratins, polypeptide hormones (e.g., ACTH and bombesin) and specific enzymes (e.g., neuron-specific enolase). Two important findings from use of these markers, as summarized by Carney (18), are that there is considerable heterogeneity in the expression of biomarkers within any one morphologic tumor type and that there is overlap in expression of markers among the different types of lung tumors. This variability in phenotypic expression among

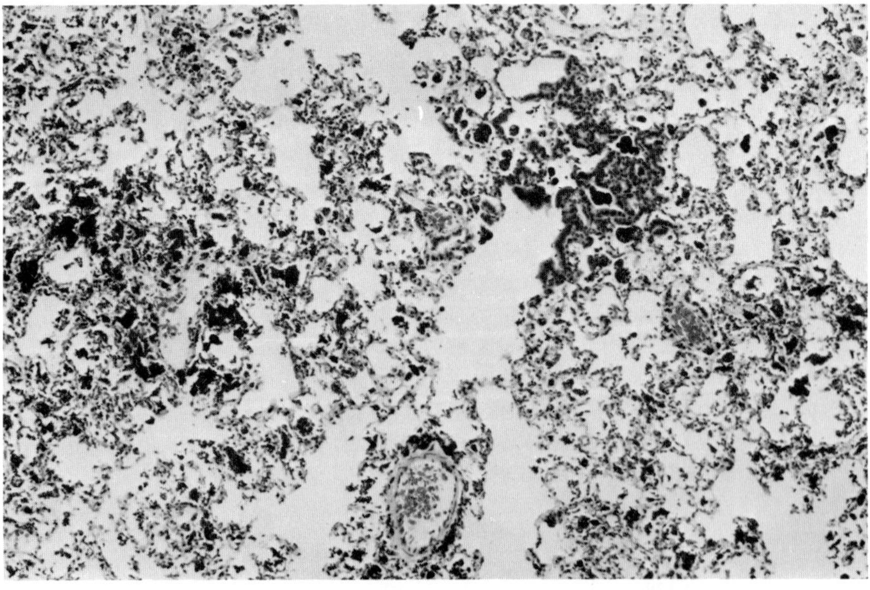

Fig. 13.11. Lung of a Syrian golden hamster exposed to unfiltered diesel exhaust. Slight bronchioloalveolar hyperplasia in association with the particle deposition. H & E, ×90.

lung tumors indicates that there is no constant relationship between the histologic type of tumor and cell of origin and hence implies that different tumors can have a common stem cell.

Increasing attention is being focused on the role of oncogene expression and amplification in tumorigenesis (19,20). As far as human lung tumors are concerned, most of the studies have been on the small-cell lung carcinoma (SCLC). Early work using transfection assays in NIH/3T3 mouse-cell lines indicated the possible importance of the *c-K-ras* oncogene (21), but this has not been substantiated (22). More recent studies using DNA hybridization techniques have implicated the *myc* family of oncogenes (particularly *c-myc* and *N-myc*) as playing an important part in the development of SCLC (18,23–26). Virtually nothing is known about oncogene activation in rodent lung tumors. Tetranitromethane-induced lung tumors of various histologic types have recently been reported to have activated *K-ras* oncogenes (27), but it is too early to draw conclusions regarding what this means relative to the role of specific oncogenes in lung tumors of humans. Although studies of oncogenes and their products have enormous potential, their relevance to risk assessment is uncertain at our current level of understanding.

In Vitro Studies

As already discussed, the types and incidence of tumors which are caused in the respiratory tissues by inhalation differ widely from species to species, including humans. This can at least partly be explained by variations in the epithelial cell type populations in different species (5). Ultrastructural variations in epithelial cells suggest differences in the biochemical activities of cells, such as their capacity for carcinogen activation and inactivation. In order to improve our understanding of the differences which exist between various species in response to a particular carcinogen, we need precise characterization, both morphologically and biochemically, of pertinent cell types in the respiratory epithelium. Since prediction and understanding of effects in humans is the final goal, this characterization must also be carried out in human cells. From cell culture studies, for instance, there is increasing awareness that, in comparison to rodent cells, human cells are much more resistant to malignant transformation by chemical carcinogens (12,28).

So far, only limited data have been published about in vitro chemical transformation of respiratory epithelial cells of various species. After treatment with nickel sulfate [29] or asbestos [30,31], human bronchial epithelial cells underwent transformation as revealed by morphological alterations, karyotypic changes, and prolonged survival. Fetal human tracheal epithelial cells demonstrated anchorage independency, slight tissue invasiveness, and prolonged survival after treatment with diethylnitrosamine [32]. In all of these cases, however, no tumor development was observed after implantation of the transformed cells into nude mice. By contrast, human fetal pulmonary epithelial cells transformed by methylcholanthrene in explant culture produced tumors resembling large-cell carcinomas when transplanted into nude mice [33]. It seems that anchorage independency or other phenotypical transformation does not necessarily lead so directly to malignancy in human epithelial cell systems as it does in most rodent epithelial cell systems. In fact, when rat tracheal epithelial cells were exposed to *N*-methyl-*N'*-nitro-*N*-nitrosoguanidine, preneoplastic cells occurred first, then they became anchorage independent, and only after an additional 11 or more weeks were they shown to be tumorigenic [34–36]. Transformation caused by the same carcinogen or benzo(*a*)pyrene in fetal Syrian hamster bronchioloalveologenic epithelial cells also required long latent periods, but the anchorage-independent cells eventually became tumorigenic [37,38]. Syrian hamster tracheal epithelial cells grown from explants treated with methylcholanthrene coated on inorganic metals also developed tumors after implantation in animals [39]. All these experiments were carried out by exposing the cells to test compounds dissolved or suspended directly in the culture media. This is an experimental condition comparable to the airway instillation of animals. These in vitro data were therefore mentioned to illustrate qualitative differences in susceptibility to malignant transformation between rodent and human cells. To make in vitro conditions quantitatively comparable to those of animal inhalation experiments, suitable gaseous or aerosol exposure chamber systems should be used [40]. There are still various critical problems to be solved, or at least improved, however, in such systems.

The reason for the observed refractoriness of human cells to chemical transformation in vitro is believed to be partly because the chromosomes are more stable and DNA repair is more rapid, proficient, and error-free in human cells than in rodent cells [11,12]. To prove the validity of this theory with regard to epithelial cells, we decided to obtain direct comparative data on in vitro responses of human and rodent cells to chemical carcinogens. Underlying this decision was our over-

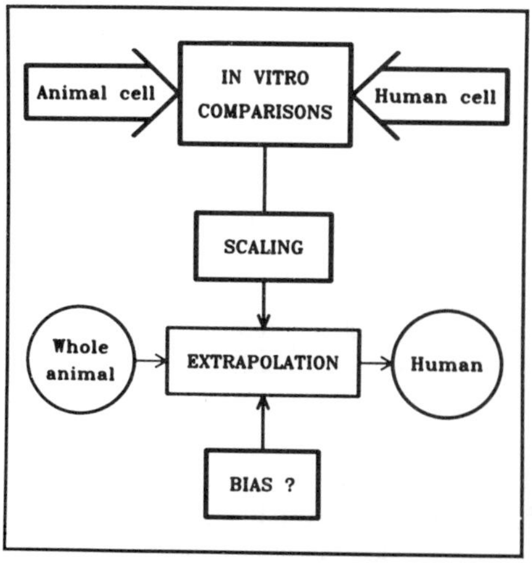

Fig. 13.12. Overall working hypothesis concerning accurate extrapolation of animal data to humans.

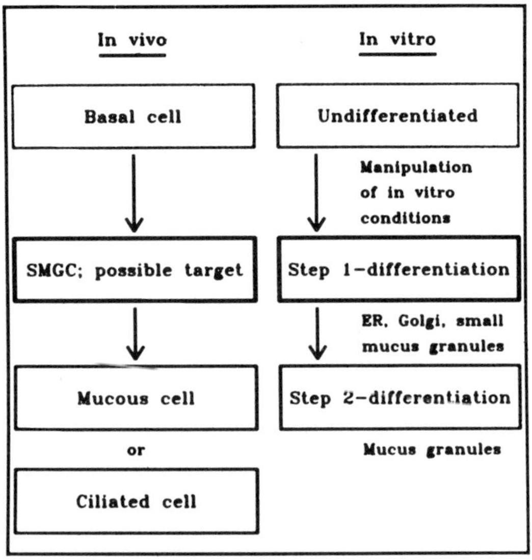

Fig. 13.13. Comparison of morphological features of hamster fetal bronchioloalveologenic epithelial cells in vitro to those of regenerating bronchiolar epithelial cells in intact hamsters.

all working hypothesis concerning accurate extrapolation of animal data to humans, which is presented schematically in Fig. 13.12.

Conventional extrapolation involves use of data from animal studies to predict effects in humans, as shown across the bottom of the figure. This affords an opportunity for considerable bias, because of the large number of assumptions which must be made in this process. Examples of possible biases are the extent of the "health conservative" approach and assumptions about threshold and low-dose extrapolation. The most important point to be made from Fig. 13.12 is that as more quantitative data on in vitro comparisons between human and animal cells becomes available for scaling purposes the unwanted influence of bias decreases.

One major drawback of cell culture systems is that, after removal from the animal and transference into an artificial culture environment, the cells rapidly lose their differentiated phenotypes, including capability for xenobiotic metabolism (41,42). Therefore, the validity of in vitro data for the in vivo state depends on how far the culture system simulates the in vivo condition. Recently, we have developed a culture system which provides to some extent both morphologically and biochemically comparable cells to those in vivo (38), although refinements are still needed.

Figure 13.13 compares some morphological features of fetal hamster bronchioloalveologenic epithelial cells cultured in our system to those of regenerating bronchiolar epithelial cells in intact hamsters. Since the capacity for carcinogen metabolism is closely associated with the extent of cellular differentiation, our efforts have been focused on the development of techniques by which the respiratory cells can either be maintained for an extended time in culture without losing differentiated phenotypes or can be stimulated to differentiate from an initially undifferentiated state.

Table 13.4. Enzyme level

Enzyme	Undifferentiated	Step 1 differentiation
NADPH cytochrome *c* reductase	Low	High
Ethoxycoumarin deethylase	Low	High

By adding hormones and growth factors to the culture medium and using collagen gel as the substratum on which the cells grow, our goal was partly achieved. Under these conditions, cells undergo step 1 differentiation, characterized by well-developed endoplasmic reticulum and Golgi apparatus, occasional small mucous granules, and an irregular cycle of stimulated DNA synthesis (38). The cells at this stage of differentiation closely resemble the "small mucous granule cells" which have been postulated to be a target of chemical carcinogens in the bronchi (43,44). Cells at this step 1 differentiation are susceptible to indirect-acting carcinogens, while cells at the undifferentiated stage are not. Step 2 differentiation, at which stage the cells produce mucous granules, is facilitated by the presence of vitamin A.

Table 13.4 shows the higher levels of NADPH-dependent cytochrome *c* reductase and ethoxycoumarin deethylase in cells at step 1 differentiation than at the undifferentiated stage.

Table 13.5 shows the much higher rates of benz(*a*)anthracene decomposition in cells at step 1 differentiation than at the undifferentiated stage.

Treatment with benzo(*a*)pyrene yielded thioguanine-resistant colonies (mutation at HPRT gene) in cells at step 1 differentiation, whereas it did not in undifferentiated cells (Table 13.6).

Anchorage-independent transformation was inducible by benzo(*a*)pyrene treatment in cells at step 1 differentiation but not in the undifferentiated cells (Table 13.7).

It was pointed out earlier in this paper that most of the bronchioloalveolar tumors in lungs of rats exposed to diesel exhaust arose from inflammatory hyperplastic and/or metaplastic foci. Similar foci were found in healing tracheal epithelia of Syrian hamsters after mechanical injury (45), and a considerable number of cells in the foci exhibited features in common with small mucous granule cells (44). Therefore, these hyperplastic/metaplastic cells in the inflammatory foci may be analogous to the cells at step 1 differentiation in vitro.

Table 13.5. Percentage of Benz(*a*)anthracene decomposed

Incubation h	Undifferentiated cells (%)	Step 1 differentiation (%)
0	–	2
22	< 2	31
48	< 4	41

Table 13.6. Colonies resistant to 6-thioguanine after treatment with benzo(*a*)pyrene

BaP (μg/ml)	Undifferentiated cells (%)	Step 1 differentiation (%)
0	< 0.003	0.003
4	< 0.005	0.013
8	< 0.005	0.615

In our cell culture system, we can therefore see some functional and morphological links to in vivo events. Using this system we have now compared Syrian hamster and human cells. Both cell lines are bronchioloalveologenic epithelial cells derived from fetuses (a female hamster fetus on day 15 of gestation and a female human fetus in week 18 of pregnancy). The culture conditions are identical for the cells of both species.

We first compared the capability for metabolism of the indirect-acting PAH, chrysene, in the cells of both species. This was done by measuring the amount of unmetabolized chrysene after various periods of incubation starting on day 8 of culture (Fig. 13.14). In both 3- and 8-day incubations, the hamster cells metabolized chrysene about 26-fold more actively than the human cells. In Fig. 13.15, the amount of critical metabolites, dihydrodiols, are compared. Essentially, all of the dihydrodiols were recovered from the water-soluble phase after incubation with β-glucuronidase/aryl sulphatase; gas chromatological analyses were done by Professors Jacob and Grimmer (Biochemisches Institut für Umweltcarcinogene, Großhansdorf, Federal Republic of Germany). Within 8 days of incubation, hamster cells produced about 3-fold more 1,2-dihydrodiol than human cells, while both hamster and human cells produced the same amount of 3,4-dihydrodiol. Since 1,2-dihydrodiol of chrysene has been regarded as the proximate carcinogen, this data suggests that the hamster cells are more susceptible to a carcinogen such as chrysene than are human cells.

High genetic stability is another factor believed to be responsible for human cell refractoriness to in vitro chemical transformation as compared with rodent cells. We set out to prove this hypothesis by examining the effects of ethylnitrosourea on the same cell lines as used for the studies of chrysene metabolism. The parameters selected for the comparison were cytotoxicity, chromatid breaks, unscheduled DNA synthesis, and 6-thioguanine-resistant mutation on the HPRT gene.

Table 13.7. Anchorage-independent transformation after treatment with benzo(*a*)pyrene

BaP (μg/ml)	Undifferentiated cells (%)	Step 1 differentiation (%)
0	~0	0.009
2	~0	0.2
4	~0	0.9
8	~0	0.8

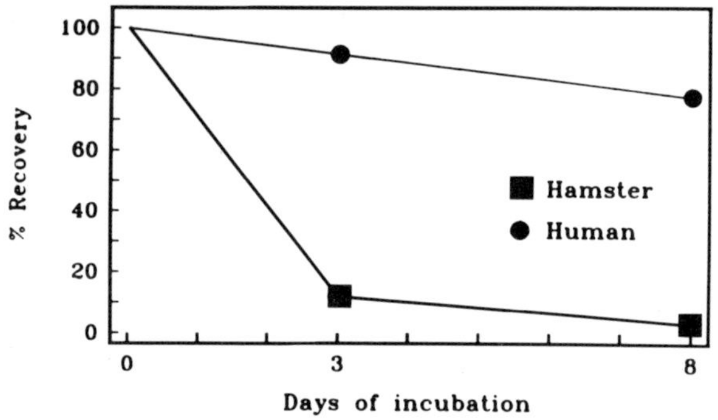

Fig. 13.14. Recovery of unmetabolized chrysene on different days of its incubation with the human and hamster fetal bronchioloalveologenic epithelial cells in vitro.

The toxicity of ethylnitrosourea (ENU) at higher doses was a little stronger in hamster cells than in human cells, although the difference was not marked (Fig. 13.16).

In Fig. 13.17, the incidence of chromatid breaks in the cells of both species is compared. At higher doses, it was much higher in hamster cells than in human cells. The incidence of sister chromatid exchange was also strikingly higher in hamster cells than in human cells at the higher dose range (data not shown).

We further compared the intensity of unscheduled DNA synthesis (UDS) in the cells of both species. Fig. 13.18 clearly indicates that the index of repair of damaged DNA was much less in human cells than in hamster cells throughout the whole dose range of ethylnitrosourea.

These data allow several interpretations. One interpretation is that the human-cell DNA was so little damaged by ethylnitrosourea that only a small amount of

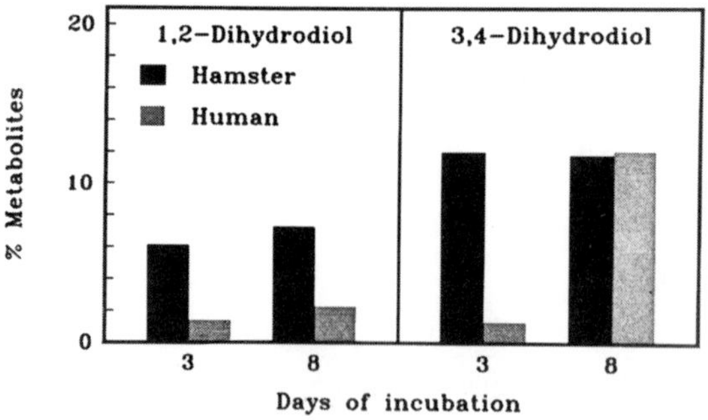

Fig. 13.15. Comparison of critical metabolites of chrysene, 1,2- and 3,4-dihydrodiols, after 8-day incubation with the human and hamster fetal bronchioloalveologenic epithelial cells in vitro.

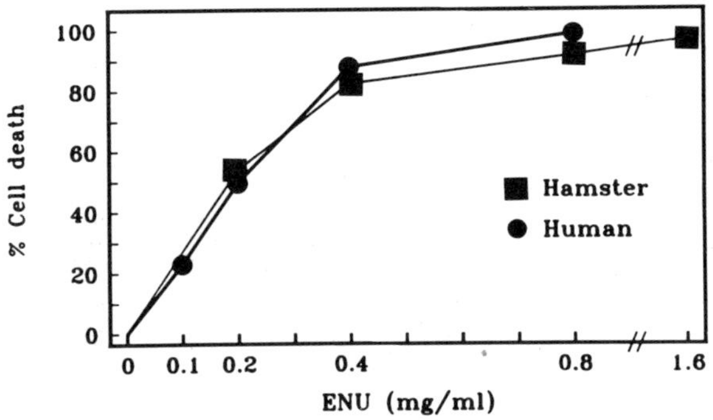

Fig. 13.16. Comparison of ENU toxicity in human and hamster fetal bronchioloalveologenic epithelial cells in vitro.

repair was needed. A second interpretation is that the mechanism of DNA repair in human cells is so precise that it is directed only toward damaged DNA sequences, whereas in hamster cells the process is more crude and large patches of DNA are excised together with damaged sequences for "repair". A third interpretation is that the human cells possess a larger thymidine pool than hamster cells (46). The fourth, unlikely interpretation is that human cells have inherently much lower activity of DNA repair as compared to the hamster cells. At present we have no specific data relative to one or other of these interpretations. In the light of data available in the literature, the first and second interpretations appear to be most plausible (47–49). The first interpretation is based on the assumption that access of damaging agents to the critical sites of DNA is much more difficult in human cells than in hamster cells. To prove this point, DNA adduct formation and the uptake of ethylnitrosourea will be investigated. As to

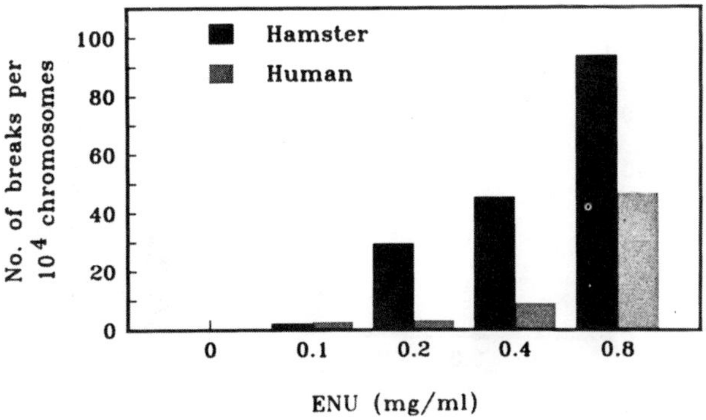

Fig. 13.17. Comparison of chromatid break frequency induced by ENU in human and hamster fetal bronchioloalveologenic epithelial cells in vitro.

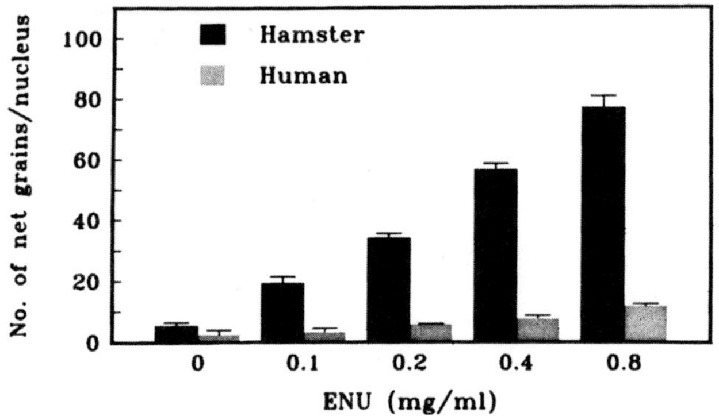

Fig. 13.18. Comparison of unscheduled DNA synthesis induced by ENU in human and hamster fetal bronchioloalveologenic epithelial cells in vitro.

the second interpretation, an experimental approach would be to demonstrate an excess of excision enzymes capable of attacking large sequences of DNA.

Ethylnitrosourea induced far more frequent mutations at the HPRT gene locus in hamster cells than in human cells (Fig. 13.19), as detected by resistance to 6-thioguanine. Since this drug resistance is the result of gene mutation caused by O^6-ethylguanine persistence (50), this and previous UDS data may indicate that the repair mechanisms in hamster cells are less efficient and more error-prone, or even more aberrant, than those in human cells.

The general conclusion from these in vitro data is that hamster cells appear to be significantly more susceptible to the genotoxicity of ethylnitrosourea than human cells. Furthermore, within a limited period of incubation with chrysene, hamster cells produced a larger amount of proximate carcinogenic metabolite than the human cells. These results may explain the greater susceptibility to in

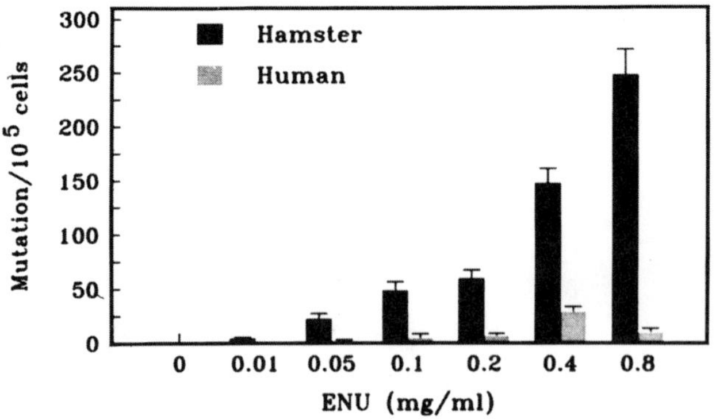

Fig. 13.19. Comparison of ENU-induced mutation at the HPRT gene locus in human and hamster fetal bronchioloalveologenic epithelial cells in vitro.

vitro chemical transformation of hamster cells over that of human cells. Complete reliance cannot be placed on in vitro comparisons, however, because it is unlikely that they would completely explain, for instance, the difference between human epidemiological evidence of carcinogenesis by heavy metals and the lack of evidence thus far in hamsters (see Table 13.3). We say this while recognizing that the relevant in vitro data is not yet available. In vivo dosimetry and the interplay of factors affecting growth and differentiation of epithelial populations in intact animals must be taken into account. Examples of the latter are epithelial-epithelial and epithelial-mesenchymal interactions, neuroendocrine influences, and the role of chronic inflammation and immune responses.

Conclusions

In a qualitative sense, there is good reason for suspecting that an inhaled agent causing tumors in the respiratory tract of the rat and/or hamster could be capable of causing tumors in humans. There are few available data, however, relevant to the quantitative relationships between the various mechanistic stages of carcinogenesis in rodents as compared to humans. Information now being developed on comparative dosimetry, toxicokinetics, and carcinogenetic mechanisms should permit some precision in the risk assessment exercise in the near future.

References

1. Mohr U, Takenaka S, Dungworth DL (1986) Morphologic effects of inhaled diesel engine exhaust on lungs of rats: comparison with effects of coal oven flue gas mixed with pyrolyzed pitch. In: Ishinishi N, Koizumi A, McClellan RO, Stöber W (eds) Carcinogenic and mutagenic effects of diesel engine exhaust. Elsevier, Amsterdam, pp 459–470 (Developments in toxicology and environmental science, vol 13)
2. Raabe OG, Yeh H-C, Newton GJ, Phalen RF, Velasquez DJ (1977) Deposition of inhaled monodisperse aerosols in small rodents. In: Walton WH (ed) Inhaled particles IV. Pergamon, Oxford, pp 3–20
3. Schreiber H, Martin DH, Pazmino N (1975) Species differences in the effect of benzo(*a*)pyrene-ferric oxide on the respiratory tract of rats and hamsters. Cancer Res 35:1654–1661
4. Brain JD, Mensah GA (1983) Comparative toxicology of the respiratory tract. Am Rev Respir Dis 128:s87-s90
5. Plopper CG, Mariassy AT, Wilson DW, Alley JL, Nishio SJ, Nettesheim P (1983) Comparison of nonciliated tracheal epithelial cells in six mammalian species: ultrastructure and population densities. Exp Lung Res 5:281–294
6. Abramson FP, Robinson D, Bai SA (1983) Relationships between propranolol plasma protein binding, glycoprotein concentration, and enzyme induction following phenobarbital administration in the dog. Biochem Pharmacol 32:2618–2620
7. Prough RA, Patrizi VW, Okita RT, Masters BSS, Jakobsson SW (1979) Characteristics of benzo(*a*)pyrene metabolism by kidney, liver, and lung microsomal fractions from rodents and humans. Cancer Res 39:1199–1206

8. Mass MJ, Kaufman DG (1983) Species differences in the activation of benzo(*a*)pyrene in the tracheal epithelium of rats and hamsters. Basic Life Sci 24:331–351
9. Schreiber H, Nettesheim P, Martin DH (1972) Rapid development of bronchiolo-alveolar squamous cell tumors in rats after intratracheal injection of 3-methylcholanthrene. J Nat Cancer Inst 49:541–554
10. Nettesheim P, Marchok A (1983) Neoplastic development in airway epithelium. Adv Cancer Res 39:1–69
11. Maher VM, Ouellette LM, Curren RD, McCormick JJ (1976) Frequency of ultraviolet light-induced mutations is higher in xeroderma pigmentosum variant cells than in normal human cells. Nature 261:593–595
12. DiPaolo JA (1983) Relative difficulties in transforming human and animal cells in vitro. J Nat Cancer Inst 70:3–8
13. Yuspa SH (1984) Mechanisms of initiation and promotion in mouse epidermis. IARC Sci Pub 56:191–204
14. Thomassen DG (1986) Role of spontaneous transformation in carcinogenesis: development of preneoplastic rat tracheal epithelial cells at a constant rate. Cancer Res 46:2344–2348
15. Brand KG, Buoen LC, Johnson KH, Brand I (1975) Etiological factors, stages, and the role of the foreign body in foreign body tumorigenesis: a review. Cancer Res 35:279–286
16. Schuller HM, Witschi HP (1987) A novel in vivo model for the induction of carcinoids and small cell cancer of the lung (meeting abstract). Toxicologist 7:19
17. Rhoads K, Mahassey JA, Sanders CL (1981) A morphometric study of rat and hamster lung following inhalation of $^{239}PuO_2$. Rad Res 88:266–279
18. Carney DN (1986) Recent advances in the biology of small cell lung cancer. Chest 89:253S-257S
19. Barbacid M (1986) Oncogenes and human cancer: cause or consequence. Carcinogenesis 7:1037–1042
20. Alitalo K, Schwab M (1986) Oncogene amplification in tumor cells. Adv Cancer Res 47:235–281
21. Yamamoto F, Nakano H, Neville C, Perucho M (1985) Structure and mechanisms of activation of *c-K-ras* oncogenes in human lung cancer. Prog Med Virol 32:101–114
22. Milici A, Blick M, Murphy E, Gutterman JU (1986) *c-K-ras* Codon 12 GGT-CGT point mutation: an infrequent event in human lung cancer. Biochem Biophys Res Comm 140:699–705
23. Chan SYT, Evan GI, Ritson A, Watson J, Wraight P, Sikora K (1986) Localisation of lung cancer by a radiolabelled monoclonal antibody against the *c-myc* oncogene product. Br J Cancer 5:761–769
24. Nau MM, Brooks BJ Jr, Carney DN, Gazdar AF, Battey JF, Sausville EA, Minna JD (1986) Human small-cell lung cancers show amplification and expression of the *N-myc* gene. Proc Nat Acad Sci USA 83:1092–1096
25. Saksela K, Bergh J, Nilsson K (1986) Amplification of the *N-myc* oncogene in an adenocarcinoma of the lung. J Cell Biochem 31:297–304
26. Wong AJ, Ruppert JM, Eggleston J, Hamilton SR, Baylin SB, Vogelstein B (1986) Gene amplification of *c-myc* and *N-myc* in small cell carcinoma of the lung. Science 233:461–464
27. Stowers SJ, Glover PL, Reynolds SH, Boone LR, Maronpot RR, Anderson MW (1987) Activation of the *K-ras* oncogene in lung tumors from rats and mice chronically exposed to tetranitromethane. Cancer Res, in press

28. Harris CC (1987) Human tissues and cells in carcinogenesis research. Cancer Res 47:1–10
29. Lechner JF, Tokiwa T, McClendon IA, Haugen A (1984) Effects of nickel sulfate on growth and differentiation of normal human bronchial epithelial cells. Carcinogenesis 5:1697–1703
30. Lechner JF, Haugen A, Trump BF, Tokiwa T, Harris CC (1983) Effects of asbestos and carcinogenic metals on cultured human bronchial epithelium. In: Harris CC, Autrup H (eds) Human carcinogenesis. Academic, New York, pp 561–588
31. Lechner JF, Tokiwa T, LaVeck M, Benedict WF, Banks-Schlegel S, Yeager H Jr, Banerjee A, Harris CC (1985) Asbestos-associated chromosomal changes in human mesothelial cells. Proc Natl Acad Sci USA 82:3884–3888
32. Emura M, Mohr U, Kakunaga T, Hilfrich J (1985) Growth inhibition and transformation of a human fetal tracheal epithelial cell line by long-term exposure to diethylnitrosamine. Carcinogenesis 6:1079–1085
33. Yoshida Y, Hattori A, Mori M (1983) Transformation of human lung cells by 3-methylcholanthrene in vitro. Gann 74:615–618
34. Steele VE, Marchok AC, Nettesheim P (1979) Oncogenic transformation in epithelial cell lines derived from tracheal explants exposed in vitro to *N*-methyl-*N'*-nitro-*N*-nitrosoguanidine. Cancer Res 39:3805–3811
35. Pai SB, Steele VE, Nettesheim P (1983) Neoplastic transformation of primary tracheal epithelial cell cultures. Carcinogenesis 4:369–374
36. Thomassen DG, Gray TE, Mass MJ, Barrett JC (1983) High frequency of carcinogen-induced early, preneoplastic changes in rat tracheal epithelial cells in culture. Cancer Res 43:5956–5963
37. Emura M, Richter-Reichhelm H-B, Böning W, Eichinger R, Schoch C, Althoff J, Mohr U (1982) A fetal respiratory epithelial cell line for studying some problems of transplacental carcinogenesis in Syrian golden hamsters. J Cancer Res Clin Oncol 104:133–144
38. Emura M, Mohr U, Riebe M, Aufderheide M, Dungworth DL (1987) Predisposition of cloned fetal hamster lung epithelial cells to transformation by a precarcinogen, benzo(*a*)pyrene, using growth hormone supplementation and collagen gel substratum. Cancer Res 47:1155–1160
39. Mossmann BT, Craighead JE (1979) Use of hamster tracheal organ cultures for assessing the cocarcinogenic effects of inorganic particulates on the respiratory epithelium. Prog Exp Tumor Res 24:37–47
40. Rasmussen RE, Crocker TT (1981) A culture system for the direct exposure of mammalian cells to airborne pollutants. In: Waters MD, Sandhu SS, Huisingh JL, Claxton L, Nesnow S (eds) Short-term bioassays in the analysis of complex environmental mixtures II. Plenum, New York, pp 119–131
41. Acosta D, Anuforo DC, McMillin R, Soine WH, Smith RV (1979) Comparison of cytochrome P-450 levels in adult rat liver, postnatal rat liver, and primary cultures of postnatal rat hepatocytes. Life Sci 25:1413–1418
42. Lake BG, Paine AJ (1982) The effect of hepatocyte culture conditions on cytochrome P-450 linked drug metabolising enzymes. Biochem Pharmacol 31:2141–2144
43. Trump BF, McDowell EM, Glavin F, Barrett LA, Becci PJ, Schürch W, Kaiser HE, Harris CC (1978) The respiratory epithelium. III. Histogenesis of epidermoid metaplasia and carcinoma in situ in the human. J Nat Cancer Inst 61:565–575
44. McDowell EM, Trump BF (1983) Histogenesis of preneoplastic and neoplastic lesions in tracheobronchial epithelium. Surv Synth Pathol Res 2:235–279

45. Keenan KP, Wilson TS, McDowell EM (1983) Regeneration of hamster tracheal epithelium after mechanical injury. IV. Histochemical, immunocytochemical and ultrastructural studies. Virchows Arch Cell Path 43:213–240
46. Yagi T, Nikaido O, Takebe H (1984) Excision repair of mouse and human fibroblast cells, and a factor affecting the amount of UV-induced unscheduled DNA synthesis. Mut Res 132:101–112
47. Warren W, Grathorn AR, Shooter KV (1979) The stability of methylated purines and of methylphosphotriesters in the DNA of V79 cells after treatment with *N*-methyl-*N*-nitrosourea. Biochim Biophys Acta 563:82–88
48. Goth-Goldstein R (1980) Inability of Chinese hamster ovary cells to excise O^6-alkylguanine. Cancer Res 40:2623–2624
49. Gerson SL, Trey JE, Miller K, Benjamin E (1987) Repair of O^6-alkylguanine during DNA synthesis in murine bone marrow hematopoietic precursors. Cancer Res 47:89–95
50. Bodell WJ, Singer B, Thomas GH, Cleaver JE (1979) Evidence for removal at different rates of *O*-ethyl pyrimidines and ethylphosphotriesters in two human fibroblast cell lines. Nucleic Acid Res 6:2819–2829
51. Hahn FF (1985) Radiation-induced squamous cell carcinoma, lung of rodents. In: Jones TC, Mohr U, Hunt RD (eds) Respiratory system. Springer, Berlin Heidelberg New York, pp 127–133
52. Heinrich U, Muhle H, Koch W, Mohr U (1985) Long-term inhalation studies with rodents. In: Homburger F (ed) Safety evaluation and regulation of chemicals 2. Karger, Basel, pp 241–250
53. Wilbourn J, Haroun L, Heseltine E, Kaldor J, Partensky C, Vainio H (1986) Response of experimental animals to human carcinogens: an analysis based upon the IARC monographs programme. Carcinogenesis 7:1853–1863
54. Liemen RA, Lee JS, Wagoner JK, Blejer HP (1976) Cancer mortality among cadmium production workers. Ann NY Acad Sci 271:273–279
55. Takenaka S, Oldiges M, König H, Hochrainer D, Oberdörster G (1983) Carcinogenicity of cadmium chloride aerosols in W rats. J Nat Cancer Inst 70:367–373
56. Thun MJ, Schnorr TM, Smith AB, Halperin WE, Lemen RA (1985) Mortality among a cohort of US cadmium production workers—an update. J Nat Cancer Inst /4:325–333
57. Goldsmith DF, Winn DM, Shy CM (eds) (1986) Silica, silicosis, and cancer. Praeger, New York
58. Heinrich U, Muhle H, Takenaka S, Ernst H, Fuhst R, Mohr U, Pott F, Stöber W (1986) Chronic effects on the respiratory tract of hamsters, mice and rats after long-term inhalation of high concentrations of filtered and unfiltered diesel engine emissions. J Appl Toxicol 6:383–395

CHAPTER 14

Experimentally Induced Emphysema and Long-Term Nitrogen Dioxide Inhalation

J. Kleinerman[1] and M.P.C. Ip[1]

For more years than I care to say, my colleagues and I have attempted to produce emphysema experimentally in laboratory animals (1–3). By emphysema I mean the disease affecting the lung parenchyma in which the air spaces are enlarged as a result of loss of tissue substance or destruction of parenchyma, but where the enlargement occurs without associated fibrosis or scarring. This enlargement of airspaces may occur with or without compromise of function.

Our major effort has involved exposure to relatively high concentrations of nitrogen dioxide (NO_2) for long periods. NO_2 is an attractive agent because (a) it and its congeners are present in cigarette smoke in high concentrations, (b) it is present in low concentrations in the polluted urban air, and (c) exposure in animals is known to produce injury to the terminal bronchioles, respiratory bronchioles, and proximal alveolar ducts. This injury may lead to bronchiolitis obliterans, an obstructive inflammatory lesion in the bronchioles.

Our early studies indicated that to produce an inflammatory and proliferative lesion in the terminal airways requires exposure to levels of 20–30 ppm for at least 5 days (4). However, despite continued exposure at this level for several weeks, when the lungs were studied histologically, we could find no evidence of bronchiolitis obliterans and no evidence of emphysema.

Clinical studies of human emphysema teach us that it is a chronic insidious disease which is rarely observed before the 5th or 6th decade of life. We therefore postulated that a long chronic exposure to the experimental agent was required for the development of emphysema in animal models. This hypothesis prompted us to develop experimental protocols of NO_2 exposure of 12 or more months. Our analysis were therefore unlike any kind of acute toxicologic study. The experimental subjects were exposed for long periods to high concentrations of NO_2. This protocol is unusual in the study of the common toxicologic agents, but it does have some resemblance to the NO_2 exposures experienced by chronic heavy cigarette smokers. This is the approach of the experimental pathologists in pursuit of a chronic respiratory disease of humans.

[1]Department of Pathology, Case Western Reserve University, Cleveland Metropolitan General Hospital, 3395 Scranton Road, Cleveland, Ohio 44109, USA.

Table 14.1. Lung volumes (LV), mean linear intercept (MLI), and internal surface area (ISA) in hamsters exposed to NO_2 for 12 months (mean ± SE)

	n	LV (ml)	MLI (mm)	ISA (cm²)
Control	6	6.38 ± 0.63	0.62 ± .02	2145 ± 44
NO_2	6	6.39 ± 0.33	0.82 ± .02*	1773 ± 51*

$*p < 0.05$

Male Syrian hamsters 90–100 g in weight were exposed in large Plexiglas chambers to 30±5 ppm NO_2 (2). Exposures were for 20–22 h/day, 7 days/week for 365 days. Comparable groups were housed in an adjacent chamber and exposed to room air. Immediately after the last day of exposure the exposed hamsters and comparable controls were sacrificed. At postmortem, the lungs of the exposed animals showed evidence of a significant increase in mean linear intercept (MLI) and a decrease in internal surface area (ISA) and in morphometrically determined elastin fiber length of the lung (Table 14.1).

These findings are consistent with those present in human emphysema of mild degree, and suggest that we had indeed induced emphysema in the hamster lungs. Because the emphysema was of limited extent, and so as to rule out the possibility that the changes represented a reversible form of overdistention, the exposures were repeated for a period of 9 months with the addition of study groups that were removed from the NO_2 after 9 months and killed after further periods of 3, 6, and 9 months in room air. The purpose of this was to determine whether the changes observed after 9 months were permanent.

The data in Table 14.2 confirm the increase in MLI and the decrease in ISA after 9 months' exposure, and indicate that these changes persist after animals are removed from the NO_2 for up to 9 months. These studies also confirm that the alterations in MLI and ISA observed after prolonged NO_2 exposure are irreversible.

Nevertheless, the changes observed in the lung parenchyma histologically after 9 months' NO_2 exposure were not characteristic of well-developed centriacinar or panacinar emphysema in humans. For this reason we required additional evidence that there had indeed been destruction of lung tissue. We proposed to look for biochemical evidence of lung tissue destruction. It is well established that in human emphysema there is a destruction of lung elastin (5). A breakdown

Table 14.2. Lung volumes, mean linear intercept, and internal surface area in NO_2-exposed hamsters after 9 months' exposure and 9 months' recovery in air (mean ± SE)

	LV (ml)	MLI (mm)	ISA (cm²)
Control	5.59 ± 0.13	0.71 ± 0.06	2434 ± 151
NO_2	5.64 ± 0.18	1.06 ± 0.02*	1762 ± 55*

$*p < 0.05$

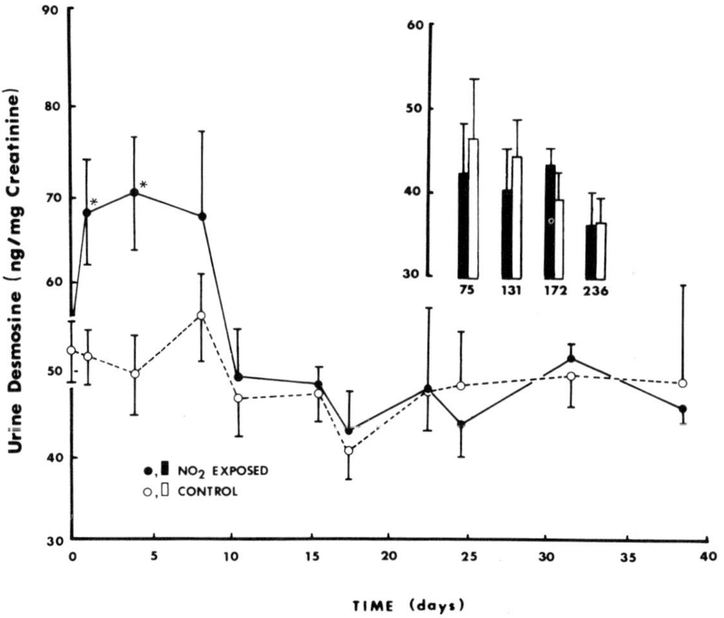

Fig. 14.1. Daily urine desmosine concentrations expressed as ng/mg creatinine during 40 consecutive days of NO_2 exposure and at 75, 131, 172, and 236 days after NO_2.

product of lung elastin is the amino acid desmosine. Desmosine is a unique and specific marker of elastolysis and is not absorbed from the gastrointestinal tract. It is excreted in the urinary tract and acts as an indicator of endogenous elastin catabolism. The daily urinary content of desmosine was determined by radioimmunoassay and related to the creatinine content of the urine (6,7). These studies were done both in NO_2-exposed and control hamsters for 236 days.

Figure 14.1 demonstrates that only during the first 9–10 days of exposure was the urinary excretion of desmosine increased significantly. This finding suggests that the elastin destruction occurs only during the first 10 days of NO_2 exposure and not thereafter. This may explain why the emphysema which occurred after the NO_2 exposure was so limited in extent. The urinary desmosine studies and the morphometric findings after NO_2 exposure indicated that in these circumstances emphysema develops early in the course of the exposure and is mild in extent. Moreover the lesion does not progress with continued exposure.

It appeared important to evaluate whether the determinants involved in the pathogenesis of emphysema were perturbed and if so, how. Our current hypothesis concerning the development of emphysema in humans is based on a balance of proteolytic and antiproteolytic substances in the lung (8). The proteolytic materials are derived mainly from the granular component of the neutrophil and the macrophage. The antiproteolytic materials are derived primarily from the plasma and consist of α1-protease inhibitor (α_1PI) and α-2-macroglobulin

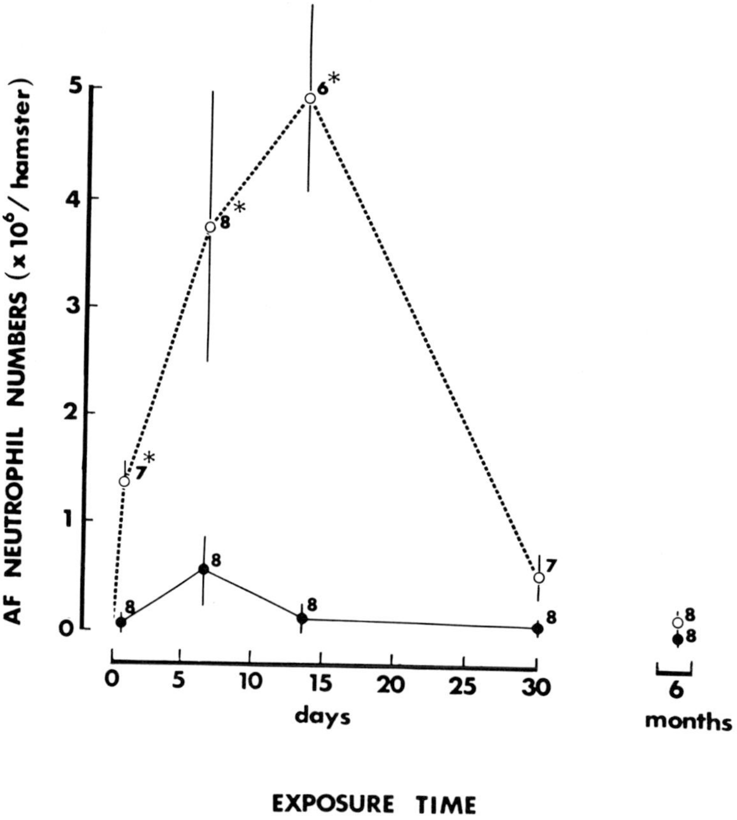

Fig. 14.2. Alveolar fluid neutrophil concentration during exposure to NO_2. The filled line and closed circle represent the controls, the dotted line and open circles the NO_2-exposed hamsters. The number at each circle is the number of animals. The vertical bar represents the standard error.

(α_2-M). We performed these studies in both NO_2-exposed and control hamsters after varying periods of NO_2 exposure. At the termination of the exposure, hamsters of both groups were lightly anesthetized with nembutal and aortic blood was obtained for study of α_1PI and white blood cell concentrations (9,10). Bronchoalveolar lavage (BAL) was performed and the lavage fluid centrifuged. The lavage supernate was analyzed for α_1PI, for elastase inhibitory capacity (EIC), and for the specific activity of α_1PI (SA). The cells were collected from the centrifuged pellet of the lavage fluid and total white cell and differential counts were performed. A separate series of studies was performed to determine the elastase content of the neutrophils and macrophages. After BAL the cell pellets were used to separate the neutrophils and macrophages and to determine the elastase content of these samples.

In Fig. 14.2 the change in the neutrophil content of the lavage fluid with time is demonstrated. The neutrophil content rises to a peak of 5 $\times$ 10^6 cells on day

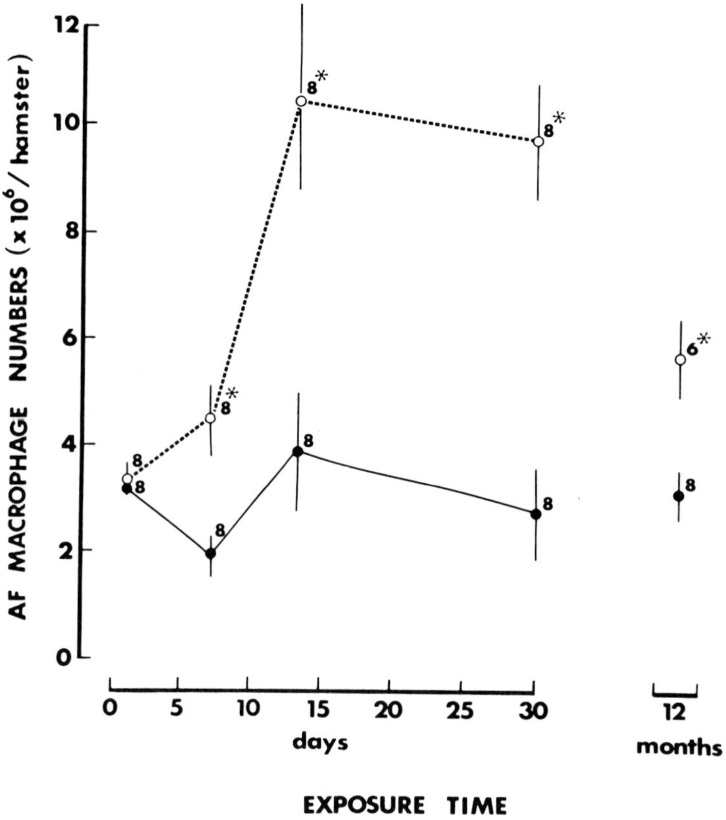

Fig. 14.3. Alveolar fluid macrophages at 7.7, 14, and 30 days and 12 months' exposure to NO_2. The filled line and closed circles represent controls, the dotted line and open circles NO_2-exposed animals. The number at each circle is the number of animals. The vertical line represents the standard error.

14 and declines thereafter. After 30 days of NO_2 it is not significantly different from control values. It remains at levels no greater than control for the remainder of the exposure.

The macrophage dynamics are somewhat different. Figure 14.3 shows that after NO_2 exposure the number of macrophages in the lavage fluid is increased after 7 days' exposure and reaches a peak value by 14 days' exposure. With continued exposure the macrophage content of the lavage fluid decreases progressively; after 12 months' exposure it is still significantly elevated but is only half the peak level.

The neutrophil elastase content increases in a pattern identical to that of the number of neutrophils and peaks at 14 days. Thereafter it decreases, until at approximately 30 days it is near control levels. The macrophage elastase rises progressively with NO_2 exposure and peaks at 14 days (9), following which it decreases slowly, but it does not reach control levels even after 12 months'

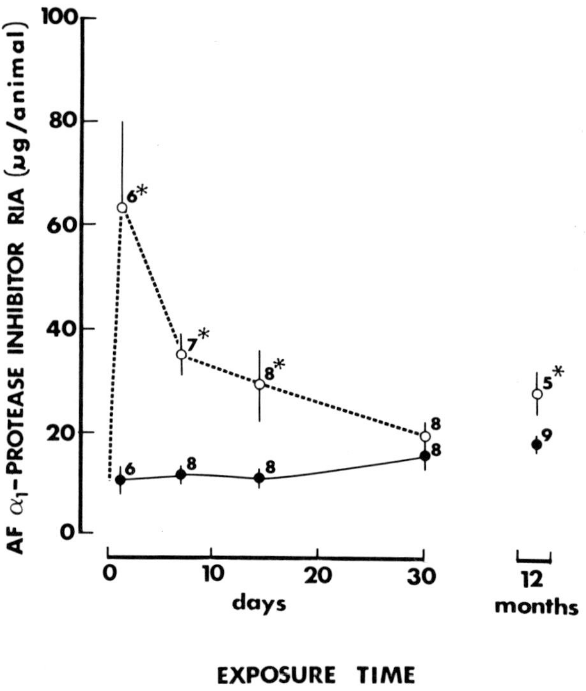

Fig. 14.4. α_1-Protease inhibitor concentration as determined by radioimmunoassay in the alveolar fluid at 1, 7, 14, and 30 days and 12 months' NO_2 exposure. The filled line and closed circles represent controls, the dotted line and open circles is the number of animals. The vertical line represents the standard error; * indicates a difference significant at $p<0.05$.

exposure. The neutrophil elastase is approximately 300 times as active as is the macrophage elastase and is by far the most important of the common leukocytes which release elastase (9).

Of the antiproteolytic proteins present in the lung, α_1PI is responsible for the greatest changes in alveolar concentrations during NO_2 exposure. Within 24 h after beginning exposure, the concentration of α_1PI in the lavage fluid is increased six-fold. With continued NO_2 exposure the alveolar concentration of α_1PI remained elevated, but there is a progressive decrease in the absolute value of alveolar α_1PI, so that after 12 months' exposure to NO_2 the concentration is only slightly—but still significantly—above control values (Fig. 14.4).

The EIC of the alveolar fluid provides an index of the functional activity of the alveolar α_1PI. It is important to evaluate the functional state of the α_1PI because in vitro studies indicate that oxidizing agents are capable of inactivating the antielastolytic activity of this protein. The data in Fig. 14.5 indicate, however, that hamsters exposed to NO_2 have increased EIC values, which are greatest during the first 7 days but persist for the entire 12 months of NO_2 exposure. There appear to be two opposing factors which affect the alveolar EIC concentration

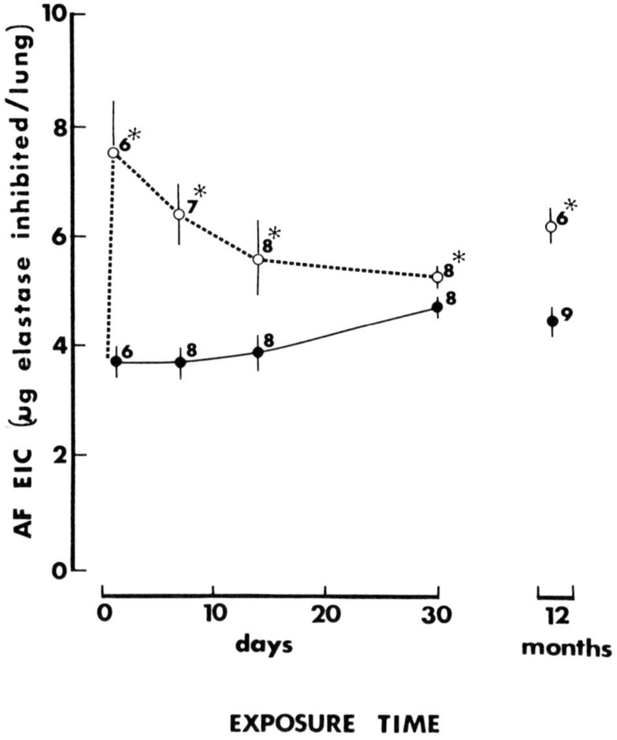

Fig. 14.5. Elastase inhibitory capacity in the alveolar fluid at 1, 7, 14, and 30 days, and 12 months after NO_2. The filled line and closed circles represent controls, the dotted line and open circles NO_2-exposed animals. The number at each circle is the number of animals. The vertical line represents the standard error; * indicates a difference significant at $p<0.05$.

during NO_2 exposure. The first is the stimulus to increase α_1PI, which probably results from increased vascular permeability of the pulmonary vessels and exudation of small amounts of serum proteins, including α_1PI into the alveolar fluid. The second factor is the oxidative effect of the NO_2 on the α_1PI (11), which in all likelihood produces a decrease in the function of alveolar α_1PI. The integrated effect is an increase in the EIC. Thc specific activity of the α_1PI is the amount of elastase inhibited per mg α_1PI. This decreased significantly during the first 7–14 days of NO_2 but increases to control levels by the 30th day of exposure. The loss of antiproteolytic activity per unit weight of α_1PI indicates that there has been some loss of functional activity of each molecule of the active protein (10). This change is likely to have resulted from the exposure of the α_1PI to the oxidizing effect of NO_2.

Table 14.3 provides a stoichiometric comparison of the values of α_1PI and elastase in the alveolar fluid after NO_2 exposure of varying duration. These data demonstrate that after each period of exposure there is an excess of α_1PI. The

Table 14.3. Estimated molar ratios of neutrophil elastase and α_1-protease inhibitor in bronchoalveolar lavage fluid after 1, 7, 14, and 30 days' NO_2 exposure

Days of NO_2	Elastase (El; pmol)	α_1 PI (pmol)	Ratio El:α_1 PI
1	13.4	1560	1:116
7	35.8	1290	1:36
14	47.4	1170	1:41
30	4.9	1060	1:216

smallest level of excess α_1PI occurs after 14 days' exposure. This data suggests that there is an excess of α_1PI present in the alveolar fluid at all times during the exposure. This circumstance would tend to minimize the likelihood of lung destruction and elastolysis from elastase at all periods of exposure.

It appears reasonable to suggest that the minimal degree of emphysema which develops as a result of the prolonged NO_2 exposure and the obvious lack of progression of the lesion is related to two pathogenetic changes. The first is the limited period following initiation of exposure when neutrophils migrate to and accumulate in the alveolar fluid. The diminished proteolytic potential associated with the decreased number of alveolar neutrophils seen in the alveolar fluid after day 21 of exposure decreases the likelihood of elastolytic injury to the lung and development of emphysema. The mechanism of the decrease in neutrophil mobilization into the alveolar fluid is not presently known. It is clear however that continued exposure to NO_2 will not elicit a continuing release of neutrophils.

While this decreased neutrophil burden may in itself be sufficient to limit any progression in lung destruction, the rapid increase in the antiproteolytic proteins in the alveolus creates an additional defense against lung destruction. The dynamic changes in concentration α_1PI within the alveolus during the early period of NO_2 exposure could result from three possible mechanisms. First, there might occur an increase in plasma levels of α_1PI as a result of lung injury and an acute phase response. This would produce an increase in circulating plasma α_1PI concentration. Our studies of the plasma α_1PI indicate that no increase occurs. Second, there may be increased synthesis of α_1PI by the lung cells or the macrophages. There is no evidence however of synthesis of α_1PI by lung tissue, and the rapid changes in α_1PI concentrations are not likely to occur as a result of synthesis and breakdown of α_1PI newly synthesized by the macrophages. We favor a third mechanism, namely, the exudation of plasma α_1PI from the pulmonary capillaries injured by the acute exposure to NO_2. The dynamic variations in alveolar α_1PI are more likely to be produced by changes in vascular permeability and resorption. The reason for the modulation in endothelial permeability during continued exposure to NO_2 is not known. It is clear however that these adaptive responses act to protect the lung tissue from progressive injury.

This analysis of the factors that are currently believed to control the development of emphysema has indicated the reason for the lack of progression of the mild emphysema associated with NO_2 exposure. It has not however allowed an understanding of how to create a more acceptable or better animal model of emphysema. Our present studies have demonstrated the need to develop new ways to increase and sustain the elastase burden of the lung while simultaneously limiting the release of α_1PI or other antielastase proteins. Additional research is required to address these critical responses.

This study has brought us to the realization that the criteria for the production of an acceptable animal model of emphysema require postulates which differ from those proposed by Robert Koch for acute infectious diseases over a century ago.

The models of chronic human disease where there is no evidence of involvement of an infectious agent require different criteria to be used. On the bases of our recent studies we propose the following criteria.

1. The experimental model must have pathologic lesions which resemble those in the human disease.
2. The functional changes present in the human disease should be produced by the animal model.
3. The pathologic lesions and functional changes should show progression with continued application of the experimental agent.
4. The experimental model must be able to be correlated with and analyzed in terms of definable pathogenetic factors.

We suggest that the application of these criteria will guide experimental pathologists or investigators to the development of reliable animal models of emphysema and other chronic human diseases.

References

1. Kleinerman J, Cowdrey CR (1968) The effects of continuous high level nitrogen dioxide on hamsters. Yale J Biol Med 405:579–585
2. Kleinerman J, Ip MPC (1979) Effects of nitrogen dioxide on elastin and collagen contents of lung. Arch Environ Health 34:228–232
3. Lam C, Kattan M, Collins A, Kleinerman J (1983) Long-term sequelae of bronchiolitis induced by nitrogen dioxide in hamsters. Am Rev Respir Dis 128:1020–1023
4. Kleinerman J (1977) Some effects of nitrogen dioxide on the lung. Fed Proc 36:1714–1718
5. Snider GL, Kleinerman J, Thurlbeck WM, Bengali ZH (1985) The definition of emphysema: report of a National Heart, Lung, and Blood Institute (Division of Lung Disease) workshop. Am Rev Respir Dis 132:182–185
6. Harel S, Janoff A, Yu SY, Hurewitz A, Bergofsky EH (1980) Desmosine radioimmunoassay for measuring elastin degradation in vivo. Am R Respir Dis 122:769–773
7. Starcher BC (1982) Antibodies to desmosine. In: Cunningham LW, Fredericksen DW (eds) Structural and contractile proteins, part A: Extracellular matrix. Academic, New York pp 588–605 (Methods in enzymology, vol 82)
8. Janoff A (1985) Elastases and emphysema. Current assessment of the protease-antiprotease hypothesis. Am Rev Respir Dis 132:417–433

9. Ip MPC, Kleinerman J and Collins J (1987) Alveolar leukocytes and protease responses with continuous vs. intermittent exposures to NO_2. In: Taylor JC, Mittman C (eds) Pulmonary emphysema and proteolysis:1986. Academic, New York, pp 507–514
10. Kleinerman J, Ip MPC, Collins J (1987) Alveolar antiprotease responses with continuous vs. intermittent NO_2 exposures. In: Taylor JC, Mittman C (eds) Pulmonary emphysema and proteolysis: 1986. Academic, New York pp 515–522
11. Dooley MM, Pryor WA (1982) Free radical pathology: inactivation of human α_1-proteinase inhibitor by products from the reaction of nitrogen dioxide with hydrogen peroxide and etiology of emphysema. Biochem Biophys Res Commun 106:981–987

CHAPTER 15

Comparisons of Respiratory Function Responses of Laboratory Animals and Humans

J.L. Mauderly[1]

Introduction

Respiratory function tests of humans are widely used as diagnostic tools, for occupational health monitoring, for epidemiological surveys, and for studying lung physiology. These tests are a rapid, noninvasive means of providing quantitative information on the functional status of the respiratory system. Measurements of the respiratory function of animals are frequently used in studies of the toxic effects of inhaled materials, basic lung physiology, and the pathogenesis of lung disease. The usefulness of these tests in animals depends on an ability to give physiological interpretation to the results and to extrapolate to humans the changes observed in animals.

This chapter focuses on the issue of whether or not respiratory function results from animals can be extrapolated to humans. The approach taken is to discuss factors contributing to differences in results obtained from animals and humans, and then to use specific examples to illustrate similarities and differences in acute, subacute, and chronic functional responses. The comparisons presented are not comprehensive; a complete review of the literature is beyond the scope of this chapter. Function testing methods will not be discussed in detail in this chapter. A recent review (30) discussed in detail the range of respiratory function assays adapted for animals, the physiological basis for the tests, and variations in methodologies. An earlier review (8) addressed these same topics briefly, and presented diagrams of representative measurement systems and some comparative results.

Role of Respiratory Function Tests

Respiratory function tests are used in toxicology to detect toxic responses, to characterize toxicant-induced lung disease, and as an aid to extrapolating findings

[1]Inhalation Toxicology Research Institute, Lovelace Biomedical and Environmental Research Institute, P.O. Box 5890, Albuquerque, NM 87185, USA.

to humans. They can be the sole indicator of response, as in the physiological detection of airway constriction (42), or might be one of many assays used to evaluate toxicity of a material (34). They might be used to detect responses at a single time (42), or be applied serially to determine the pathogenesis of progressive lung disease (34). Much is known about interrelationships among impaired respiratory function, symptoms of respiratory illness, clinical lung disease, and occupational disability in people. Information from toxicological studies and studies of structure-function relationships in experimentally induced lung diseases are adding confidence to our interpretation of functional alterations in animals. We have much yet to learn about the specificity of the relationship between alterations in lung structure and measured changes in respiratory function of both humans and animals. However, our present understanding is sufficient to make reasonable predictions of human functional responses from animal data.

It must be understood that respiratory function tests are not an alternative to histopathological observation; rather, the two are complementary (30). It is possible for either morphological or functional changes to exist in the absence of detectable changes in the other. Conversely, one can sometimes predict with good accuracy changes in one endpoint from changes observed in the other. Functional and morphological evaluations are best used together in order to understand both the injuries produced and their implications for human health.

Adaptation of Respiratory Function Tests for Animals

Scope of Tests Applied to Animals

In general, all respiratory function tests applied to humans either have been applied to animals, or could be (8,30). The scope of these assays ranges from simple measurement of respiratory frequency to rank the irritant potentials of inhaled chemicals (3), to comprehensive evaluations of breathing patterns, dynamic and static lung mechanics, forced airflow limitation, intrapulmonary gas distribution, and alveolar-capillary gas exchange to describe lung disease in detail (18). Animal size is not an absolute limitation. Both of the preceding examples (3,18) used small rodents, and subjects as large as ponies are readily measured in the laboratory (27). The lack of voluntary cooperation of animals during testing need not be a severe limitation, nor are anesthesia or sedation necessarily required. Measurements have been performed without sedation and with minimal restraint on hamsters, rats, guinea pigs, rabbits, dogs, and ponies at the Lovelace Inhalation Toxicology Research Institute, Albuquerque, NM (26,27,31). The tests need not be invasive, and can be applied repeatedly throughout the subject's life span with no detectable ill effects (33). Oral–tracheal catheters are readily placed in subjects as small as mice (28), obviating the need for tracheostomy, and noninvasive methods for measuring breathing mechanics of conscious animals which tolerate esophageal catheters poorly (2,39) can obviate the need for the intrapleural catheters frequently used in guinea pigs (42).

Differences in Measurements of Humans and Animals

Methodological Differences

All measurements of respiratory function of animals require some modification of techniques used for humans, and the effects of methodological differences on the results must be considered when extrapolating between species. Measurements of conscious animals require some restraint even of trained or conditioned subjects (26,27,31,42), and precautions are necessary to avoid artifacts due to restraint, such as chest wall restriction from slings or exposure tubes, or compression of the trachea by seals around the neck. External attachments to the airway, such as masks and breathing valves, can introduce dead space or airflow restriction which would alter the respiratory pattern. Excitement-induced artifacts in respiration are a concern for conscious animals.

Anesthesia is an abnormal physiological state. Data from anesthetized animals do not represent normal values for conscious animals, and there are few data from anesthetized humans for direct comparison to data from animals. In general, the respiratory function of anesthetized animals is altered by lung disease in a manner similar to that observed in conscious subjects, when compared to baseline or control data collected under identical conditions. Changes in lung volumes, mechanics, gas distribution, and gas exchange caused by altered lung structure are seldom eliminated by anesthesia. In contrast, caution must be used in interpreting function changes mediated by reflex mechanisms, such as sensory irritation or airway reactivity. It must also be remembered that tracheal catheters prevent measurement of flow resistance and reflex responses in the upper airway.

Many function tests require specialized breathing maneuvers, such as controlled inhalation and exhalation and breath-holding, which are done voluntarily by humans. These movements are induced in animals by applying positive and negative pressures either to the airway (8) or the body surface (36) during apnea induced by inflation reflex or paralytic drugs. The airway pressure and body surface pressure techniques have been compared and discussed in detail (30). Both produce useful information, but the airway technique gives the faster response and the better simulation of rapid voluntary movements. The use of airway pressures might appear as an obvious artifact, compared to voluntary movements; however, the pressure gradients applied to the lung are the same in both cases, and both theory (41) and practice (see pp. 253–256) show that results are comparable.

Anatomical-Physiological Differences

Consideration of differences in the structure of the respiratory systems of humans and animals is a key step in extrapolating respiratory function results between species. A review of the literature in this area is not attempted here: the reader is referred to an excellent series of published papers (47) resulting from a workshop on comparative lung biology held by the US National Institutes of

Health in 1982. One of the most important structural differences is the highly compliant (flaccid) chest wall of rodents, compared to the stiffer chest wall of larger animals and humans. The implications of this difference are illustrated by the examples given on pp. 250–256.

Differences in Sensitivity to Inhaled Materials

Species differences in sensitivity to inhaled toxicants must be considered when comparing respiratory function responses of animals and humans. Some differences in sensitivity might be caused by the different respiratory system structures of animals and humans, while others appear related to receptor-reflex or metabolic differences. Interspecies differences in sensitivity are particularly troublesome when comparing acute functional responses, but can also influence chronic responses. When possible, functional responses should be compared on the basis of similar underlying structural changes. If the sensitivities (dose-time-response relationships) of humans and animals to an inhaled material result in different types or extents of lesions, the respiratory function data from animals can still be very useful if it is known that identical lesions cause identical functional changes in both species.

Comparisons of Functional Responses of Animals and Humans

Representative respiratory functional responses of humans and animals are compared below. The comparisons are semiquantitative, since few published data allow direct quantitative comparisons between animals and humans. An attempt was made to limit comparisons to those in which the lesions underlying the functional changes are known to be similar in humans and animals. The body of literature meeting the requirement of similar inhalation exposures or similar structural changes in both humans and animals, and including actual data for functional changes, is surprisingly limited.

Acute Responses to Inhaled Materials

Animals have been used extensively to examine the acute (immediate) effects of inhaled gases, vapors, and particles. The functional parameters typically measured include the breathing pattern (respiratory frequency, tidal volume, and minute volume) and dynamic lung mechanics (dynamic lung compliance and airway resistance). The goal of these studies is usually to develop dose-response information for setting standards for short-term exposures, and less often for studying mechanisms of action. The functional responses are often mediated by reflex alterations of respiratory control and airway smooth muscle tone, rather than from tissue injury. Mice and guinea pigs are the species most commonly used. In addition to studies of oxidants, acid aerosols, and chemicals acting as sensory irritants, as described below, considerable work has been done with isocyanates (23).

Ranking of Chemicals as Sensory Irritants

Many chemicals cause irritation of the eyes and upper respiratory tract upon contact. This action has been termed "sensory irritation" and is presumed to result from stimulation of the trigeminal nerve in the nasal passages and cornea (3). Inhalation of these materials causes a reflex inhibition of respiration in mice and rats, involving reduction of both respiratory frequency and tidal volume (7). Measurements of the respiratory frequency of mice during short-term exposures have been used to construct concentration-response curves allowing the ranking of a variety of chemicals as sensory irritants (3,4).

No direct comparison of human and animal responses will be attempted here. Alarie (4) addressed the issue by comparing published information on human responses to 11 chemicals to responses predicted at progressive multiples of the RD_{50}, the concentration of chemical producing a 50% reduction in the respiratory frequency of mice. He reported a good correspondence between predicted and observed responses. He also demonstrated a close correlation between threshold limit values proposed for human exposures on the basis of responses in mice and the threshold limit values set by observations in humans. Results to date suggest that the mouse assay is useful for predicting responses of humans to sensory irritants.

Effect of Ozone on Breathing Pattern

The effects of oxidant gases on respiratory function of humans and animals have previously been compared in detail (29). The effects of nearly identical exposures to ozone on the breathing pattern of guinea pigs and humans will be compared here as an example of transient airway irritation.

Bates and Hazucha (5) exposed ten healthy, nonsmoking men to 0.75 ppm ozone for 2 h, with the subjects alternately resting or exercising lightly. Respiratory function was measured at 0.5-h intervals during and after the exposure. Murphy et al. (38) exposed ten conscious young adult male guinea pigs to 0.68 ppm ozone for 2 h and measured respiration during and after the exposure. The respiratory frequency increased, while tidal volume decreased, in both humans and guinea pigs (Fig. 15.1). The magnitudes of the responses were remarkably similar. At the end of the 2-h exposure, frequency was increased to 135% and 144% of baseline and tidal volume was decreased to 73% and 72% of baseline values in humans and guinea pigs, respectively.

Acute Airway Constriction from Sulfuric Acid

Constriction of airway smooth muscle by either direct or reflex effects is a common response to inhaled irritating materials. This response is manifested subjectively as dyspnea and functionally as increased resistance to airflow. If the constriction occurs in lower airways, it is often reflected by an increase in dynamic lung compliance (42). The response is typically transient and disappears soon after exposure ends. If a greater response occurs on repeated

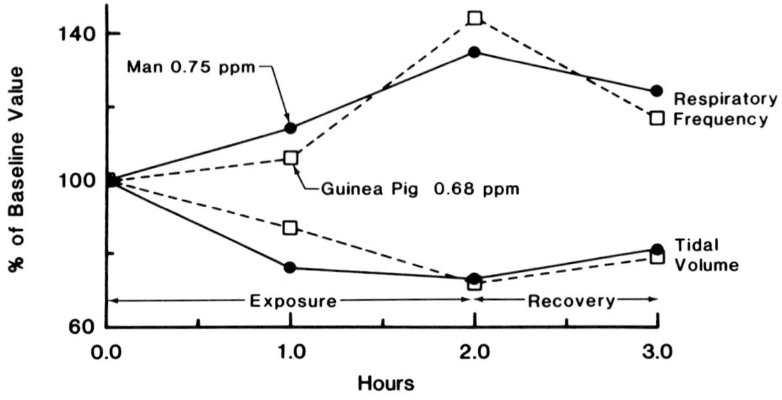

Fig. 15.1. Effects on respiratory frequency and tidal volume of 2-h exposure of humans (5) and guinea pigs (38) to similar concentrations of ozone. Data are mean values plotted as percentages of preexposure baseline values.

exposure to the same material, "specific sensitization" to the material is considered to have occurred. Sensitization to isocyanates is an example (23). The acute effects of inhaled sulfuric acid on airflow resistance of naive men and guinea pigs during exposure are compared here as an example of a response to inhaled irritant particles.

Sim and Pattle (43) measured the airway resistance of healthy men after 30 min exposure to 3–39 (mean = 21) mg/m³ aerosol of sulfuric acid having a particle size of 1.5 μm. The exposures caused eye and nose irritation and coughing, which was reduced enough at 10 min after exposure to allow measurements. At that time, resistance was increased to 143–250% of normal (Fig. 15.2). Silbaugh et al. (42) exposed Hartley guinea pigs for 1 h to 24–48 (mean = 38) mg/m³ of sulfuric acid aerosol with a particle size of 1.0 μm, and measured dynamic lung compliance and airway resistance at 15-min intervals. After 30 min exposure, the

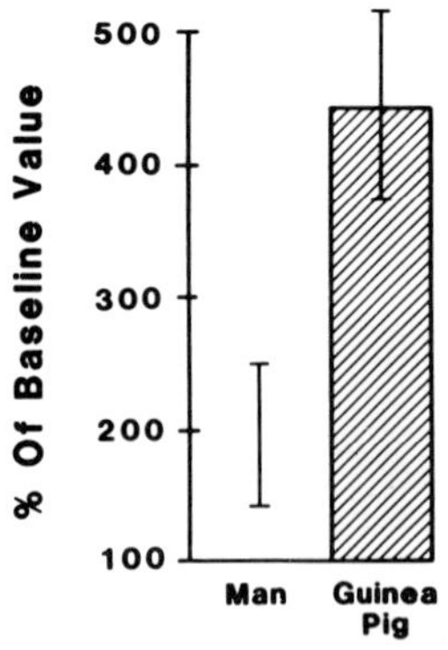

Fig. 15.2. Effect of 30-min inhalation exposures to sulfuric acid aerosols on airway resistance of men (43) and guinea pigs (42). The brackets enclose the range of responses of men, and the bar for guinea pigs represents the mean ± SE, both plotted as percentages of preexposure baseline values.

animals had become dyspneic, compliance was reduced, and resistance was increased to a mean of 446% of the baseline value (see Fig. 15.2). The finding of approximately twice the degree of response in guinea pigs at approximately twice the level of human exposure suggests that men and guinea pigs respond similarly to sulfuric acid.

Subacute Responses to Inhaled Oxidants

Subacute functional responses, those that occur within hours to days after inhalation of toxic materials, usually result either directly or indirectly from cellular injury. Three examples, all involving oxidant gases, are presented here.

Effect of Ozone on Airway Reactivity

An increase in airway reactivity caused by inhaled toxicants is a special case of a subacute functional response. Although the increased reactivity is thought to be related to epithelial injury and influx of inflammatory cells (37), the functional change that is measured is not a direct result of this injury. The change that is measured is the increase in bronchoconstriction caused by an inhaled or injected bronchoactive drug. Resistance to airflow is often normal after exposure to the oxidant and before administration of the bronchoconstrictor. An increase in response to a bronchoactive drug, rather than to the inhaled toxicant itself, is termed "nonspecific sensitization." Nonspecific sensitization can be induced by a variety of materials, is usually transient, and, unlike the specific sensitization caused by materials such as isocyanates (23), does not have an immunological mechanism.

The increases in nonspecific airway reactivity observed in humans, dogs, sheep, and guinea pigs in seven studies are illustrated in Fig. 15.3. Golden et al. (15) exposed eight healthy, nonsmoking human subjects to 0.6 ppm ozone for 2 h during oral breathing at rest in a large chamber. They assessed airway reactivity immediately and at 1 day and 1 week after exposure by measuring airway resistance after inhalation of histamine aerosol. The response to histamine was nearly doubled immediately after exposure and was then progressively reduced (but still elevated from baseline) at 1 day and 1 week. Gordon and Amdur (16) exposed Hartley guinea pigs to 0.8 ppm ozone for 1 h and measured airway resistance after subcutaneous injection of histamine at 1 h after exposure. The increase in resistance was almost identical to that obtained in humans by Golden et al (15). Murlas and Roum (37) exposed Hartley guinea pigs to 3.0 ppm ozone for 1 h and measured specific airway resistance during intravenous injection of acetylcholine at 2 h, 1 day and 2 days after exposure. In contrast to the preceding studies, the acetylcholine dose to double specific resistance was only slightly increased at 2 h, then peaked at 1 day. A similar pattern was observed in dogs by Lee et al. (24), who exposed healthy mongrels to 0.7 ppm ozone for 2 h and measured the increase in airway resistance caused by inhaled histamine aerosol at 1 h, 1 day, and 5 days after exposure. The response to histamine peaked at 1 day, and then

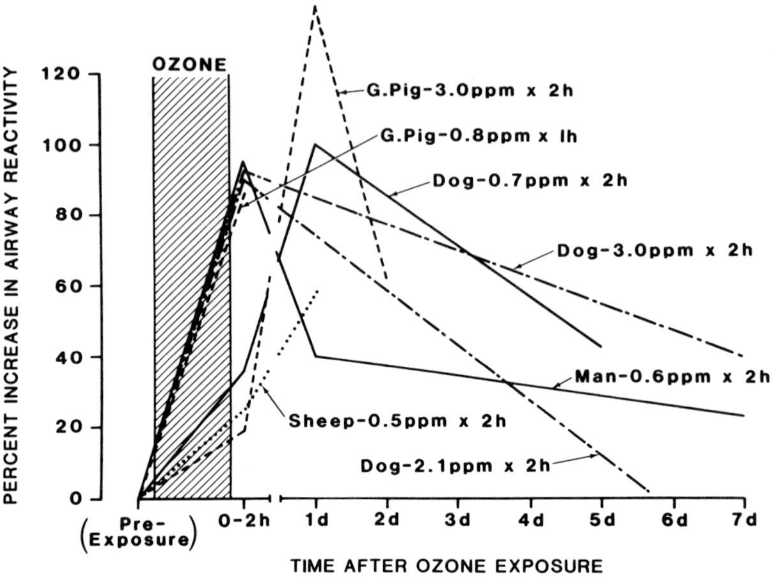

Fig. 15.3. Effect of 1- to 2-h inhalation exposures of men (15), dogs (10,24,69), sheep (1), and guinea pigs (16,37) on airway responses to bronchoactive drugs. The ordinate scale represents the percentage change from the magnitude of preexposure baseline responses to bronchoprovocation challenge. Responses were expressed as changes in airway resistance, specific airway resistance, or the drug concentration producing a preselected level of response.

decreased. Two other studies demonstrated responses in dogs that were nearly identical to that of humans. Holtzman et al. (19) exposed mongrels to 2.1 ppm ozone for 2 h and measured the concentration of acetylcholine in an aerosolized solution that caused a preselected increase in airway resistance at 1 h and 1 week after exposure. The response was nearly doubled (concentration halved) at 1 h and was slightly less than baseline at 1 week. Fabbri et al. (10) exposed mongrels to 3.0 ppm ozone for 2 h and used an identical approach to measure the acetylcholine aerosol response concentration at 1 h and 1 week after exposure. They also found a doubled response at 1 h, and a decreased, but still elevated, response at 1 week. Abraham et al. (1) exposed eight female sheep to 0.5 ppm ozone for 2 h via a tracheal catheter and measured airway resistance during inhalation of carbachol aerosol immediately and at 1 day after exposure. The response of the sheep to carbachol was elevated 25% above the baseline response immediately after ozone exposure, and was elevated 58% at 1 day after exposure.

The above results illustrate several points. First, a variety of methods have been used to assess nonspecific airway reactivity, including both inhaled and injected bronchoactive drugs. Second, responses very similar to those of humans have been obtained in animals. In the above comparison, humans and guinea pigs had

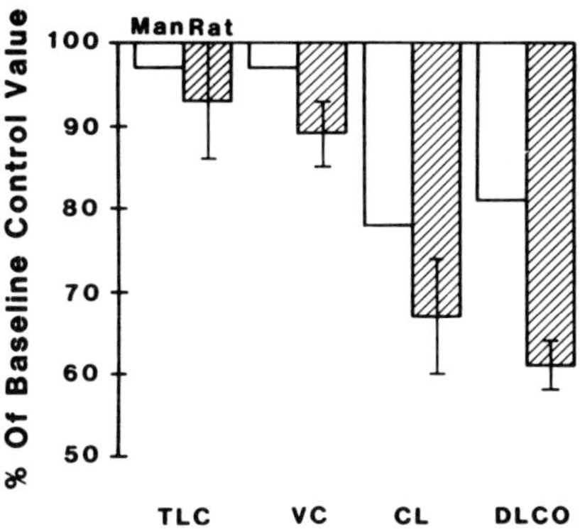

Fig. 15.4. Effects on respiratory function of a man (6) and rats (17) of breathing one atmosphere of oxygen for 48 h. TLC, total lung capacity; VC, vital capacity; CL, dynamic (man) or quasistatic (rat) lung compliance; DLCO, carbon monoxide diffusing capacity. Bars for the man indicate the percentage of the preexposure baseline value. Bars for the rats indicate the mean ± SE percentage of values from unexposed control rats.

peak responses of identical magnitude at 1 h after exposure to ozone at 0.6 and 0.8 ppm, respectively. Third, responses can vary, both between and within species. In two studies, dogs had responses similar to humans, but at higher exposure concentrations. This would suggest that dogs are less sensitive to the induction of airway reactivity than humans and guinea pigs. Fourth, some differences in response are presently difficult to explain. The sheep study, one dog study, and one guinea pig study demonstrated peak responses at 1 day after ozone exposure, rather than immediately. The sheep and dogs were exposed to ozone via a tracheal catheter, eliminating exposure of the upper airways, while the other studies used exposures by mouth. Although it is tempting to suggest an effect of exposure route, the guinea pigs that had a delayed response were exposed by mouth. It is not possible to explain the reasons for the differences at this time. To improve extrapolation, animal studies should be done using exposure and challenge methods as similar as possible to those used for humans.

Oxygen Toxicity

Humans exposed to 100% (one atmosphere) of oxygen for periods longer than a few hours develop respiratory distress, which is reversible upon return to air breathing. The structural changes consist of inflammation and edema at the alveolar level. Oxygen toxicity has been well studied, and similar lesions are known to occur in similarly exposed animals.

Caldwell et al. (6) evaluated the respiratory function of human subjects after exposure to 98% oxygen at one atmosphere for 30–74 h. Subject no. 2, a 28-year-old male, was exposed for 48 h. Harkema et al. (17) exposed 4-month-old rats to 100% oxygen at one atmosphere for 48 h and examined correlations between respiratory function and morphological changes. Selected functional changes of the man and the rats are compared in Fig. 15.4. Qualitatively identical reductions in lung volumes, lung compliance, and alveolar-capillary gas exchange (carbon monoxide diffusing capacity) were observed in the two species. The changes were greater in the rats, reflecting their greater sensitivity to oxygen toxicity. This is consistent with the finding (in the same studies) that prolongation of exposures to 72 h and beyond resulted in mortality among rats, but the human subjects were not seriously injured. This comparison illustrates that alveolar inflammation and edema cause similar functional changes in humans and rats.

Nitrogen Dioxide-Induced Lung Edema

Exposure to high concentrations of nitrogen dioxide causes cell death, inflammation, and edema at the alveolar level, much like that caused by oxygen. Accidental exposures of humans, such as when welding in enclosed spaces or working in enclosed silos, have yielded data on functional changes, although the exposure concentrations are rarely known. The principal life-threatening effect is the impaired gas exchange caused by alveolar edema.

Jones et al. (21) reported four cases of known or suspected accidental exposure to nitrogen dioxide. Subject no. 2 was a 35-year-old shipyard worker who developed symptoms after using an oxyacetylene torch in an enclosed fuel tank. Although the exposure was probably not limited to nitrogen dioxide, the results were typical, including elevated respiratory frequency (200% of normal), coughing which produced yellow sputum, and radiographic evidence of edema. The subject's subsequent improvement of gas exchange was monitored by repeated measurements of carbon monoxide diffusing capacity, which returned to normal by 2 weeks after exposure (Fig. 15.5). Johnson et al. (20) exposed dogs for 6 h to 69 ppm nitrogen dioxide and evaluated symptoms and respiratory function. As in humans, the respiratory frequency was elevated (240% of baseline), and the dogs coughed and produced yellow sputum. Respiratory function tests demonstrated a marked gas exchange impairment, including a reduced carbon monoxide diffusing capacity (see Fig. 15.5). The diffusing capacity returned to normal by 2 weeks after exposure, in parallel to resolution of the edema as observed in dogs by serial killing. The similarities of the magnitude and time course of the changes in carbon monoxide diffusing capacity of the human subject and the dogs after nitrogen dioxide exposure are striking.

Chronic Lung Disease

Studies of respiratory function changes in chronic (long-term, irreversible) lung diseases of laboratory animals typically involve serial measurements of a spectrum of function endpoints and serial evaluations of histopathology in order to describe the pathogenesis of the disease. Two examples (fibrosis and emphysema) are presented here, in both of which common animal "models" of human lung disease are compared to the human counterpart. There has been consider-

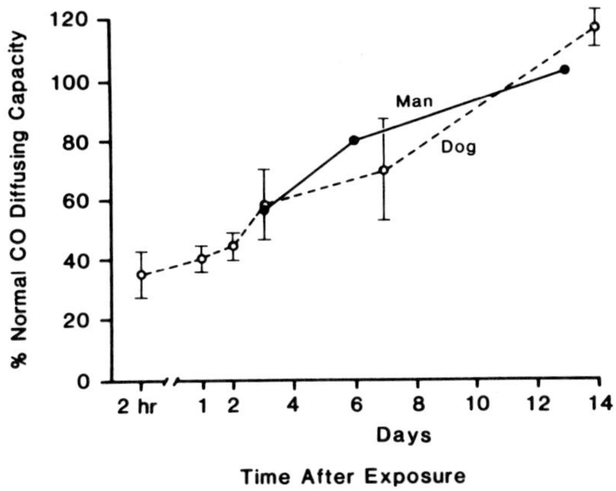

Fig. 15.5. Recovery of gas exchange efficiency, as reflected by carbon monoxide diffusing capacity, of a man (21) and dogs (20) after inhalation of high concentrations of nitrogen dioxide. The ordinate represents the percentage of predicted (human) or baseline (dog) values.

able work on bleomycin-induced fibrosis and enzyme-induced emphysema as animal models of representative human chronic lung diseases. Caution must be exercised, however, in extrapolating information obtained using these models to humans, as both animal models "model" only a very limited subset of the human populations with fibrosis or emphysema. The examples presented here provide a comparison between structure-function correlates in man and rats, the species most commonly used in long-term inhalation toxicological studies which include respiratory function tests. These models also illustrate the need to consider both physiological and methodological differences in comparing results from animals and humans.

Chronic Interstitial Fibrosis

Pulmonary fibrosis, the most common restrictive lung disease of humans, has many etiologies and occurs in a variety of histological forms. Pulmonary fibrosis is also a common sequela in long-term studies of inhaled materials in animals, such as in studies of inhaled radionuclides (32) and diesel exhaust (33) at the Lovelace Inhalation Toxicology Research Institute, Albuquerque, NM. Intratracheal instillations of bleomycin have been used to induce a model of chronic lung fibrosis in hamsters (44,46) and rats (9). A patchy, peribronchiolar fibrosis with persistent infiltration of leukocytes is achieved after an initial inflammatory stage. The administration of high concentrations of oxygen for a short time after bleomycin instillation results in a more diffuse distribution of the fibrosis (46). Although the bleomycin model produces a disease similar to that of some human patients, it does not closely model the diffuse interstitial fibrosis that occurs in several human syndromes. The present comparison uses a report of human fibrosis in which the histological features were similar to those of the animal model, and which also presented physiological data.

Fulmer et al. (12) reported cases of idiopathic pulmonary fibrosis selected from patients with fibrotic lung diseases referred to the US National Institutes of Health. The cases were selected on the basis of clinical, radiographic, physiological, and histopathological (biopsy) criteria. They presented respiratory function data for 23 subjects. Six nonsmokers with high fibrosis scores were selected for the present comparison. These subjects included three men and three women ranging in age from 27 to 66 years (mean = 51) and having dyspnea during exertion of 0.5–5.0 years duration. Varying degrees of interstitial fibrosis were observed by lung biopsy, and there were interstitial and alveolar cell infiltrates of lymphocytes and macrophages, but few neutrophils or eosinophils. No vasculitis or granulomas were present, there were no mineral deposits, and cultures were negative for microorganisms.

Pino et al. (40) instilled 1.6 units of bleomycin in 0.4 ml saline intratracheally into three male and three female 12-week-old F344 rats and then exposed the rats continuously to 85% oxygen (0.7 atmosphere) for 72 h. Respiratory function was measured as previously reported (17) at 90 days after instillation, and the rats were then killed for histopathological analysis. The rats were not dyspneic at rest; no observations were made during exercise. Lesions consisted of patchy interstitial fibrosis, predominantly near airways and subpleurally, with a diffuse, mild increase in alveolar septal collagen. There was mild interstitial and alveolar infiltration of mononuclear cells (lymphocytes and macrophages), with few neutrophils.

Values for respiratory function parameters reported for the human subjects are compared in Fig. 15.6 to corresponding data from the rats. Lung volumes, including total lung capacity, vital capacity, and functional residual capacity (FRC), were reduced in humans. Similar reductions in total lung capacity and vital capacity were observed in rats, but FRC was not reduced (the slight increase was not significant at $p < 0.05$). Gas exchange was impaired (reduced carbon monoxide diffusing capacity) and lung elastic recoil was increased (reduced lung compliance) in both species. There was no evidence of substantial airflow obstruction in either species. The volume expired by the human subjects in 1 s was reduced in proportion to the forced vital capacity; thus, the percentage of vital capacity expired in 1 s was normal. The forced-flow rates of rats were not reduced in proportion to their reduced vital capacity; thus, the percentage of vital capacity expired in 0.1 s was slightly increased above that of controls.

Figure 15.6 shows that similar reductions of maximal lung inflation (reduced total lung capacity and vital capacity), impairments of alveolar-capillary gas exchange (lower carbon monoxide diffusing capacity), and increases in lung elastic recoil (lower compliance) occur in humans and rats with similar types of fibrosis. The slight increase in FRC of the rats was accompanied by an increase in residual volume (not shown), and both were similar to increases in these volumes in bleomycin-treated rats reported by Costa et al. (9). To reconcile the increased FRC of rats with the decrease seen in humans, both methodological and physio-

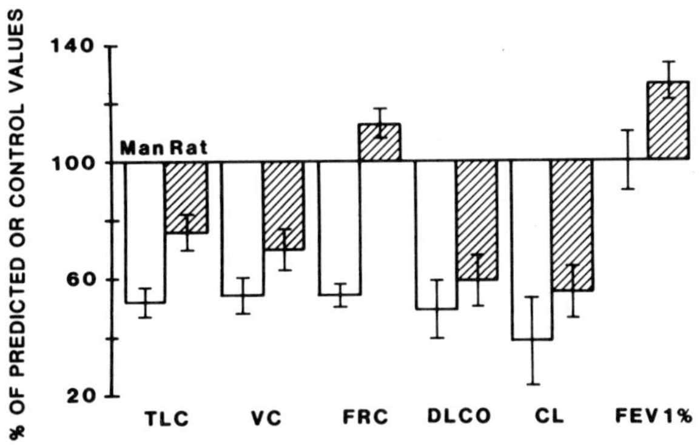

Fig. 15.6. Effects of pulmonary fibrosis on respiratory function of human subjects (12) and rats (40). TLC, total lung capacity; VC, vital capacity; FRC, functional residual capacity; DLCO, carbon monoxide diffusing capacity; CL, static (human) or quasistatic (rat) lung compliance; FEV1%, percentage of forced vital capacity exhaled in 1.0 s (human) or 0.1 s (rat). Bars represent the mean ± SE of the predicted normal (human) or untreated control (rat) values.

logical differences must be considered. The parameter termed "FRC" of rats is the relaxed lung volume of the anesthetized subject, in contrast to the end-expiratory volume of conscious humans. Different mechanisms set the level of FRC in rats and humans (14), and, while conscious humans breathe at an FRC similar to the relaxed lung volume, conscious rats are thought to breathe at an FRC that is higher than the relaxed lung volume. Although the mechanism is uncertain at this time, one possibility is that the relaxed volume measured in anesthetized rats is fixed at a higher than normal level by the development of fibrosis, while the conscious rats breathe at a volume that is higher (the conscious FRC). The slightly higher percentage of forced vital capacity expired per unit of time in rats than in humans suggested that there was a slight small airway component to the disease of man that paralleled their decreased lung volume, in contrast to the observation of no airway involvement in the rats. This would result in a normal volume-specific flow in humans, but an increase in rats.

Uncomplicated Emphysema

Pulmonary emphysema is a common chronic obstructive lung disease in humans, most frequently accompanied by chronic bronchitis as part of the chronic obstructive disease complex caused by cigarette smoking. Emphysema uncomplicated by disease of the conducting airways is infrequent in humans, occurring most often in subjects with α_1-antitrypsin deficiency. Emphysematous lesions, accompanied by other structural changes, have been observed in lungs of animals in inhalation toxicological studies, such as after chronic exposure to nitrogen dioxide (11) and diesel exhaust (33). Uncomplicated pulmonary emphysema of humans is frequently modeled in animals by instillation or inhalation of proteo-

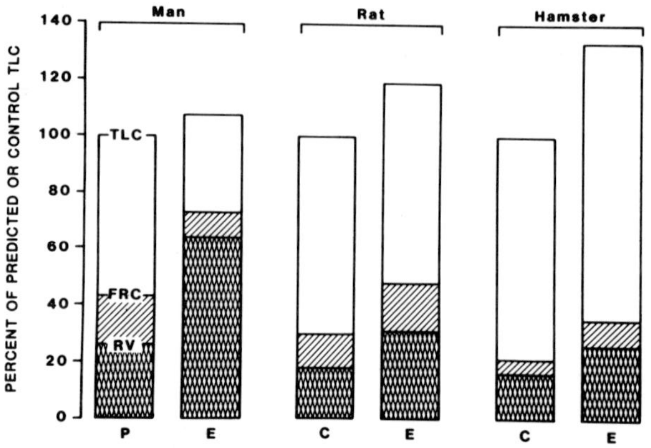

Fig. 15.7. Effects of pulmonary emphysema on lung volumes of two human subjects (unpublished data, see text), rats (25), and hamsters (22). TLC, total lung capacity; FRC, functional residual capacity; RV, residual volume; P, predicted; E, emphysema; C, control. Volumes are plotted as percentages of predicted normal (human) or untreated control (rat, hamster) total lung capacity.

lytic enzymes, such as papain, porcine pancreatic elastase, or neutrophil-derived elastase (45). The enzyme-induced emphysema of animals is a reasonable model for the uncomplicated emphysema of humans, but does not model the disease complex most common in man.

Emphysema is defined as the dilation of alveolar spaces and disruption of alveolar spetae, and is thought to result primarily from damage to elastic fibers. The resulting reductions of lung elastic recoil and alveolar surface area are manifested by several changes in respiratory function. The loss of elastic recoil causes a shift to the left of the lung pressure-volume curve, which were shown to be similar in humans, dogs, rats, and hamsters (29). The change in the pressure-volume relationship is also reflected by an increase in lung compliance, the slope of the pressure-volume curve. The loss of surface area reduces gas exchange efficiency and is reflected by a reduced carbon monoxide diffusing capacity in both humans and animals (29). The loss of elastic recoil also alters lung volumes. Total lung capacity is increased because of the lowered recoil pressure at maximal inflation. The FRC is increased because there is less inward recoil of the lung to counterbalance the outward recoil of the chest wall. Residual volume is increased because the loss of support of small airways causes an earlier collapse during maximal exhalation.

The effects of emphysema on lung volumes of human, rat, and hamster are compared in Fig. 15.7. There were no published data from which to plot all the subdivisions of lung volume for human subjects with uncomplicated emphysema. Data for two men, 43 and 51 years old and having emphysema due to α_1-antitrypsin deficiencies, were provided by Dr. W.I. Christensen of the Lovelace Medical Center, Albuquerque, NM. Values for these subjects are compared to values predicted for men of the same age and height. Lung volumes of 15 young adult male F344 rats at 3 weeks after instillation of 1.0 IU porcine pancreatic elastase per 100 g body weight are compared to values for 15 matched controls (25). Lung volumes of five young adult male Syrian hamsters at 3 weeks after instillation of 0.1 mg porcine pancreatic elastase per 100 g body weight are compared to values from 12 matched controls (22).

Emphysema caused qualitatively similar changes in the lung volumes of the three species. The changes in the rodents were of similar magnitude, but were quantitatively different from those in humans. It must be recognized that the human subjects were symptomatic and had advanced disease, while the disease in the rodents was subtle. The greater increase in FRC and residual volume in the men likely resulted from their stiffer chest wall, which exerted a greater outward force on the flaccid lung than would have occurred in the rodents. The greater increase in total lung capacity of the rodents likely resulted from the use of a standardized inflation pressure, in contrast to dependence on muscle strength and voluntary effort in humans. Again, the chest wall offers little resistance to inflation in rodents.

Another manifestation of the loss of lung elastic recoil is a loss of radial traction on small, membranous airways. This distending force tends to keep the airways open during forced exhalation, and the loss of radial traction in emphysema promotes airway collapse and flow obstruction. Maximal expiratory flow-volume (MEFV) curves of normal and emphysematous humans, dogs, rats, and hamsters are compared in Fig. 15.8. Gelb et al. (13) reported physiological data for several patients in whom emphysema was confirmed by biopsy. Subject no. 6 in that report, a 79-year-old male, had panlobular emphysema, and his MEFV curve is compared to a mean curve for age-matched nonsmokers. Mink (35) reported MEFV curves from six mongrel dogs in which emphysema was produced by repeated instillation of papain, and for five saline-instilled control dogs. The data for rats are from a recent, unpublished study at the Lovelace Inhalation Toxicology Research Institute, Albuquerque, NM. The MEFV curves from 16 male F344 rats at 19 months after instillation of 0.5 IU porcine pancreatic elastase per 100 g body weight are compared to curves from 16 matched saline-instilled controls. Snider et al. (45) reported MEFV curves for hamsters at 4 weeks after instillation of 200 μg porcine pancreatic elastase, and for saline-instilled controls. The MEFV curves of all of the animals were measured during anesthesia by positive-negative airway pressures. Since forced expiratory flow is volume-dependent, the curves were plotted on the basis of absolute lung volume, in order to compare flows of normal and emphysematous subjects at the same lung volumes.

Emphysema affected the MEFV curves of humans and animals similarly, although differences in curve shape and location are apparent. Flows at each lung volume were reduced by emphysema, demonstrating the obstructive effects of the disease. Both total lung capacity (highest volume) and residual volume (lowest volume) were increased in the animals, consistent with the description given above, but not in humans. These volumes are typically increased in

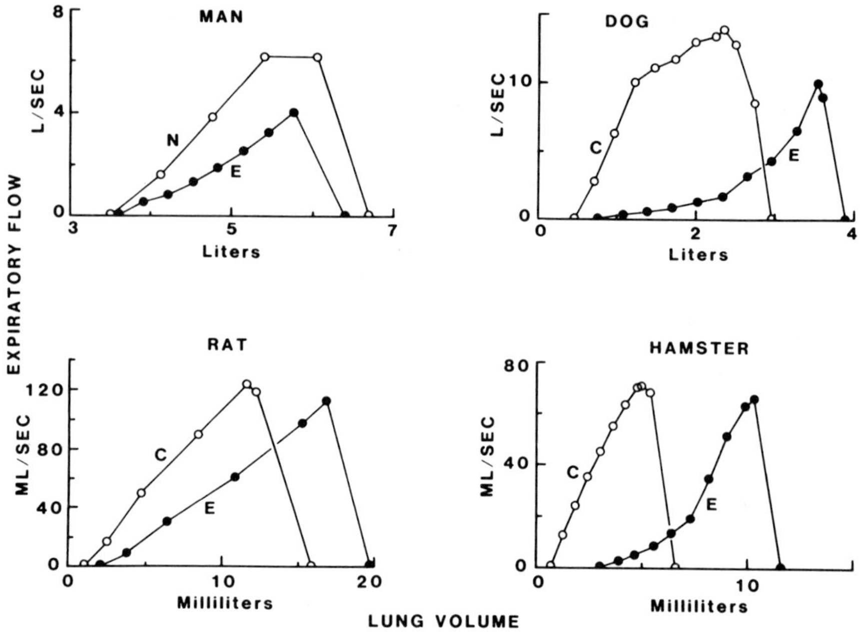

Fig. 15.8. Effects of pulmonary emphysema on maximal expiratory flow-volume curves of a man (13), dogs (35), rats (unpublished data, see text), and hamsters (45). N, predicted normal; C, untreated conrol; E, emphysema. Flows (ordinate) and volumes (abscissa) are in absolute units, so that emphysema-related differences in lung volumes can be seen.

humans, as shown in Fig. 15.7, and it must be remembered that the human curve is for only one subject measured at one time. Peak expiratory flow was substantially reduced in human and dog, but not in rat and hamster. This difference might also be related to differences in chest wall stiffness. The movement of both the lung and chest wall must be accelerated to reach peak flow, and lung elastic recoil adds to the initial acceleration of normal subjects. The slower acceleration, and resulting lower peak flow, might be more accentuated in species with stiff chest walls which resist movement than in rodents with their more flexible chests.

Summary

Respiratory function assays are a useful tool for studies of the toxicology of inhaled materials. A broad spectrum of respiratory function tests have been adapted for use with animals, and a considerable body of data on animal lung function exists in the literature. The tests can be used for a variety of purposes, ranging from measurement of a single parameter, to detect a preselected response, to comprehensive evaluations of function at a level of sophistication equal to that of human testing. The body of literature allowing direct comparisons between structure-function correlates of humans and animals is very limited. The comparisons that can be made at this time suggest that lung structural changes which are similar in humans and animals will result in similar changes in respiratory function. Apparent differences in response can largely be ascribed to interspecies differences in sensitivity to inhaled materials, and to differences in measurement technique. When these factors are considered, there appears to be little difference in the relationship between altered respiratory system structure and function in humans and animals.

Acknowledgments. The author gratefully acknowledges the assistance of numerous members of scientific and technical staff of the Lovelace Inhalation Toxicology Research Institute who have contributed to the studies described herein, have participated in continuing discussions of comparative lung physiology and pathology, and have provided helpful comments on this manuscript. The research was supported by the Office of Health and Environmental Research, US Department of Energy, under contract no. DE-AC04-76EV01013, and by the Health Effects Institute under Agreement 83-13 with the US Department of Energy. It was conducted in facilities fully accredited by the American Association for Accreditation of Laboratory Animal Care.

References

1. Abraham WM, Januszkiewicz AJ, Mingle M, Welker M, Wanner A, Sackner M (1980) Sensitivity of bronchoprovocation and tracheal mucous velocity in detecting airway responses to ozone. J Appl Physiol 48:789–793
2. Agrawal KP (1981) Specific airway conductance in guinea pigs: normal values and histamine-induced fall. Respir Physiol 43:23–30
3. Alarie Y (1973) Sensory irritation of the upper airways by airborne chemicals. Toxicol Appl Pharmacol 24:29–297
4. Alarie Y (1981) Dose-response analysis in animal studies: prediction of human responses. Environ Health Perspect 42:9–13
5. Bates DV, Hazucha M (1973) The short-term effects of ozone on the human lung. In: Proceedings of the conference on health effects of air pollutants, Natl Acad Sci, Nat Res Council, 3–5 Oct 1973, pp 507–540
6. Caldwell PRB, Lee WL, Schildkraut HS, Archibald ER (1966) Changes in lung volume, diffusing capacity and blood gases in men breathing oxygen. J Appl Physiol 21:1477–1483
7. Chang JCF, Steinhagen WH, Barrow CS (1981) Effect of single or repeated formaldehyde exposure on minute volume of $B6C3F_1$ mice and F-344 rats. Toxicol Appl Pharmacol 61:451–459
8. Costa DL (1985) Interpretation of new techniques used in the determination of pulmonary function in rodents. Fundam Appl Toxicol 5:423–434
9. Costa DL, Lehmann JR, Slatkin DN, Popenoe EA, Drew RT (1983) Chronic airway obstruction and bronchiectasis in the rat after intratracheal bleomycin. Lung 161:287–300

10. Fabbri LM, Aizawa H, Alpert SE, Walters EH, O'Byrne PM, Gold BD, Nadel JA, Holtzman MJ (1984) Airway hyperresponsiveness and changes in cell counts in bronchoalveolar lavage after ozone exposure in dogs. Am Rev Respir Dis 129:288–291
11. Freeman G, Crane SC, Furiosi NJ, Stephens MJ, Moore WD (1972) Covert reduction in ventilatory surface in rats during prolonged exposure to subacute nitrogen dioxide. Am Rev Respir Dis 106:563–579
12. Fulmer JD, Roberts WC, von Gal ER, Crystal RG (1979) Morphologic-physiologic correlates of the severity of fibrosis and degree of cellularity in idiopathic pulmonary fibrosis. J Clin Invest 63:665–676
13. Gelb AF, Gold WM, Wright RR, Bruch HR, Nadel JA (1973) Physiologic diagnosis of subclinical emphysema. Am Rev Respir Dis 107:50–63
14. Gillespie JR (1983) Mechanisms that determine functional residual capacity in different mammalian species. Am Rev Respir Dis 128[Suppl]:S74–S77
15. Golden JA, Nadel JA, Boushey HA (1978) Bronchial hyperirritability in healthy subjects after exposure to ozone. Am Rev Respir Dis 118:287–294
16. Gordon T, Amdur MO (1980) Effect of ozone on respiratory response of guinea pigs to histamine. J Toxicol Environ Health 6:185–195
17. Harkema JR, Mauderly JL, Hahn FF (1982) The effects of emphysema on oxygen toxicity in rats. Am Rev Respir Dis 126:1058–1065
18. Harkema JR, Mauderly JL, Gregory RE, Pickrell JA (1984) A comparison of starvation and elastase models of emphysema in rats. Am Rev Respir Dis 129:584–591
19. Holtzman MJ, Fabbri LM, O'Byrne PM, Gold BD, Aizawa H, Walters EH, Alpert SE, Nadel JA (1983) Importance of airway inflammation for hyperresponsiveness induced by ozone. Am Rev Respir Dis 127:686–690
20. Johnson WK, Mauderly JL, Hahn FF (1982) Lung function and morphology of dogs after sublethal exposure to nitrogen dioxide. J Toxicol Environ Health 10:201–221
21. Jones GR, Proudfoot AT, Hall JI (1973) Pulmonary effects of acute exposure to nitrous fumes. Thorax 28:61–65
22. Karlinsky JB, Goldstein RH, Catanese A, Snider GL (1986) Young hamsters are more resistant than adults to endotracheally instilled porcine pancreatic elastase. Exp Lung Res 11:229–243
23. Karol MH (1986) Respiratory effects of inhaled isocyanates. CRC Crit Rev Toxicol 16:349–379
24. Lee LY, Bleecker ER, Nadel JA (1977) Effect of ozone on bronchomotor response to inhaled histamine aerosol in dogs. J Appl Physiol 43:626–631
25. Likens SA, Mauderly JL (1982) Effect of elastase or histamine on single-breath N_2 washouts in the rat. J Appl Physiol 52:141–146
26. Mauderly JL (1974) The influence of sex and age on the pulmonary function of the beagle dog. J Gerontol 29:282–289
27. Mauderly JL (1974) Evaluation of the grade pony as a pulmonary function model. Am J Vet Res 35:1025–1029
28. Mauderly JL (1977) Bronchopulmonary lavage of small laboratory animals. Lab Anim Sci 27:255–261
29. Mauderly JL (1984) Respiratory function responses of animals and humans to oxidant gases and to pulmonary emphysema. J Toxicol Environ Health 13:345–361
30. Mauderly JL (1987) Effect of inhaled toxicants on pulmonary function. In: McClellan RO, Henderson RF (eds) Concepts in inhalation toxicology. Hemisphere, Washington DC (in press)

31. Mauderly JL, Tesarek JE, Sifford Linda J, Sifford Lorna J (1979) Respiratory measurements of unsedated small laboratory mammals using nonrebreathing valves. Lab Anim Sci 29:323–329
32. Mauderly JL, Muggenburg BA, Hahn FF, Boecker BB (1980) The effects of inhaled 144-cerium on cardiopulmonary function and histopathology of the dog. Radiat Res 84:307–324
33. Mauderly JL, Gillett NA, Henderson RF, Jones RK, McClellan RO (1987) Relationships of lung structural and functional changes to accumulation of diesel exhaust particles. In: Ann Occup Hyg (in press)
34. McClellan RO (1986) Health effects of diesel exhaust: a case study in risk assessment. Am Ind Hyg Assoc J 47:1–13
35. Mink SN (1984) Expiratory flow limitation and the response to breathing a helium-oxygen gas mixture in a canine model of pulmonary emphysema. J Clin Invest 73:1321–1334
36. Moorman WJ, Lewis TR, Wagner WD (1975) Maximum expiratory flow-volume studies on monkeys exposed to bituminous coal dust. J Appl Physiol 39:444–448
37. Murlas CG, Roum JH (1985) Sequence of pathologic changes in the airway mucosa of guinea pigs during ozone-induced bronchial hyperreactivity. Am Rev Respir Dis 131:314–320
38. Murphy SD, Ulrich CE, Frankowitz SH, Xintras C (1964) Altered function in animals inhaling low concentrations of ozone and nitrogen dioxide. Am Ind Hyg Assoc J 25:246–253
39. Pennock BE, Cox CP, Rogers RM, Cain WA, Wells JH (1979) A noninvasive technique for measurement of changes in specific airway resistance. J Appl Physiol 46:399–406
40. Pino MV, Hahn FF, Pickrell JA (1984) Bleomycin-induced pulmonary fibrosis in Fischer-344 rats. In: Guilmette RA, Medinsky MA (eds) Inhalation toxicology research institute annual report, LMF-113. Lovelace Biomedical and Environmental Research Institute, Albuquerque, NM, pp 372–376. NTIS, Springfield
41. Rodarte JR, Rehder K (1986) Dynamics of respiration. In: Macklem PT, Mead J (eds) Mechanics of breathing, part 1: the respiratory system. American Physiological Society, Bethesda, pp 131–144 (Handbook of physiology, sect 3)
42. Silbaugh SA, Wolff RK, Johnson WK, Mauderly JL, Macken CA (1981) Effects of sulfuric acid aerosols on pulmonary function of guinea pigs. J Toxicol Environ Health 7:339–352
43. Sim VM, Pattle RE (1957) Effect of possible smog irritants on human subjects. J Am Med Assoc 165:1908–1913
44. Snider GL, Hayes JA, Korthy AL (1978) Chronic interstitial pulmonary fibrosis produced in hamsters by endotracheal bleomycin. Am Rev Respir Dis 117:1099–1108
45. Snider GL, Lucey EC, Stone PJ (1986) Animal models of emphysema. Am Rev Respir Dis 133:149–169
46. Tryka AF, Godleski JJ, Skornik WA, Brain JD (1983) Progressive pulmonary fibrosis in hamsters. Exp Lung Res 5:155–171
47. Tyler WS, Coalson JJ, Stripp B (1983) Comparative biology of the lung. Am Rev Respir Dis 128(2):1–91

Part V
Risk Assessment of Airborne Toxicants

CHAPTER 16

Population Studies in Risk Assessment: Strengths and Weaknesses

M.R. Becklake[1]

519 275

Population Studies: A General Introduction to their Scope

Epidemiology is defined as the study of the distribution and determinants of health-related events (including illness and related phenomena) in populations (1). It has also been described as occurrence research involving the study of "occurrence parameters, their determinants and modifiers of relations" (2). The determinants considered are usually classified as host and environmental factors. In the context of inhalational toxicology, the focus is obviously on the latter, in particular on airborne pollutants capable of entry into and retention within the respiratory tract for a sufficient period of time to evoke a biologic response (3). In this presentation, the emphasis will be on human populations, though the approaches and methods can also obviously be applied to animal populations, and to phenomena other than those of medical interest.

The *time frame of study* required to include the biologic response(s) of interest obviously varies with the nature of the putative agent(s) as well as the intensity of exposure, and this must influence all aspects of a population study: design, target population, the methods of measurements used for exposure as well as for the response variables, and approach to analysis (3). For gases and vapors, the time frame is usually short, measured sometimes in seconds, more often in minutes or hours (3); examples are exposure to the oxides of nitrogen and to acutely irritant gases such as SO_2 and NH_4. For such agents, the study design will either be experimental (involving, for instance, controlled low-level exposure, similar to animal exposure studies), or, if the exposure has been uncontrolled, as, for instance, accidental past exposure in the workplace, one of the other study designs developed for chronic disease epidemiology may be applicable (3). For pollutants such as the mineral dusts or fibers, the time frame is usually much longer, measured in years or decades; examples are exposure to mineral fibers

[1]Departments of Medicine and of Epidemiology and Biostatistics (Pulmonary Research Laboratory), McGill University, 1110 Pine Ave West, Montreal, Quebec H3A 1A3 Canada.

such as asbestos and dusts such as silica (3), and for this type of study the techniques of chronic disease epidemiology are also more appropriate.

In this presentation, the emphasis will be on chronic effects and the illustrative examples taken from chronic disease epidemiology with particular reference to asbestos exposure. This agent was chosen because in addition to being the area of personal experience of the author (4–6), asbestos is responsible for both malignant and nonmalignant ill-health effects, and so provides a literature which is not only extensive (7) but is also rich in examples of a wide variety of study approaches with lessons applicable to other fields. It is also a topical issue of considerable public concern (8–10).

Seminal Research Questions in Inhalational Toxicology Susceptible to Study Using Epidemiologic Methods

The research questions which can be addressed in human population studies can be grouped under 3 general categories. The first (*Is there an ill-health effect associated with exposure to the agent(s) and/or occupation(s) in question?*) is relevant in the identification of new hazards. If the ill-health effect is acute and/or severe enough to result in the ready identification, the corrective steps (removal or neutralization of the toxic material) can often be simply and effectively achieved (3). Likewise, if the ill-health effect is sufficiently unusual [e.g., mesothelioma in relation to exposure to crocidolite asbestos mining in the North West Cape, South Africa (6)], the association with exposure may be accepted as causal from the outset without further study. If the ill-health effect under consideration is also common in nonexposed populations, e.g., lung cancer, then further studies are needed, addressing the second seminal research question (*Is the effect dose-related and what are the time trends?*). Studies designed to bring out exposure-response relationships are necessary to build up the case for causality (11) as well as to provide information relevant to risk assessment and management (12–15), discussed in more detail below. These first two seminal research questions may be answered by appropriately designed analytic studies. The effectiveness of risk management can be assessed by industrial hygiene and environmental monitoring (personal and station), but less attention has been paid to the more important though less easily studied component of the third seminal research question on how to evaluate the efficacy of the steps taken in risk management (*Has the institution of environmental controls resulted in improvement in health status of those exposed?*). Thus in general, evaluation studies are based on the experimental design (see Fig. 16.1), of which the randomized control trial, usually of drugs, but also of treatments, is the most common example (3). Such studies are not feasible in industrial toxicology to assess the effect of controls on health, and epidemiologists have shown less creativity in exploiting nonexperimental designs to address this important issue of evaluation (16). For instance, in the context of occupational exposure to asbestos, despite the

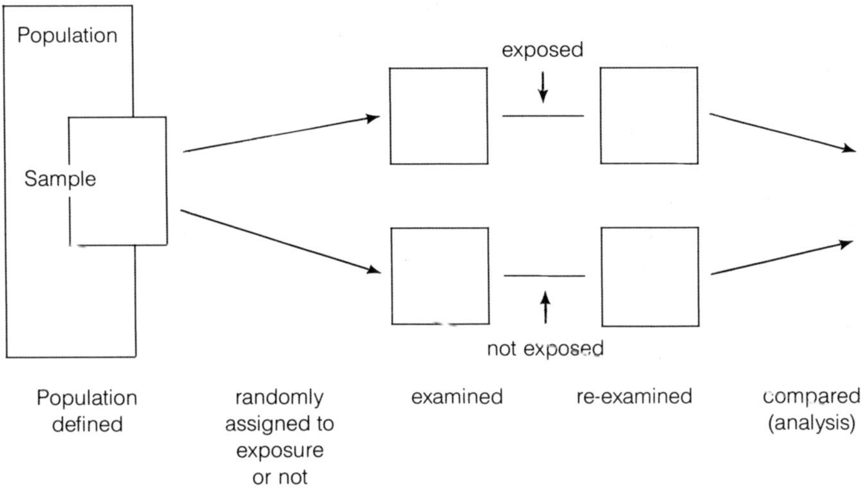

Fig. 16.1. The experimental design. Listed at the bottom of the diagram are the steps in a study following the experimental design; most epidemiologic studies use a less than complete experimental design, the randomized control trial (RCT) being the exception.

introduction of environmental controls from the late 1960s, with further stringency introduced in the 1970s (17) and proposed for the 1980s (18), few studies (19,20) have attempted to evaluate the very important issue of whether implementation of these workplace standards has reduced the risk to human health (5,6). In part, this is technical, due to a change in the industrial hygiene technology used to measure airborne asbestos dust [fiber counts have replaced particle counts (21)]. As a result, there is serious doubt about the comparability of past and current measurements of pollution (22), and so of exposure-response relationships.

The Design of Population Studies

Key to scientific study is use of the experimental design shown in Fig. 16.1, a design in which the researcher has control over all phases of the study. This includes the opportunity to study a complete population (or to sample from it by a random procedure), assignment to exposure or not (also by a random procedure), examination before and after exposure, and complete follow-up of all individuals, exposed or not. Population studies, whether in the context of inhalational toxicology or in any other context, usually fall short of this. Thus, selection from the general population into various occupations is seldom random [workers tend to be healthier than those who do not enter the job market (23)], and the same is true of the entry to jobs with exposures, often heavier physically than other jobs. Clinical data describing preexposure status is rarely available, and follow-up is seldom complete. Thus, with the exceptions mentioned above [i.e., short-term exposure studies to low controlled levels of pollutants (3)], study design in population studies is nonexperimental, a compromise between the nature of the health event to be studied, the population(s) in whom the study can be carried out, and the available information on who was (or is) at risk, and their past health status.

The main study designs (see Table 16.1) are: (a) *cohort* or *longitudinal*, generally used to study occurrence rates, particularly those which can be clearly defined, e.g., death; (b) *cross-sectional*, generally used to study occurrence rates of a chronic disease process for which the precise moment of onset cannot be specified, e.g., asbestosis; and (c) *case-control*, an approach closer to that of clinical medicine, in that the argument starts from the individual(s) with a recognized ill-health effect (cases) and contrasts the occurrence of exposure in cases compared to that of a sample of the general (base) population (controls) from which the cases were drawn. This approach is particularly suitable for the study of infrequent occurrences [e.g., mesothelioma, a rare tumor with an incidence rate of 1–2 per million in nonasbestos-exposed populations (6)]. It also has the advantage of practicality and economy of effort; the key to its success lies in the wise choice of the procedure used to select controls (2,16). Stratification or matching, for instance, on age and smoking within a cohort mortality study of lung cancer in asbestos workers (24), provides additional strength in dealing with the distribution of the determinant under study (in this example, asbestos exposure) in relation to confounders (2).

Population: Base, Sample, and Sample Size

The population base in inhalational toxicology studies is usually one or more workforces, made up of individuals naturally or self-selected into the industries and/or occupations with the exposure of interest; those currently at work, those who were at work in the past, and retirees may all be included in the study base, depending on the occurrence chosen for study (3). Selection factors into and out of industries are many, are not infrequently health-related, and invariably result in bias, termed the "healthy worker effect" (1). Originally described in relation to mortality experience (23), the effect is probably applicable to other biological characteristics (25). Compared to the general population, those at work are likely to be above average in fitness, above average in general health, and above average in withstanding the particular type of target organ response which their exposure entails. If the base population is large, and the outcome measurements complex and time-consuming, the researcher may resort to sampling, preferring fewer quality measurements to a larger number of less precise ones (17).

Miettinen (2) makes the distinction between scientific occurrence research, concerned with explaining relationships (for instance, is the risk of lung cancer increased with increasing intensity of exposure to asbestos?) and particularistic research (for instance, in a given asbestos mining workforce, how many individ-

Table 16.1. Contrasting arguments in cohort and case-control studies[a]

	Occurrence (response)	
	Present	Not
Exposure		
Present	A	B
Not	C	D

[a]Cohort (and cross-sectional studies) argue from exposure to response, i.e, horizontally across the table; occurrence rates are compared in exposed (A/A+B) and nonexposed (C/C+D) subjects; case-control studies argue from the occurrence of a response to its association (or not) with exposure, i.e., vertically down the table; exposure rates are compared in cases (A/A+C) and controls (B/B+D).

uals have an asbestos-related disability requiring use of health care facilities?) Workforce-based research studies can often provide both types of information, scientific (relevant to risk assessment) and particularistic (relevant to the public and personal health issues in members of the workforce).

Sample size, an important determinant of the power of a study, is seldom a matter of choice for the researcher in this field, who must use the population at hand, i.e., the workforce(s) with the relevant exposure. For this reason, negative studies need careful scrutiny; if the sample size and/or number of expected events was small, only large relative risks could have been detected (13).

Health-Related and Exposure Measurements

Issues related to the characterization and measurement of health-related events are no different for inhalational toxicology studies than for any other type of population study; these are treated in detail elsewhere (2,3,26). Important aspects in measurement include careful definition (conceptual and operational) of the health outcome of interest (Table 16.2), even if such definitions do not correspond to the usual clinical definitions of the same outcome (27–29). Ordinal (qualitative) as well as quantitative scales are often useful and can be, particularly if well formulated, biologically credible. Standard indices enhance comparability of study results with published data and should be employed wherever possible and appropriate. The most frequently used tools for measurements of morbidity in inhalational toxicology studies are the respiratory symptom questionnaire, lung function tests, and the chest radiograph, each of which has been specifically adapted for use in population studies (3).

Exposure measurements are, however, the key to successful inhalational toxicology studies, and the extent to which they are quantitative rather than qualitative [and measured using currently applicable industrial hygiene techniques (8)],

Table 16.2. Examples of conceptual and operational definitions of health-related measurements

Conceptual definition	Possible operational definitions
Chronic bronchitis	(i) Answers yes to the question[a] "Do you usually bring up phlegm from your chest?" (ii) Increased ratio of mucus gland to bronchial wall thickness (Reid index).
Asbestosis	(i) Reading of 1/0 or more for small irregular opacities on the chest radiograph.[b] (ii) Presence of basal crepitations on clinical examination. (iii) Both of the above.
Mesothelioma	(i) As recorded on the death certificate. (ii) Based on pathologic review.[c]

[a]Based on the ATS standardized respiratory symptom questionnaire (27).
[b]Reading may be based on 1 or more readers using the ILO classification (28).
[c]Usually including reference to a mesothelioma panel (29).

determines the scientific value of a given study, particularly for risk assessment (3,8,12,13). Ideally, for instance, exposure measurements for asbestos, or indeed for any other inhaled pollutant, should take into account duration, intensity, quality (particle or fiber, size and shape, biologic potency), and exposure profile (short bursts of high exposure versus long-term low exposure), as well as host factors which might modify any of the above, e.g., use of masks, mouth versus nose breathing, and job stress (3). For past occupational exposures, use may be made of job history, matched to available industrial hygiene measurements, and it may be possible to take into account some of the modifiers listed above (30,31). Peak and short-term heavy exposures can also be modelled (31), though not quantitatively. Cumulative exposure indices (30) almost certainly involve misclassification resulting in attenuation of exposure-response relationships (32). Nevertheless, most studies of asbestos-exposed populations have shown exposure-response relationships for both nonmalignant and malignant outcomes (3–6). However as already indicated, it was in relatively few that the exposure measurements were of sufficient quality and precision to make the results suitable for standard setting.

An additional complication in the case of asbestos arises from the differences in biological activity of different fiber types. Evidence for such a biologic gradient varies with the outcome, being least for asbestosis, strongest for mesothelioma, and variable for lung and other cancers (4–6,8–10,22). The ingenious use of comparison rates for mesothelioma vis-à-vis excess lung cancers in workforces exposed to different fiber types has greatly strengthened this evidence (33). However, even this evidence is qualitative (based on amount of different types of fiber used in a given plant or industry), not quantitative (based on direct measurement of different fiber types in the airborne pollution cloud).

Balancing the Strengths and Weaknesses of Epidemiologic Data in Risk Assessment

Risk assessment has been described as "the scientific process by which we estimate the probability that some harm will come to an individual or a population as a result of exposure to a substance or a situation" (12). It comprises four steps: (a) qualitative assessment of the hazard (in the case of asbestos exposure, recognized ill-health effects include fibrosis of the lungs and pleura, as well as cancer of these organs); (b) quantitative assessment of the hazard (based on exposure response information); (c) establishing who is at risk (number of individuals exposed and to what levels); and (d) from the above, estimating the probability of exposed individuals being affected. *Risk management* is the use of this information to make policy decisions (12). In the case of asbestos exposure, this involves setting workplace and environmental standards, and/or proposing other steps to control human exposure, e.g., banning the use of certain or all fibers.

The criteria for the first two steps in risk assessment are purely scientific and no different from those used by the scientist writing a review article in a given field or preparing the background for a research protocol. Published reports are evaluated systematically, each component (design, population, measurements, analysis) being examined for strengths and weaknesses (12,13). Disagreements in interpretation and synthesis are a feature of the battleground of scientific thought, and in the real world no study is flawless, and few are without some bias. It is thus the overall judgement of the scientific reader which will determine whether or not, on balance, the findings should be accepted and incorporated into the knowledge base. Information from different sources is then synthesized; in the case of inhalational toxicology, particularly for certain chronic outcomes like cancer, this will first involve establishing causality. This is done on the basis of the now familiar criteria originally formulated by Doll and Hill (11), criteria which include consistency in the demonstration of clear associations between outcome and exposure (with dose-response relationships including a negative effect with withdrawal) in studies free of bias carried out by different researchers in different exposed populations. Dose-response relationships based on qualitative measurements of exposure provide valid evidence for establishing causality; however, quantitative measurements using established industrial hygiene methods are required for generalizability (which includes use of the information in risk management), and for the establishment of workplace and/or environmental control levels.

Lessons from the Asbestos Example

There are several lessons for the scientific community from their involvement with asbestos, lessons directly linked with the process of synthesis and interpretation of scientific data and how their strengths and weaknesses are dealt with.

The first relates to the complexity of the agent and its biological effects; not one, but several mineralogic fiber types are involved, with differences in physical and chemical composition, and also, as it turns out, with differences in biologic potential (4–6,8–10). As a result, between-workforce differences in disease rates for what appeared at first to be equivalent exposure doses are probably due not to imperfect science, as originally implied (34), but due to differences in the nature of the airborne particles to which different workforces are exposed. Thus, in addition to fiber type differences, chemical and physical, there are differences in the fiber shape and size characteristics of particles released in different industrial processes, e.g., mining and milling compared to cement manufacture and textile weaving (3–5). Understanding how these differences relate to biologic potential still challenges scientific elucidation and also has implications for control, including risk management.

A second lesson, already referred to, relates to changing industrial hygiene technology for measurement of airborne dust levels. Earlier measurements in the 1960s using the midget impinger focused on particles (now considered a surrogate measure for the active agent); these gave way to fiber counts (probably the active form of the agent) in the 1970s (21). However, there was no responsibility, implicit or legal, to provide parallel measurements from the same sampling sites over a period of time to establish equivalences (21). Such studies as are available indicate that there are no simple conversion factors (21,22). This makes it difficult to compare results of the earlier health studies using millions of particles per cubic foot as the scale for the exposure measurement with later studies using fibers per milliliter. Also related to industrial hygiene technology is another lesson, the need to validate in practice exposure assessment algorithms, rather than bypass established technology (21).

A third lesson relates to what has been described as the "disconnection between what science can prove and what public officials need to know to make necessary decisions" (12). Indeed the quotation itself indicates an aspect of the problem, since the scientific method proceeds by rejection, not proof, of hypotheses. The issue was one of extrapolation, to provide estimates of risk at low levels of exposure, such as might occur to those who work or study in buildings in which asbestos has been used in construction [median exposures range from approximately 0.00005 to 0.0005 fibers/ml (21)], from workplace exposures which are orders of magnitude greater [current legislated standards vary from 2 to 0.5 fibers/ml in different jurisdictions (17), and of course past levels were much higher (30)]. Several estimates of risk have been offered based on different assumptions (8,33). One, considered defensible (21), estimates an excess of 0.25 deaths per year per million exposed for a 6-year period, compared to 1200 for long-term smoking and 10 for playing high-school football (33). It is unlikely that the large-scale, low-level exposure studies called for by some (13) are feasible or affordable; they also call for detection probably beyond the achievable limits of current methodology.

What part should the scientist working in the field of epidemiology play in this arena? There can be no doubt that providing a sound information base remains the most powerful offering. Thus, the epidemiologist's first task is meticulous documentation of occurrences and their determinants in populations, with reporting in reviewed scientific journals for scrutiny, comment, and criticism. In contrast to much other data in inhalational toxicology, epidemiologic data in this field are usually based on human rather than animal studies, thus avoiding the need for extrapolation from one species to another. They are therefore likely to remain of key importance in the assessment and management of human risk, and the need to synthesize and summarize data in the public domain with a view to developing policy will continue. Scientists are often hesitant to enter this debate, particularly in their own field: nonscientists less so. Circumstances may force this to change, and it is in this belief that the present chapter is offered. Certainly future public debate on current issues in inhalational toxicology is likely to increase, not decrease, and the lessons learned from the case of asbestos may be applicable or prove valuable in the study and management of other toxic or potentially toxic inhaled agents.

Acknowledgment. This work was supported by the Medical Research Council of Canada. Dr. Becklake is a Career Investigator of the Medical Research Council of Canada.

References

1. Last JM (ed) (1983) Dictionary of epidemiology. Oxford University Press, New York
2. Miettinen OS (1985) Theoretical epidemiology: Principles of occurrence research in medicine. Wiley, New York, pp 1–359
3. Becklake MR (1985) Epidemiologic studies in human populations. In: Witschi HP, Brain JD (eds) Toxicology of inhaled materials. Springer, Berlin Heidelberg, New York, pp 115–147 (Handbook of experimental pharmacology, vol 75)
4. Becklake MR (1976) Asbestos-related diseases of the lungs and other organs: Their epidemiology and implications for clinical practice. Am Rev Respir Dis 114:187–227
5. Becklake MR (1982) Asbestos-related diseases of the lungs and pleura: Current clinical issues. Am Rev Respir Dis 126:187–194
6. Becklake MR (1983) Occupational lung disease: Past record and future trends using the asbestos case as an example. Clin Invest Med 6:305–317
7. Peters GA, Peters BJ (1980) Source book on asbestos diseases: Medical, legal, and engineering aspects. Garland STPM Press, New York, pp A1-K18
8. Dupre JS (chairman) (1984) Report of the Royal Commission on matters of health and safety arising from the use of asbestos in Ontario. Queen's Printer for Ontario, Toronto, pp 1–920
9. Acheson ED, Gardner MJ (1979) The ill-health effects of asbestos on health. In: Asbestos, vol 2. Final report of the advisory committee. Health and Safety Commission. Her Majesty's Stationery Office, London, pp 7–84
10. Acheson ED, Gardner MJ (1983) Asbestos: the control limit for asbestos (an update). Health and Safety commission. Her Majesty's Stationery Office, London, pp 1–26
11. Doll R (1984) Occupational cancer: problems in interpreting human evidence. Ann Occup Hyg 28:291–305

12. Alm AL (1985) Introductory remarks. Toxicol Ind Health 1:1–5
13. Erdreich LS, Burnett C (1985) Improving the use of epidemiologic data in health risk assessment. Toxicol Ind Health 1:65–81
14. Davis DL, Mandula B, Van Ryzin J (1985) Assessing the power and quality of epidemiologic studies of asbestos exposed populations. Toxicol Ind Health 1:93–110
15. National Academy of Science (1984) Asbestiform fibers: nonoccupational health risks. National Academy Press, Washington, pp 1–334
16. McDonald JC (1981) Epidemiology. In: Weill H, Turner-Warwick M (eds) Occupational lung diseases: research approach and methods. Dekker, New York, pp 373–404
17. McDonald JC (1980) Aspects of the asbestos standard. In: Gee BGL, Morgan KWG, Brooks SM (eds) Occupational lung disease. Raven, New York, pp 139–149
18. Environmental Protection Agency (1986) Asbestos: proposed mining and import restrictions and proposed manufacturing importation and processing prohibitions. Federal Register 51:3737–3759
19. Berry G, Gilson JC, Holmes S, Lewinsohn HC, Roach SA (1979) Asbestosis: a study of dose response relationships in an asbestos textile factory. Br J Ind Med 36:98–112
20. Cordier S, Theriault G, Provencher S (1984) Radiographic changes in a group of chrysotile miners exposed to low asbestos dust concentrations. Br J Ind Med 41:384–388
21. Corn M (1986) Asbestos and disease: an industrial hygienist's perspective. Am Ind Hyg Assoc J 47:515–523
22. Doll R, Peto J (1985) Asbestos: effects on health of exposure to asbestos. Health and Safety Commission, London, Her Majesty's Stationery Office, 1–58
23. Weed DL (1986) Historical roots of the healthy worker effect. J Occup Med 28: 343–347
24. McDonald JC, Liddell FDK, Eyssen GE, McDonald AD (1980) Dust exposure and mortality in chrysotile mining, 1910–75. Br J Ind Med 37:11–24
25. Ernst P, Dales R, Nunes F, Becklake MR (1987) Health selection may be determined by airway reactivity in a dusty work environment. Chest 91:273 (abstract)
26. Abramson JH (1979) Survey methods in community medicine (2nd edn). Churchill Livingston, Edinburgh, pp 1–220
27. Ferris BG (1978) Epidemiology standardization project. Am Rev Respir Dis 118:6(Part2):1–120
28. International Labour Office (1980) ILO U/C International classification of radiographs of pneumoconiosis. ILO, Geneva. (Occupational health and safety series no. 22, revised)
29. Craighead JE (chairman) (1982) Asbestos-associated diseases. Arch Path Lab Med 106:541–597
30. Gibbs GW, Lachance M (1972) Dust exposure in the chrysotile mines and mills of Quebec. Arch Environ Health 24:189–197
31. Copes R, Thomas D, Becklake MR (1985) Temporal patterns of exposure and nonmalignant pulmonary abnormality in Quebec chrysotile workers. Arch Environ Health 40:80–87
32. Monson RR (1980) Occupational epidemiology. CRC Press, Boca Raton, pp 95–96
33. Hughes JM, Weill H (1986) Asbestos exposure-quantitative assessment of risk. Am Rev Respir Dis 133:5–13
34. Brodeur P (1985) Outrageous misconduct: The asbestos industry on trial. Pantheon, New York, pp 1–374

CHAPTER 17

Human Clinical Exposure Studies: Body Box or Pandora's Box?

M.J. Utell[1]

Introduction

The development of air quality standards or assignment of risk for acute and/or chronic inhalation of low-level environmental air pollutants is complex. Typically, the database for these exercises arises from three separate arenas: the epidemiologic study, animal exposures, and human inhalation studies. Each possesses unique advantages but also carries significant limitations. For example, the epidemiologic study examines the "real world" but then struggles with real-world problems: such important confounders as cigarette smoking, socioeconomic status, and occupational factors, as well as the difficulties in characterizing exposure. This is contrasted with inhalation studies in animals which allow remarkable precision in quantifying exposure duration and concentration, a wide variety of physiological, biochemical, and histological endpoints, and the opportunity to examine extremes of the exposure-response relationship. Often, however, consideration of these studies in the standard-setting process is constrained by difficulty in extrapolating from animals to humans, and occasionally exclusion results from unrealistic exposure design.

This presentation will focus on a third and complementary approach, the carefully controlled quantitative study of exposed humans. Human clinical studies create atmospheric conditions in laboratory settings which are considered relevant to ambient pollutant atmospheres and document any health-related effects which result from breathing the atmospheres. Advantage is taken of the highly controlled environment to identify responses to individual pollutants and characterize exposure-response relationships as well as to examine interaction between pollutants per se or with other environmental variables such as exercise, humidity, or temperature. Insofar as individuals with acute and chronic respiratory diseases can participate in exposure protocols, a special opportunity emerges to study susceptible populations. Unfortunately, this approach also has limitations: for practical and ethical reasons, studies must be limited to small groups

[1]University of Rochester, Rochester, NY 14642, USA.

presumably representative of larger populations, to short durations of exposure and to pollutant concentrations that are expected to produce only mild and transient responses. Furthermore, endpoint assessment is invariably pulmonary function; to date, too little emphasis has been placed on developing alternative methodologies. Despite these limitations, the establishment of adverse health effects based partially on controlled human exposures has become a reality.

In the following presentation, we examine the entry and growth of the clinical study in the field of risk assessment using three timeframes, the past, the present, and the future. From the past, we review the methodologies and technologies that are the foundation for today's sophisticated studies. In the present, we concentrate on defining exposure-response relationships for healthy and susceptible populations and clarifying the "lowest dose" at which reproducible effects occur. To examine the strengths and weaknesses of the current approach, selected results from studies with three criteria pollutants are presented. For the future, we will recommend a slight change in course with a more vigorous effort to link our understanding of pollutant-induced injury with new assessment techniques. The tools are emerging and sensitive, and more specific "markers" await identification.

The Past: Methodologies and Technologies

Before proceeding with our chronology, we would emphasize that the proposed "past," "present," and "future" are not sharply demarcated periods. The overlap acknowledges that the inhalation technologies and pulmonary methodologies have been available for some time, but that a dynamic process allows for modification and development.

Inhalation Facilities

The number of studies on simulated gaseous and particulate pollutants has greatly increased during the past decade. Much of the technology needed for clinical inhalation studies was developed earlier but utilized either for particle deposition and retention studies or assessment of the physiology of bronchoconstriction. However, with the pioneering studies of Amdur et al. (1) using face masks and of Bates et al. (3) in developing a chamber for exposing humans, the era opened for clinical inhalation studies.

These two types of technologies remain the standards in modern clinical investigations and were reviewed recently by Morrow and Utell (18). Despite growing sophistication in pollutant monitoring and control, the basic exposure designs have undergone little change.

In brief, individual units incorporate mouthpiece or face mask exposures and typically use commercially available nebulizers which are widely used in pulmonary function laboratories or inhalation therapy. These are economic, compact systems relatively easy to design and adaptable to permit exercise during the exposure. Furthermore, such systems provide an opportunity to obtain quantitative information about the exposure, even to the extent of estimating dose. Unique limitations to individual units are the artificial ventilatory patterns induced by the mouthpiece, exclusion of the highly effective nasal filter for particles and gases, and the requirement for relatively short exposures. In addition, the assessment of responses requires discontinuation or interruption of the exposure.

In comparison, the chamber-type exposure "immerses" the individual in the highly controlled, synthetic atmosphere with or without an added pollutant. Obviously, there are important distinctions between chamber and environmental exposures, primarily related to the complex mixtures of pollutants occurring in the outdoors. Yet there exist special opportunities available only in the chamber setting, i.e., normal activities, intermittent peak levels, and unencumbered measurements of breathing. Several of these features are essential to studies lasting many hours because they allow the subject freedom of motion and comfort while still providing sufficient control of the exposure. Using inductive plethysmography, the subject's total ventilation can be measured. Thus, the chamber study comes closer to the dosimetric approach achieved with the mouthpiece exposure. Finally, the response measurements can be made while the chamber exposure continues.

Although pollutant-induced bronchoconstriction is enhanced at rest using the mouthpiece exposure system, differences in response become less pronounced with greater exercise levels as the normal physiological switch from nasal to oral ventilation occurs at higher ventilatory rates (approximately 35 L/min) (11,19).

Measuring the Response

Pulmonary physiology and pulmonary function testing underwent explosive growth from the mid-1950s through the mid-1970s. This early development of standard tests impacted greatly upon the emergence of clinical studies. More recent contributions in the field of pulmonary function testing (with the exception of airway reactivity) have often emphasized standardization and quality assurance rather than new test development. Today virtually every clinical study of the effects of inhaled pollutants on the lung relies on standard measurements of pulmonary function. In general, measurements of flow rates, lung volumes, or airway resistance are made before, during, and after the exposure of volunteers to selected pollutants and compared with the results obtained from sham exposure or preexposure values. The level of change of pulmonary function after exposure, then, relates to the potency of the pollutant.

Because pulmonary tests poorly discriminate regional airway effects, this lack of response specificity limits the differentiation of large airway, small airway, and gas exchange region effects. However, it is clear that tests could be preselected to more effectively evaluate the site of pollutant uptake or deposition. It is equally clear that investigators rarely consider the suitability of their measurement technique to the targets they propose to assess.

A large variety of pulmonary function measurements are incorporated into controlled clinical studies. The measurement of resistance to airflow is regarded as an important investigative and clinical tool. Both airway resistance and total thoracic resistance measurements are used in air pollutant studies. Measurements of airway resistance (or conductance) are most widely applied; these require a body plethysmograph ("body box"). Airway resistance is principally of use in the diagnosis of airway obstruction and in the evaluation of its reversibility. The relative sensitivity of airway resistance to narrowing of upper airways, central airways, and peripheral airways is of great importance. Because most of the airway resistance in normal subjects is located in large, central airways, it has been claimed that airway resistance should be useful in identifying the predominant site of flow limitation. Diseases that produce significant flow obstruction in large airways (asthma) tend to elevate airway resistance more than diseases involving peripheral airways. Although controversy remains regarding the major site of airflow resistance in the lung, the effects of gases absorbed or particles deposited in upper or central airways are best detected by measurements of airway resistance. This measurement proves ideal for the very soluble gases.

Certainly the most commonly evaluated parameters in controlled exposure studies are measurement of forced vital capacity (FVC), forced expiratory volume in 1 s (FEV_1), and maximal flow-volume curves. An earlier review (26) indicated that over the past few years, 90–95% of pollutant exposure studies evaluated responses with at least one of these tests. They are easy to perform, and only small changes in FVC or FEV_1 are detectable in the same subject studied repeatedly on the same day or consecutive days. Although the FEV_1 is probably not as sensitive as closing-volume or partial flow-volume loops in detecting changes in peripheral airways, its reliability and reproducibility make it a measurement of choice. Changes in FEV_1 reflect alterations either in the central or the more peripheral airway. Reductions in lung volumes such as the FVC following pollutant exposures are more characteristic of restrictive than obstructive changes. The measurement of FVC and FEV_1 are most sensitive in detecting alterations induced by particles or gases deposited in the conducting or peripheral airways.

The diffusing capacity is the only noninvasive, readily available test of lung performance that provides information on the gas exchange function of the lung in distinction to mechanical properties. In contrast to spirometric measurements, alterations in diffusing capacity are rarely examined in controlled clinical studies. Although there are large differences in diffusing capacity from individual to individual, the test is easily performed, quickly repeated, and demonstrates excellent reproducibility. However, its usefulness in controlled clinical studies may be limited because it is influenced both by changes in lung volume and by exercise. Since exercise itself may increase the diffusing capacity, any marginal reduction in this parameter resulting from inhalation of a pollutant could be negated. Despite these limitations, given the few options for assessing insoluble, nonreactive gases, this is a measurement which warrants further evaluation.

The measurement of airway reactivity has generated intense interest in the past few years. Although the ability of certain substances to produce bronchospasm when inhaled by asthmatics was recognized as early as the late 1940s (7), the introduction of this technique into studies of health effects of air pollutants is comparatively recent. The role of reactivity testing in clinical studies was recently examined by Sheppard (24). Two reasons for inclusion of these measurements were identified. First, when the major effect of exposure to a specific pollutant is bronchoconstriction, airway reactivity testing permits determination of the inherent baseline airway responsiveness of the subject. In earlier studies in our laboratory at the University of Rochester (27), we related changes in pulmonary function following inhalation of a pollutant to the inherent reactivity of the volunteer's airway. We examined in asthmatic subjects the relationship between baseline airway reactivity assessed by the response to carbachol and responsiveness to an inhaled sulfuric acid aerosol. High correlation was found between the decrease in specific airway conductance after exposure to low concentrations of carbachol and the reduction in specific airway conductance after inhalation of 1000 $\mu g/m^3$ sulfuric acid. Although baseline airway reactivity identified responders to the acidic aerosols, this relationship between baseline airway tone and responses to the gaseous pollutant sulfur dioxide or ozone has shown a much weaker correlation.

In addition, development of an acute change in airway responsiveness after pollutant exposure may be a sensitive marker of airway injury or inflammation. Holtzman et al. (9) studied the effects of ozone on airway reactivity in dogs and concluded that the acute induction of increased reactivity was due to injury to airway epithelial cells, with subsequent recruitment of neutrophils into the airway wall. Airway reactivity following ozone has also been linked to the recruitment of neutrophils in healthy humans (23). Similar to its sensitivity in stable asthma, increased airway reactivity may be a more sensitive indicator of pollutant-induced defects than standard pulmonary function tests. Although the sensitivity of the measurement seems clear, its reproducibility needs further evaluation. However, if airway hyperreactivity is ultimately shown to be a risk factor in the development of obstructive airway disease, then alteration in airway response after acute exposure to pollutants should acquire additional significance.

The Present: Analysis of Results from Controlled Clinical Studies

With development of appropriate exposure units, sophisticated monitoring equipment, and suitable physiological measurements, the controlled clinical study entered the present decade. Given the high costs and ethical constraints, relatively few laboratories became involved. State-of-the art research emerged along the following lines: (a) development of exposure-response relationships based exclusively on pulmonary function, with emphasis on contrasting healthy and susceptible populations; (b) establishment of the "lowest concentration" at

Table 17.1. Physical characteristics, behavior, and clinical findings with three pollutant gases

Pollutant	Characteristics	Uptake site	Clinical findings
Sulfur dioxide	Soluble	Upper airways	Asthmatic sensitivity > normal; effects on airway resistance; lowest effect level 0.25–0.40 ppm
Ozone	Insoluble highly reactive	Entire airway	Asthmatic sensitivity = normal; effects on FEV_1; lowest effect level 0.12–0.18 ppm
Nitrogen dioxide	Relatively insoluble and reactive	Distal airway	Asthmatic sensitivity > normal but variable reduction in FEV_1; lowest effect level ~0.3 ppm

which individual pollutants provoked reproducible responses; and (c), when feasible, development of protocols to examine "mechanisms" of pollutant-induced lung injury. The results of studies with sulfur dioxide, ozone, and nitrogen dioxide, all criteria pollutants in the United States and regulated by the US Environmental Protection Agency, will be used to illustrate the strengths and weakness of the approach. For each, we will briefly: (a) outline uptake of the inhaled gas, (b) summarize key clinical findings, (c) examine the relationship between uptake and effect on lung function, and (d) speculate as to potential impact on the regulatory process (Table 17.1).

Sulfur Dioxide

Sulfur dioxide (SO_2) and sulfuric acid aerosols are released during the combustion of fossil fuels. SO_2 is soluble in water and readily absorbed upon contact with the moist surfaces of the nose and upper airway passages. Although SO_2 is almost completely removed by nasal absorption under resting conditions in humans, penetration to the lower respiratory tract increases with exercise and increased ventilation associated with the shift from nasal to oral breathing at a ventilation of approximately 35 L/min (19). In addition, SO_2 in combination with hygroscopic particles will enhance penetration of the pollutant in the airway.

Since SO_2 alone or in combination with particles is primarily absorbed in the upper airways during exercise exposures, techniques are needed to measure the bronchoconstrictor response characteristic of this segment of the respiratory tract. In fact, measurements derived from the "body box" have proven ideal for this task. Studies by several investigators (6,13) have demonstrated that airway (or respiratory) resistance is the most sensitive parameter in evaluating responses to the highly soluble gas SO_2. Incorporating moderate to heavy levels of exercise, these investigators found significant group mean changes in specific airway resistance for asthmatics exposed to 0.4–0.6 ppm SO_2. In some individuals, changes in specific airway resistance were observed at levels as low as 0.25 ppm with heavy exercise. SO_2 provides a model for linking pollutant properties with assessment techniques. The pollutant is absorbed in the upper airway; the clinical tool, the body box, effectively measures the upper airway response.

A clinical study will generate highly useful data for the risk assessment process only if satisfactory measures of airway injury, inflammation, or reflex change are available. Such is the case for SO_2. At least two major findings will likely impact directly on the regulatory process: (a) asthmatics are now known to represent a sensitive population and probably are an order of magnitude more sensitive to SO_2 than normal populations, and (b) some SO_2-sensitive asthmatics are at risk of experiencing significant bronchoconstriction when inhaling SO_2 concentrations of 0.40–0.50 ppm or greater, when performing moderate exercise.

Ozone

Ozone, an oxidant formed in the atmosphere from complex photochemical reactions, is perhaps the most thoroughly studied of the criteria pollutants. It is the major component of photochemical smog. In contrast to SO_2, ozone is a relatively insoluble gas; however, it is highly reactive and can react with virtually every type of biological substance. Because of its unusual stability–reactivity characteristics, tracking its deposition in the respiratory system is far more complex than for SO_2. However, observations from modeling and experimental studies together provide information on sites of uptake in the airway. Morphological studies from animals reveal that ozone is absorbed along the entire respiratory tract; it penetrates further into the peripheral airways as inhaled ozone concentration increases (8). Although there are differences in the anatomy of the respiratory tract between experimental animals and humans, the junction between the conducting airways and the gas exchange region, i.e., the transitional airways, is the site most severely damaged by ozone exposure in animals. The dosimetry model simulations given by Miller et al. (15) predict that the maximal tissue uptake occurs at the region of predominant morphological damage in animals. Similar ozone uptake in humans is predicted from the model (16). However, it is apparent that nasopharyngeal absorption can lessen the quantity of ozone delivered to the lungs, since exposure of isolated upper airways to ozone has resulted in 50–75% ozone removal (28).

Insofar as ozone is absorbed along the entire airway, volunteers exposed to this gas should predictably manifest a variety of alterations in lung function. McDonnell et al. (14) have found changes in FEV_1 at ozone levels as low as 0.12–0.18 ppm, when exposure is combined with heavy exercise. Avol et al. (2) confirmed these findings in a study of competitive cyclists who exercised continuously in a chamber containing various ozone concentrations for 1 h. Furthermore, exposure during exercise of the same subjects to ambient Los Angeles air containing a mean of 0.15 ppm ozone (as well as the local oxidants and particles) caused symptoms and spirometric changes similar to those observed at 0.16 ppm ozone in the chamber environment. This demonstrates that the pulmonary effects of inhalation of ozone observed in chamber experiments are representative of the effects of exposure to natural ambient pollution with a dominant pollutant. However, not all pulmonary responses show the same sensitivity to ozone exposure. Indeed, higher ozone levels were required to produce measurable increases in specific airway resistance during exercise, for example.

It is evident with ozone that clinical studies have contributed to the understanding of mechanisms and the analysis of risk. The body box may be relegated to a lesser role with this pollutant but other standard pulmonary function measures have successfully filled the gap. Although the precise sites and dosimetry of inhaled ozone require further clarification, the sensitivity of spirometric measurements suggest an effect in central or peripheral airways. A summary of the major findings from clinical studies likely to impact on the regulatory process include the following:

1. That low concentrations of ozone ranging from 0.12–0.18 ppm cause impairment of lung function in healthy exercising volunteers
2. The equal sensitivity to ozone of normal and asthmatic individuals
3. The considerable intersubject variability in the magnitude of spirometric changes induced by a given ozone exposure, but the highly reproducible response to ozone in individuals
4. The development of "adaptation" with sequential ozone exposures

Nitrogen Dioxide

In contrast to consensus emanating from studies with SO_2 and ozone, acute controlled studies with nitrogen dioxide (NO_2) have generated conflicting data. The characteristics of NO_2 are different from those of SO_2 or ozone; it is a relatively insoluble, less reactive gas than ozone that penetrates to the peripheral lung with its major site of injury at the terminal bronchioles. Exercise results in the delivery of a greater quantity of NO_2 to the alveolar region than that delivered in the resting state (20). Miller et al. (17) predict that with exercise, 15 times more NO_2 is delivered to pulmonary tissue at maximal tidal volumes than at resting tidal volumes. Their model also indicates approximately 75–80% uptake at the respiratory tissue level during exercise. Bauer et al. (5) measured NO_2 deposition and reported total deposition (uptake) of NO_2 increased from 72% at rest to 87% during exercise during oral breathing.

If changes in pulmonary function induced by NO_2 result in part from increased peripheral uptake and deposition during exercise, measurements of airway resistance (most sensitive to change in central airways) may have been relatively insensitive to these changes. In fact, airway conductance (reciprocal of resistance) is rarely altered after NO_2 exposure. In studies of asthmatics exposed

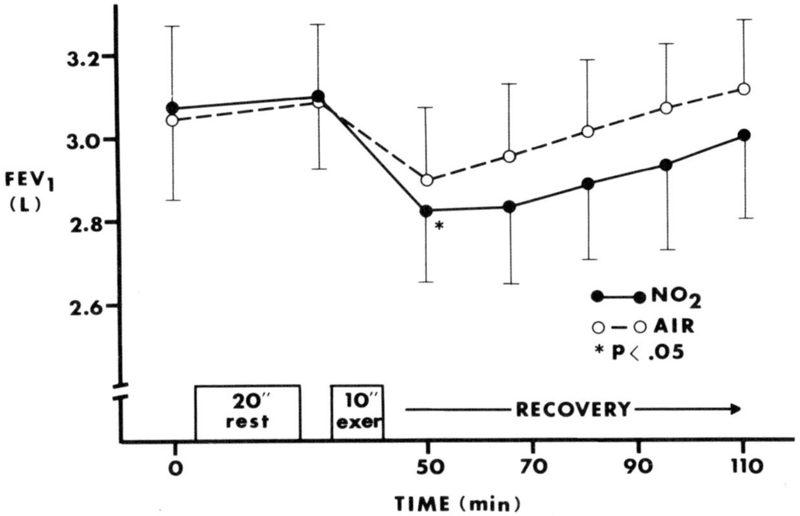

Fig. 17.1. Changes in FEV_1 after inhalation of 0.3 ppm NO_2 for 20 min at rest [ventilation at 8.1 ± 0.7 l/min (SE)] followed by 10 min of exercise (ventilation at 30.4 ± 1.4 liter/min) in 15 asthmatics. Data are mean values; bars represent $\pm$ 1 SEM. *Change in FEV_1 from baseline after NO_2 exposure compared to change in FEV_1 from baseline after air exposure: $p < 0.05$ by paired t test.

to NO_2 concentrations of 0.1 ppm and 0.2 ppm, increased airway reactivity to carbachol or methacholine has been inconsistently observed. In our laboratory, Bauer et al. (5) found that a 30-min exposure to 0.3 ppm NO_2 inhaled via a mouthpiece produced reductions in flow rates in exercising asthmatics compared to exercising in clean air (Fig. 17.1). Although airway function returned to baseline during a 1-h recovery period, isocapnic cold air hyperventilation enhanced airway hyperreactivity in the NO_2-exposed asthmatics (Fig. 17.2). Furthermore, a preliminary report from Roger et al. (22) of the US Environmental Protection Agency using an environmental chamber with unencumbered breathing and a similar protocol confirmed these findings; they observed that 0.3 ppm NO_2 caused decrements in pulmonary flow rate in moderately exercising, naturally-breathing asthmatics. Unfortunately, the status of NO_2 effects becomes more complicated as both Bauer et al. (4) and the EPA group (D. Horstman, personal communication) have had difficulty replicating their initial findings. Furthermore, Linn et al. (12) found no alteration in lung function of asthmatic volunteers at NO_2 concentrations as high as 4.0 ppm.

The explanation for the inconsistent findings with NO_2 is uncertain. It is unlikely that the mode of exposure accounts for the variability. Roger et al. (22) performed their initial studies in a chamber but with different exposure durations. Recently, Bauer et al. (4) observed a group of asthmatics that were equally responsive to 0.3 ppm NO_2 whether exposed by mouthpiece or in a chamber.

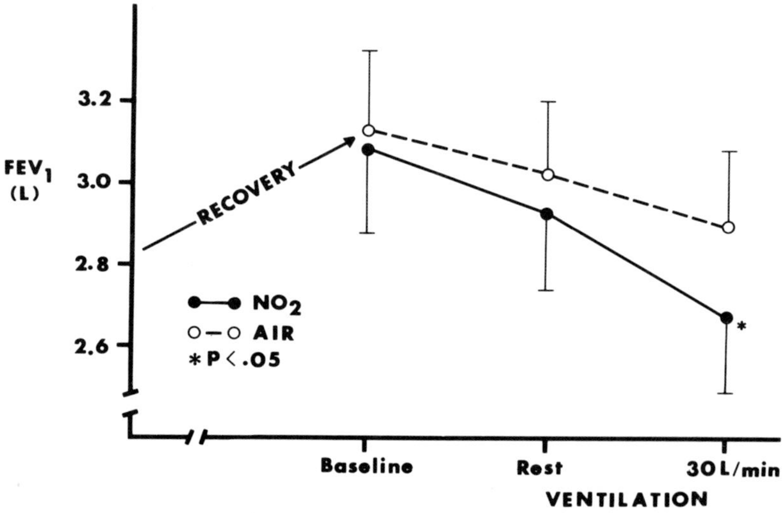

Fig. 17.2. Changes in FEV_1 with isocapnic cold air inhalation following 1-h recovery from NO_2 inhalation in asthmatics. Data are mean values; bars represent ±1 SEM. *Change in FEV_1 from baseline after NO_2 exposure compared to change in FEVI from baseline after air exposure: $p<0.05$ by paired t test.

Perhaps the variability results mostly from differences in subject characteristics. Additionally, it reflects an inability to measure changes in the terminal airways at the site of NO_2 uptake and injury. Although Bauer et al. examined changes in diffusing capacity after NO_2 exposure, few effects were noted. The influence of exercise on the diffusing capacity may limit its sensitivity as previously discussed above. For this pollutant, clinical study has served to open Pandora's box. In assessing effects of NO_2, the body box has not achieved the success it claimed with SO_2 or ozone, undoubtedly because it is a "nonideal" tool. Even though the clinical studies have failed to achieve a consensus, there are interesting clues that may impact on the regulatory process: (a) that, as a group, asthmatics appear more responsive to NO_2 than healthy volunteers, and (b) that the threshold for asthmatic responses to NO_2 is probably close to the 0.3 ppm level, but confirmation awaits development of more specific assessment techniques.

The Future: Considerations for New Directions

It would be difficult to overstate the contributions made by controlled clinical research to the setting of ambient air quality standards in the United States. These standards are promulgated by the US Environmental Protection Agency as mandated in the US Clean Air Act. Clinical research has played a major role in the identification of groups likely to be susceptible to air pollution, especially the asthmatic. Furthermore, the approach has been remarkably effective in defining a range of levels at which changes in airway function predictably occur.

Widespread use of airway function measurements has been made with far less attention to possible nasal, alveolar, or systemic actions. This consideration has created a number of related informational gaps which can generally be described as deficits in the investigative armamentarium for detecting possible health-related effects of inhaled pollutants. It is evident that more pulmonary function measurements alone are unlikely to unravel the uncertainties, as with NO_2. We commented upon the inconsistency in human experimental studies with NO_2 and conclude that the measurements often lack sensitivity and appropriateness for the presumed sites of NO_2 action, since NO_2 is known to injure the small airways but pulmonary function studies are most sensitive at detecting changes in the caliber of large airways. Alveolar assessments are more complex but may be highly germane in the case of NO_2.

The adaptation of new clinical investigative tools such as bronchoalveolar lavage (BAL) should permit new approaches to the mechanisms of pollutant-induced effects. BAL offers unique opportunities to assess responses to toxic agents and to develop markers of exposure or injury. Developed by Reynolds and Newball in the early 1970s (21), it permits serial samples to be obtained from the fluid lining the epithelial surface of the lower respiratory tract, as well as a representative sample of the effector cell populations that make up the inflammatory response. The technique is a simple extension of fiberoptic bronchoscopy. To date, BAL has been used in clinical studies to link airway reactivity to ozone and airway inflammation (23). In subjects demonstrating increases in airway reactivity to methacholine after 0.6 ppm ozone exposure, retrieved neutrophils increased as assessed by BAL. Other markers of inflammation such as prostaglandins were assayed and also increased (23). In preliminary studies in our laboratory (25), we found that low-level NO_2 exposure elevated enzyme levels and the protein α_2-macroglobulin in lavage fluid. In addition, BAL provides an opportunity to explore normal host defense mechanisms. For example, Smeglin et al. (25) found less efficient viral inactivation by alveolar macrophages obtained by BAL from NO_2 than air-exposed subjects. One can envision an array of cellular, immunological, and biochemical studies directed at host defenses.

Unquestionably, additional tools utilized in clinical investigation are available for incorporation into controlled pollutant studies. Nasal lavage, nasal biopsies, aerosol probes, and measurements of bronchoalveolar permeability with radiolabelled aerosols, for example, should provide new methodologies. To date, limited application of these techniques has appeared, but, when utilized, they can provide fascinating insights. For instance, the preliminary observations by Kerhl et al. (10) indicated that ozone exposure increased respiratory epithelial permeability as measured by radiolabelled diethylenetriaminepentaacetate (DTPA) aerosols.

Keeping in mind that subject selection tends to exclude those potentially at greatest risk and many of the responses evaluated in clinical research may not be optimal, it would seem prudent to avoid overinterpreting the "no-effect" or so-called negative study. Methodological development may eventually permit evaluation at the site of action.

Conclusions

Controlled clinical studies provide a means for examining responses to air pollutants, especially those identified from epidemiologic studies. Exposures have been performed either in environmental chambers or by mouthpiece and the responses assessed mainly by changes in respiratory mechanics. To date, clinical studies with air pollutants have identified susceptible populations, characterized exposure-response relationships, and examined "lowest-effect" levels. With some pollutants, however, it is probable that the most sensitive site of action has not been evaluated because the methodology required was inadequate, too invasive, or nonexistent. The adaptation of new clinical investigative tools such as bronchoalveolar lavage, nasal lavage, and measurement of bronchoalveolar permeability with radiolabelled aerosols, permit new approaches to the study of mechanisms of pollutant-induced effects. Although the body box has specific limitations, it would be difficult to overstate its contribution to controlled clinical studies which have impacted so dramatically on the assessment of risk and setting of air quality standards.

Acknowledgments. The author greatly appreciates the helpful review and discussions with Dr. Paul E. Morrow. He also acknowledges support of the human studies of air pollutants at The University of Rochester by the Health Effects Institute in Cambridge, Massachussetts (contract nos. 83-9 and 84-3), the National Institute of Health (grant NIEHS R01ES02679), the Division of Research Resources (grant RR 00044), and the Biomedical Research Division of General Motors Corporation in Warren, Michigan.

References

1. Amdur MO, Silverman L, Drinker P (1952) Inhalation of sulfuric acid mist by human subjects. Arch Ind Hyg Occup Med 6:305–313
2. Avol EL, Linn WS, Venet TG, Shamoo DA, Hackney JD (1984) Comparative respiratory effects of ozone and ambient oxidant pollution exposure during heavy exercise. J Air Pollut Control Assoc 34:804–809
3. Bates DV, Bell G, Burnham C, Hazucha M, Mantha J, Pengelly LD, Silverman F (1972) Short-term effects of ozone on the lung. J Appl Physiol 32:176–181
4. Bauer MA, Utell MJ, Morrow PE, Speers DM, Gibb FR (1985) Route of inhalation influences airway responses to 0.30 ppm nitrogen dioxide in asthmatic subjects (abstract). Am Rev Respir Dis 131:A171
5. Bauer MA, Utell MJ, Morrow PE, Speers DM, Gibb FR (1986) Inhalation of 0.30 ppm nitrogen dioxide potentiates exercise-induced bronchospasm in asthmatics. Am Rev Respir Dis 134:1203–1208

6. Bethel RA, Erle DJ, Epstein J, Sheppard D, Nadel JA, Boushey HA (1983) Effect of exercise rate and route of inhalation on sulfur-dioxide induced bronchoconstriction in asthmatic subjects. Am Rev Respir Dis 128:592–596
7. Curry JJ (1945) The action of histamine on the respiratory tract in normal and asthmatic subjects. J Clin Invest 25:785–791
8. Dungworth DL, Castleman WL, Chow CK, Mellick PW, Mustafa MG, Tarkington B, Tyler WS (1975) Effect of ambient levels of ozone on monkeys. Fed Proc Fed Am Soc Exp Biol 34:1670–1674
9. Holtzman MJ, Fabbri LM, O'Byrne PM, Gold BD, Aizawa H, Walter EH, Alpert SE (1983) Importance of airway inflammation for hyperresponsiveness induced by ozone. Am Rev Respir Dis 127:686–690
10. Kehrl H, Vincent L, Kowalsky R, Horstman D, McCartney W, O'Neil J, Bromberg P (1986) Ozone-induced increased respiratory epithelial permeability correlates with FEV_1 decrements (abstract). Am Rev Respir Dis 133:A215
11. Kirkpatrick MB, Sheppard D, Nadel JA, Boushey HA (1982) Effect of the oronasal breathing route on sulfur dioxide-induced bronchoconstriction in exercising asthmatic subjects. Am Rev Respir Dis 125:627–631
12. Linn WS, Solomon JC, Trim SC, Spier CE, Shamoo DA, Venet TG, Avol EL, Hackney JD (1985) Effects of exposure to 4 ppm nitrogen dioxide in healthy and asthmatic volunteers. Arch Environ Health 40:234–239
13. Linn WS, Venet TG, Shamoo DA, Valencia LM, Anzar UT, Spier CE, Hackney JD (1983) Respiratory effects of sulfur dioxide in heavily exercising asthmatics. Am Rev Respir Dis 127:278–283
14. McDonnell WF, Horstman DH, Hazucha MJ, Seal E, Haak ED, Salaam S, House DE (1983) Pulmonary effects of ozone exposure during exercise: dose-response characteristics. J Appl Physiol 45:1345–1352
15. Miller FJ, Menzel DB, Coffin DL (1978) Similarity between man and laboratory animals in regional deposition of ozone. Environ Res 17:84–101
16. Miller FJ, Overton JH, Jaskot RH, Menzel DB (1985) A model of the regional uptake of gaseous pollutants in the lung, I: the sensitivity of the uptake of ozone in the human lung to lower respiratory tract secretions and to exercise. Toxicol Appl Pharmacol 79:11–27
17. Miller FJ, Overton JH, Meyers ET, Graham JA (1982) Pulmonary dosimetry of nitrogen dioxide in animals and man. In: Schneider T, Grant L (eds) Air pollution by nitrogen oxides. Proceedings of US-Dutch international symposium on NO_X. Elsevier, Amsterdam, pp 377–386
18. Morrow PE, Utell MJ (1986) Technology and methodology of clinical exposures to aerosols. In: Lee SD, Schneider T, Grant LD, Verkerk PJ (eds) Aerosols: research, risk assessment and control strategies. Proceedings of the second US-Dutch international symposium. Lewis, Chelsea, MI, pp 661–669
19. Niinimaa V, Cole P, Mintz S, Shephard RJ (1980) The switching point from nasal to oronasal breathing. Respir Physiol 42:61–71
20. Overton JH (1984) Physiochemical processes and the formulation of dosimetry model. J Toxicol Environ Health 13:273–294
21. Reynolds HY, Newball HH (1974) Analysis of proteins and respiratory cells obtained from human lungs by bronchial lavage. J Lab Clin Med 84:559–573
22. Roger LJ, Horstman DH, McDonnell WF, Kehrl H, Seal E, Chapman RS, Massaro EJ (1985) Pulmonary effects in asthmatics exposed to 0.3 ppm NO_2 during repeated exercise (abstract). Toxicologist 5:70

23. Seltzer J, Bigby BG, Stulbarg M, Holtzman MJ, Nadel JA, Ueki IF, Leikauf GD, Goetzl EJ, Boushey HA (1986) O_3-induced change in bronchial reactivity to methacholine and airway inflammation in humans. J Appl Physiol 60:1321–1326
24. Sheppard D (1985) Measurement of airway responsiveness in studies of health effects of air pollution. In: Frank R, O'Neil JJ, Utell MJ, Hackney JD, Van Ryzin J, Brubaker PE (eds) Inhalation toxicology of air pollution: clinical research considerations. American Society for Testing and Materials, Philadelphia, pp 53–59
25. Smeglin AM, Roberts NJ Jr, Morrow PE, Utell MJ (1986) Effect of 0.6 ppm nitrogen dioxide on human alveolar macrophage inactivation of virus (abstract). Am Rev Respir Dis 133:A216
26. Utell MJ (1986) Measurements of central and peripheral pulmonary function to assess responses to air pollutants: an overview. In: Frank R, O'Neil JJ, Utell MJ, Hackney JD, Van Ryzin J, Brubaker PE (eds) Inhalation toxicology of air pollution: clinical research considerations. American Society for Testing and Materials, Philadelphia, pp 43–52
27. Utell MJ, Morrow PE, Speers DM, Darling J, Hyde RW (1983) Airway responses to sulfate and sulfuric acid aerosols in asthmatics. Am Rev Respir Dis 128:444–450
28. Yokoyama E, Frank R (1972) Respiratory uptake of ozone in dogs. Arch Environ Health 25:132–138

CHAPTER 18

Occupational Exposure Standards in Europe: History, Present Status, and Future Trends

D. Henschler[1]

If occupational exposure standards are defined as quantitatively determinable upper limits of airborne contaminants in the working area, established to protect the health of the worker, their introduction into occupational hygiene occurred rather late. The history of occupational disease from exposure to chemicals dates back, according to definitive reports, to more than 23 centuries ago when Hippocrates first described lead intoxication in plumbers. The history of occupational standards has just completed one century. K.B. Lehmann was the first to publish, in 1886, work substantiating health-based upper limit concentrations for short-term and long-term exposure to some common occupational toxicants (1). He performed field studies as well as animal experiments under standardized conditions, always analyzing the prevalent exposure concentrations with the chemical methods of those days. He must be given credit for introducing the quantitative approach into occupational hygiene, long before others adopted what now constitutes our prevailing system of prevention of impairment to the health of the worker in chemical workplaces.

From 1919 onwards, K.B. Lehmann was joined in these activities by a toxicologist, F. Flury, who introduced a theoretical concept for explaining concentration–effect relationships for some pulmonary irritants and for a certain type of systemically active noxious gas (2). By 1938, these two authors had proposed some 100 exposure limits for gases, vapors, and suspended particulates, mostly for irritants and organic solvents (3,4). In the early 1950s, a new European initiative was launched. H.B. Oettel tried to call together experts from various countries to establish exposure limits similar to the threshold limit values (TLVs) in the United States, to be applied on a supranational level and called maximum concentrations at the workplace (MAK-Werte), but failed to achieve consensus. Nevertheless, some European countries with rapidly growing industrial production and chemical innovation and development felt obliged to introduce exposure standards to protect the health of the worker. Some copied the US TLV List.

---

[1]Institute of Toxicology, University of Würzburg, Versbacher-Str 9, D-8700 Würzburg, FRG

Germany developed its own list of MAK values from 1968 on. Holland (5) and Sweden (6) followed with their own systems of standards in 1979. The USSR developed a different type of exposure limit, starting in the 1920s (7). This list, with regular revisions, is used in part or in total by several Eastern countries.

Efforts to establish internationally accepted occupational exposure limits have been made several times by the World Health Organization (WHO) (8), the International Labor Organization (ILO) (9), and the European Economic Community (EEC) (10), as well as by an Italian scientist, Vigliani (11). All have been unsuccessful so far, due to major differences in tradition, scientific concepts, industrial and social structures, and medical systems, to mention just a few reasons. Recently, the EEC prepared a limited list of exposure standards for discussion, compiled from several national lists but restricted to chemicals where no major differences exist between countries (12).

Scientific Criteria

Health-orientated exposure limits are based on thresholds of toxic effects. The threshold of a toxic effect may be defined as the lower end of a regular dose-effect or dose-response curve, indicating a dose or a concentration below which no harmful response will result or will be determinable with the methods given. The first statement in the scientific literature of the existence of such a no-effect dose is generally ascribed to Paracelsus who, in his famous Carinthian Defences (Third Defence) stated that "anything may be poison and nothing may be without poison; it is the dose which makes a thing non-poison" (13) (he did not say "drug," as is frequently misquoted; rather with the term "thing" he obviously had in mind every potentially harmful factor in the human environment) (14).

There are purists who oppose this pragmatism by claiming that every reactive molecule within a living system will lead to a biological change and it might just be a matter of definition whether or not this may or may not be considered impairment of health. But such scientists overlook the basic fact that toxicologists have long been in a position to discriminate between reversible and irreversible effects, and that (complete) reversibility is one prerequisite for assuming the existence of thresholds of effects. Two examples, one for each category, have decisively influenced the systems of setting occupational exposure limits.

The very first demonstration of the relationship between concentration, time of exposure, and toxic effect of an inhalable toxicant was performed in Germany in 1915 with phosgene, with experimental animals which were exposed to varying concentrations (c) over varying periods of time (t). The data obtained on death or survival led Flury (15) to establish the equation

$$c \times t = \mathrm{E} = \text{constant}$$

which says that there is a constant effect (E) resulting from identical products of concentration and time, irrespective of the magnitude of the factors. One can also deduce from this equation that each fraction of an exposure adds to all the others and that nothing is lost in the total balance; hence, a threshold or no-effect level does not exist. Phosgene may be taken as the prototype of covalently interacting chemicals causing irreversible effects, and the hyperbolic curve characteristic of the $c \times t$ equation has, on principle, been confirmed for carcinogens (16).

The other type of relationship was established with hydrocyanic acid which—as we now know (17)—interacts noncovalently with some metal-containing biochemical pigments by completely reversible complex formation, and is enzymically detoxicated (18). Flury concluded from the data obtained in inhalation experiments (19) that a definite concentration exists below which the toxic criterion—in this case, death—will not occur however long exposure may be, due to an elimination factor or factors (e) which may be subtracted from the exposure concentration value:

$$(c - e) \times t = \mathrm{E} = \text{constant}.$$

From this equation, a threshold can be deduced.

Due to the imprecision of methods for determining that type of threshold of effects, to uncertainties in interspecies variation, and to individual differences in susceptibility to toxic reactions, an experimentally determined threshold can only be taken as a first approach. The finally accepted tolerance level has to be set at a lower concentration; the difference between these two is often called the "safety margin."

There are some well-defined conditions for setting health-based standards which may be summarized as follows:

1. The toxic effect must be reversible.
2. The elimination characteristic (reversion) of a biological change must be zero order to guarantee absence of accumulation, or
3. If a certain alteration of biological states is considered to be tolerable, it must not exceed a well-definable steady-state level in the course of a work shift, or—in some cases with long-acting chemicals—over longer periods of time.
4. A minimum of knowledge of the toxic mechanism or mechanisms is necessary to be sure of meeting the above conditions.

These criteria constitute an ideal. Only too often the relevant data to fulfill these requirements are partly or even completely lacking, and so standards have to be set on a rather arbitrary basis. These insufficiencies are inherent in the systems as practised in the past and present.

Insufficiencies

One of the major disadvantages of the system is an ongoing controversy as to what should be regarded as the state of health, or as a toxicologically significant deviation from it. Neither on a national nor on an international level have we succeeded in establishing consistent definitions of health. Instead of trying to achieve this, pragmatic case-to-case evaluations have governed the scene. Even if a globally accepted definition of health could be agreed upon, it would change with time, because of improvements in scientific instruments to determine the normal and deviations from normal, and—hand in hand with this—because of increasing expectations of and postulates for higher degrees of safety and security in our prospering societies. A realistic view of these items will, however, reveal that the negative effect on one population as compared to another due to differences in definitions of health is fairly insignificant—if identifiable at all.

Much more relevant seems to be the fact that for the majority of existing standards the database is insufficient. Most exposure limits are based just on descriptive morphologic data from short-term exposure in just one animal species. Pharmacokinetic information, which is certainly one of the most important elements of risk evaluation of systemic toxicants, is available for only a very limited number of compounds, and experiments to elucidate the mechanism of toxic actions are exceptions rather than the rule. A review of the database of some 180 compounds compiled in the German MAK List (20) reveals less than 10% for which the database may be considered satisfactory. One way out of this dilemma would be to declare the majority of insufficiently documented exposure levels "preliminary." This is of course rigorously opposed by formalists in regulatory agencies who want a standard to be firm and definite. But once a standard is taken as definite it is in no-one's primary interest to continue investigations for an improvement of the database. Seen from this point of view, the declaration of "preliminary" is a better alternative for protection of the health of the worker, because it implies a plea to scientists in academia, in industry, and elsewhere to do more work in order to substantiate a proposed standard or change it in the appropriate direction.

Traditionally, human data have taken precedence over animal data because interpretation of them is not hampered by the difficulty of extrapolating from one species to another which may be more or less sensitive. Apart from some exceptions, however, there is no scientific justification for considering human data more relevant than animal data, simply because exposure assessment in well-planned and well-conducted laboratory experiments is much better and much more representative than in the usual type of field studies. More important seems to be that the majority of today's chemicals are newly introduced and human data are not available for them at all. Also, it should not be overlooked that improvements of protective measures in the workplace are diminishing exposure concentrations and numbers of individuals at exposure, thus reducing the possibility of obtaining quantitative data to establish or validate an exposure limit. In addition, the general movement from cure towards prevention as observed in health policies strengthens the importance of animal experiments which aim at the prediction of adverse effects from chemicals in humans before the chemicals are introduced into general use. The present difficulties in overcoming uncertainties in the extrapolation process will be reduced by the extent to which we perform case studies with the ever-increasing numbers of novel chemicals, the more so when we include specific studies on pharmacokinetics and mechanisms of toxic effects.

Other insufficiencies of the concept may be seen in the lack of satisfactory strategies to regulate short-term peak exposures and exposure to mixtures of occupational chemicals. Limitation of short-term exposure by introducing simple "ceiling values" lacks a scientific basis, and is difficult to comply with using the majority of existing analytical techniques. Alternative systems based on pharmacokinetic and mechanistic considerations, such as that recently introduced in Germany (21), need probation under field conditions. In handling mixed exposures we are confronted with one of the desert areas of toxicology. A very naive approach was proposed long ago: it adds up the fractions of the proportions of limit values of the single components of a mixture, claiming that compliance is achieved if the sum does not exceed the statistical unit, or 100%. This method lacks any scientific background and neglects simple rules of toxicological dose-response relationships. There is an urgent need for developing sound concepts to evaluate toxic effects of mixtures of compounds as a basis for setting safe standards.

Occupational Carcinogens: Alternative Risk Evaluation

The first lists of occupational exposure limits did not mention carcinogenic materials or processes, although occupational cancer from exposure to chemicals was described by P. Pott as early as 1775 (22), and other important landmarks such as the detection of bladder cancer in dye-stuff production workers (23), chromate and nickel cancers, and others followed. The first mention of occupational carcinogens occurred in the German MAK List in 1958, with just three entries. An upsurge of the number of carcinogens listed took place in the early 1970s, starting with an exponential increase and then shifting towards characteristic linear accumulation in the 1980s.

Traditionally, occupational carcinogens have been subdivided, according to the origin of relevant data, into "human" and "animal" carcinogens. Rapid progress in modern short-term tests for carcinogens, as well as in the understanding of mechanisms of carcinogenicity and structure–activity relationships, however, enforced a reevaluation of this classical system. In 1974, the German List introduced a new system which has been copied by some other countries, and by recent EEC legislation:

A1. Working materials capable of inducing malignant tumors as shown by experience with humans.

A2. Compounds which in the Commission's opinion have proven so far to be unmistakably carcinogenic in animal experimentation only, under conditions comparable to those for possible exposure of a human being at the workplace, or from which such a comparability can be deduced.

B. Compounds which are justifiably suspected of having carcinogenic potential and which urgently need further investigation to confirm or reject the suspicion.

On the basis of this classification system, an ever-increasing number of proven or suspected carcinogens has been filed. At present, more than 150 compounds are listed under one of the above categories. This amounts to one-third of the present list of occupational toxicants. One can easily predict that in a few years the 50% level will be exceeded.

There are several reasons for this fulminant development: more and more whole animal lifetime studies are being conducted with maximum tolerated doses, ending up with equivocal results which are interpreted as sufficient evidence for a carcinogenic risk to humans; the rapid increase in the use of short-term in vitro mutagenicity tests, positive results of which are taken as justifiably predictive of a carcinogenic potential of the compounds being tested; and the development of most in vitro and in vivo test systems to such a level of hypersensitivity that they yield slightly positive results under extreme exposure conditions which will never prevail in the normal living conditions of human beings. A more systematic review of the insufficiencies of present screening tests for carcinogenicity has been published elsewhere (24).

Thresholds for Carcinogens: Do They Exist?

Early toxicologists called on to produce exposure limits did not differentiate between reversible and irreversible effects, and between carcinogens and non-carcinogens. Therefore, the lists of exposure standards in the 1950s and 1960s contained threshold values for occupational carcinogens and some national lists have continued to publish "health-based" exposure limits for some carcinogens. However, present scientific knowledge does not provide evidence for the existence of thresholds for typical carcinogens, for a variety of reasons:

1. All lifetime animal carcinogenicity studies on a quantitative level have failed to reveal evidence of the existence of a threshold of effect.
2. Molecular biological theories of cancer induction indicate the absence of zero effect (or risk) even at lowest levels of exposure.
3. Epidemiological studies cannot, on principle, exclude risks of cancer.
4. Efforts to differentiate between genotoxic and epigenetic effects, and to postulate thresholds for the latter are not well-based so long as we lack precise knowledge of epigenetic mechanisms; and even then there would remain the fundamental difficulty of proving the negative—the nonoccurrence of effects in a biological system, in this case the exclusion of interference with the genetic material.

There is a possibility that for certain types of carcinogens, presently called "promoters," thresholds might exist and might be scientifically justifiable. However, we still lack a sound understanding of the modes of action of these compounds and cannot envisage a common denominator for all promoters. Rather, there seems to be a variety of different mechanisms of promoting activities. In addition one encounters clear-cut organ and tissue specificities the reasons for which are not understood at all. This situation impedes efforts to introduce generally applicable criteria or rules for setting health-based standards for carcinogens. This does not, however, exclude single cases where sufficient knowledge of the underlying mechanisms and dose-response relationships may allow the identification of a threshold.

Nevertheless, the ever-increasing number of proven or suspected carcinogens for which as low as possible or zero exposure is recommended or postulated has produced a serious crisis for conventional regulating measures. Moreover, the whole system of safety assessment and safety evaluation is losing credibility. One way out of this dilemma would be the acceptance of a certain residual risk from handling carcinogenic substances and an approach which balances health risk against socioeconomic benefit.

A Substitute: Tripartite Compromise

Everybody acknowledges the need for a practical guide on how to control exposure to carcinogens at the workplace which goes further than just forbidding production, importation, and use of the indicted chemicals. Germany was the first country to introduce another type of standard: technical guiding concentrations (TRK-Werte). These are maximum concentrations on a time-weighted average basis which should not be exceeded according to a given chemical-analytical protocol. The criteria for setting such a standard are: acceptance of a residual cancer risk; technological feasibility; chemical-analytical feasibility; socioeconomic compatibility; and the expectation that compliance with this standard will reduce risk as compared to setting no limit at all. Of course this type of standard cannot be established by scientists but needs technical, economic, and social expertise, as well as tripartite compromise. Hence, TRK-Werte are established by another committee which consists of representatives from all social groups involved. The acceptability and credibility of these limit values is strengthened by publishing documents which make the emphasis placed on the different decision elements completely transparent.

Pros and Cons of Exposure Limits

The existing system of occupational exposure limits is rightly credited with having decisively reduced occupational disease caused by chemicals. No better alternative is or will be conceivable in the foreseeable future. Once an exposure limit has been established, employers and health and technical inspectors are forced to analyze workplace atmospheres which, taken in the long run, yield a database for the reevaluation of the validity of the standard and the enforcement of changes if necessary. As a consequence, exposure limit values have undergone a process of continuous reduction in the course of many years.

However, this tendency has encouraged critics to question the whole system, arguing that the experience of a certain amount of damage to health is needed before a lowering of the standard can be induced. There is some truth in this statement, but the more carefully one looks into specific situations at the workplace, the more one encounters noncompliance with the standards as the cause of reported harm. The first and best approaches to an improvement of the system should be seen in the creation of better databases by means of more toxicological investigations, in practicing more caution in the process of setting standards, and in more intense analytical surveillance, rather than in a fundamental change in today's philosophy of safety evaluation and regulation.

References

1. Lehmann KB (1886) Experimentelle Studien über den Einfluß technisch und hygienisch wichtiger Gase und Dämpfe auf den Organismus. Arch Hyg 5:1
2. Flury F (1921) Über Kampfgasvergiftungen. Z Ges Exp Med 13:1
3. Flury F, Zernik F (1931) Schädliche Gase. Springer, Berlin
4. Lehmann KB, Flury F (1938) Toxikologie und Hygiene der technischen Lösemittel. Springer, Berlin
5. Zielhuis RL, Notten WRF (1979) Permissible levels for occupational exposure: basic concepts. Int Arch Occup Environ Health 42:269
6. Holmberg B, Westlin A (1979) Considerations in the decision of the Swedish occupational health standard for VCM. Ann NY Acad Sci 329:201
7. Ismerow NPH (1974) Principles underlying the establishment of air quality standards in the USSR. WHO Chron 28:255
8. WHO (1980) Programme of action on worker's health. Revised medium-term programme 1979-1984. OCH/80.2. Geneva
9. ILO (1980) Occupational exposure limits for airborne toxic substances, 2nd edn. ILO, Geneva
10. EEC (1978) Entschließung des Rates vom 29. Juni 1978 über ein Aktionsprogramm der Europäischen Gemeinschaften für Sicherheit und Gesundheitsschutz am Arbeitsplatz. Amtsblatt der Europäischen Gemeinschaften Nr C 165/2, 11 July 1978
11. Vigliani E (1977) Methods used in Western European countries for establishing maximum permissible levels of harmful agents in the working environment. Fondazione Carlo Erba, Milano
12. EEC (1986) Vorschlag für eine Richtlinie des Rates zur Änderung der Richtlinie 80/1107 EWG zum Schutz der Arbeitnehmer vor der Gefährdung durch chemische, physikalische und biologische Arbeitsstoffe bei der Arbeit. Amtsblatt der Europäischen Gemeinschaften Nr C 164/04, 2 July 1986
13. Paracelsus, ThB von Hohenheim (1538) Epistola dedicatera St. Veit/Kärnten (3. Defension)
14. Deichmann WB, Henschler D, Holmstedt B, Keil G (1986) What is there that is not poison? A study of the Third Defense by Paracelsus. Arch Toxicol 58:207
15. Flury F (1921) Über Kampfgasvergiftungen. I: Über Reizgase. Z Ges Exp Med 13:10
16. Druckrey H (1943) Quantitative Grundlagen der Krebserzeugung. Klin Wochenschr 22:532
17. Warburg O (1927) Über die Wirkung von Kohlenoxyd und Stickoxyd auf Atmung und Gärung. Biochem Z 189:354
18. Lang K (1933) Die Rhodanbildung im Körper. Biochem Z 259:243

19. Flury F, Heubner W (1919) Über Wirkung und Entgiftung eingeatmeter Blausäure. Biochem Z 95:249
20. Henschler D (ed) (1972-1987) Toxikologisch-arbeitsmedizinische Begründung von MAK-Werten. VCH, Weinheim
21. Henschler D, zur Mühlen T, Drope E (1979) Begrenzung von Konzentrationsspitzen der Exposition gegenüber gesundheitsschädlichen Arbeitsstoffen (Kurzzeitwerte). Arbeitsmed Sozialmed Präventivmed 14:191
22. Pott P (1775) Chirurgical observations: the cancer of the scrotum. Carnegy, London
23. Rehn L (1895) Blasengeschwülste bei Anilinarbeitern. Arch Kli Chir 50:588
24. Henschler D (1985) Carcinogenicity testing—existing protocols are insufficient. Trends in pharmacological sciences, Federation of European Societies of Toxicology Supplement, November 1985

CHAPTER 19

Current Approaches for Determining Workplace Exposure Limits in the USA

T.R. Lewis[1]

Introduction

There are a number of national organizations within the United States of America which are engaged in the development and issuance of occupational exposure guidelines or the promulgation of health standards. Some are independent non-governmental entities; others are of governmental origin. Each has its specific purposes and modus operandi. Accordingly, while there are generic similarities in the approaches for determining workplace exposure limits in the United States, there are also finite differences in the philosophies, organizational structures, and chartered mandates of the organizations active in such endeavors. Such differences may result in numerical variances in occupational exposure limits assigned to the same chemical by various organizations. However, all have been deemed adequate, within the framework of the various organizations, to protect the health of the worker throughout his or her lifetime.

Factors Affecting Exposure Limits

Key issues with an impact on the numerical value assigned to an occupational exposure limit include but are not limited to: (a) whether or not the limit is intended to protect all members of the workforce, including those with genetic or acquired hypersusceptibilities to chemical insult; (b) the margin of safety applied to the principal health risk, e.g., cancer versus sensory irritation; (c) the existence or nonexistence of safe levels (thresholds or no effect levels) for known or suspected occupational carcinogens; and (d) the duration and magnitude of excursion or short-time exposure limits to protect against sensory or respiratory irritation, chronic or irreversible tissue damage, narcosis, or intensive odor.

---

[1]National Institute for Occupational Safety and Health, 4676 Columbia Parkway, Cincinnati, OH 45226, USA

There are other cogent issues that the limit-setting organization must address. These include:

1. The concept of nuisance particulates and at what concentrations or exposure conditions they pose a health hazard
2. The reliability, efficacy, and justification of respiratory protection in lieu of meeting occupational exposure limits solely by engineering controls
3. The adequacies and inadequacies of existing methodologies to determine the additive and synergistic toxicologic effects of concurrent exposures to mixtures of chemical substances
4. The specifics of cutaneous absorption and the delineation of the relative health risks from dermal exposures
5. The relative merits of environmental and biological monitoring of workers exposed occupationally to substances in the work-place
6. The assessment of differing toxicities of metals and metal-containing substances due to their solubility in biological fluids and nature of the chemical bond
7. The adequacy of odor detection as a deterrent to exposures which may pose a significant health risk
8. The frequency of monitoring to determine adherence to the occupational exposure limit
9. The desire to limit exposures to achieve worker comfort rather than protect against health hazards.

Nongovernmental Organizations Involved with Exposure Limits

Among the nongovernmental organizations that have proposed guidelines for permissible occupational exposure guides are the Threshold Limit Values (TLV) Committee of the American Conference of Governmental Industrial Hygienists (ACGIH), the American Industrial Hygiene Association (AIHA), the American Society for Testing Materials (ASTM), and the American National Standards Institute (ANSI). Of these, the TLV Committee of the ACGIH has had the greatest national and international impact.

The ACGIH TLV Committee

The TLV Committee was organized in 1942 and, as its initial effort, compiled a table of 63 toxic substances with their "maximum allowable concentrations (MACs)." This list was comprised of exposure limits from 26 various state, county, and city departments of industrial hygiene within the United States of America (1). In 1946, the TLV Committee developed its initial independent list of occupational exposure guidelines, which included MACs for 131 chemical substances and 13 mineral dusts. In 1946, the TLV Committee also introduced the policy that this list be revised annually (2). In 1948, the term "MACs" was changed to "TLVs."

The period from 1946 to the present has been characterized by dynamic activities and innovative approaches by the TLV Committee in establishing occupational exposure guides. This has resulted not only in a steady increase in the number of substances to which the Committee has assigned TLVs, but also in changes in existing TLVs as new data dictate. Additional policies and practices, notably in the preface and appendices of the TLV booklet, have enhanced protection of the worker by those who follow the TLV Committee's recommendations.

Presently, there are 25 persons associated with the TLV Committee on Chemical Substances, 17 members and 8 consultants, all of whom volunteer their time and services without pay. The Committee is divided into four Subcommittees: Inorganics and Dusts, HOC (organic compounds containing only hydrogen or hydrogen and oxygen), Misco (organic compounds containing elements other than oxygen), and Cancer. The first three Subcommittees are responsible for the selection of compounds, development of new TLVs, review and update of existing TLVs, and development and revision of TLV documentations (3). The Subcommittee on Cancer advises the other Subcommittees of substances in industrial use which have proven to be carcinogenic in humans or which are suspect as a potential carcinogen for humans.

It is the policy and practice of the TLV Committee that all TLVs, existing or newly proposed, will have a written documentation, supported by referenced sources, which contains information relevant to the health hazards posed by the substance, and a clearly stated summary describing precisely the basis for the assigned TLV value. Such limits are based upon relevant industrial experience, human data, and results from animal experimentation. The written documentations are not intended as literature reviews on the substances, but rather as professional evaluations and judgments of the most relevant data for establishing a healthy workplace environment. Responsibility for particular substances is assigned by the Subcommittee chairperson to individuals for the development of documentation which will support a recommended TLV. In addition, the Subcommittee will consider draft documentations prepared by outside sources. Draft documentations are reviewed by the full Subcommittee for their technical accuracy and completeness and for the validity of the bases of the proposed TLV.

Ad hoc working groups are also formed to address special areas of interest or need, such as the concept or means of protection of the hypersusceptible worker, the utilization of TLVs to protect against adverse health effects in populations besides the work force, the application of TLVs to novel or extended work shifts, and issues raised by individuals corresponding with the Committee about specific TLVs or actions and positions taken by the Committee.

Recommendations of the Subcommittees and working groups, along with supporting documentation, are critiqued, discussed, and voted upon (Committee members only, not consultants). These activities culminate in recommendations for additions or retention of substances on the Notice of Intended Changes list, where the values are placed for a minimum of 2 years to permit comment. The Subcommittees also recommend to the full Committee the transfer of TLVs from the Notice of Intended Changes to the adopted list of TLVs.

The full Committee critiques, discusses, and votes upon the Subcommittee's recommendations, culminating in recommendations for both the Notice of Intended Changes list and the adopted list of TLVs. Recommendations from the plenary Committee are communicated by the Committee chairperson to the ACGIH Board of Directors for review and to the Conference membership for approval at the annual meeting of the American Industrial Hygiene Conference in May of each year.

In a further refinement of a previously adopted policy and practice, the ACGIH has recently proposed new procedures for particle size-selected threshold limit values, since many health hazards posed by aerosols are dependent upon the particle size (4). Different particle-size distributions of the same substance will cause major changes in deposition in different regions of the respiratory tract. Differences in the distribution of inhaled aerosols will determine different doses within the respiratory tract and have an impact on the site, probability, and nature of the associated diseases. Recommendations were made by the ACGIH Air Sampling Procedures Committee that three particulate mass fractions were applicable to workplace sampling (5). Inspirable particulate mass (IPM) would be used for substances hazardous anywhere in the respiratory tract; thoracic particulate mass (TPM) would be used for substances hazardous within the lung airways and the gas exchange region; and respirable particulate mass (RPM) for substances hazardous only to the gas exchange region of the lung.

Other Nongovernmental Organizations

A second nongovernmental organization which recommends occupational exposure guidelines is the American Industrial Hygiene Association's Workplace Environmental Exposure Level Guides (WEELs) Committee (6). This Committee was established by the AIHA in 1976. There are currently 32 members on the Committee, four of whom are toxicologists. The other 28 members are industrial hygienists. The substances selected as candidates for existing or future WEEL Guides are chemicals which have no current exposure guidelines established by other organizations. Similarities to the procedures utilized by the ACGIH include the availability of documentations for completed WEEL Guides, the utilization of the skin notation, and definitions of exposure categories. AIHA WEEL Guides, however, may have excursion levels defined as a 1–30 min time-weighted average (TWA), e.g., WEELs for lithium hydroxide and lithium oxide are defined as a short-term TWA of 1 mg/m^3, 1 min. WEELs are often guides based on experiences rather than exclusively on the results of animal experimentation conducted under conditions relevant to the workplace, e.g., inhalation exposures. Toxicity data and human experience are obtained on a voluntary basis from both producers and users. By 1986, approximately 40 WEELs had been established by the AIHA Committee.

A second activity of the American Industrial Hygiene Association relating to the issuance of occupational exposure guidelines is the publication of a series of information bulletins, called Hygienic Guides. The purpose of the Hygienic Guides, which were initiated in 1955, is to provide authoritative and substantiated information on the toxicity of common industrial chemicals and materials. Each guide lists the recommended maximum allowable exposure concentration for both short- and long-term exposures. These recommended exposure limits are primarily those offered by other organizations; in those cases where values are not available they are developed by AIHA. All the guides are being updated and revised by a Committee of 18 under a new format developed in 1976 and initially seen as published documents in 1978. Fifteen Hygienic Guides were revised in 1986; an additional 25 are scheduled for revision in 1987. A date is included at the end of a Hygienic Guide indicating when the literature search was terminated.

Other private organizations which have played a role, or are active in recommending occupational exposure limits, are the American Society for Testing and Materials (ASTM) and the American National Standards Institute (ANSI). Standard practices developed by ASTM must be reviewed every 5 years to maintain their status. In their initial development, these standards are open for broad commentary by interested parties and adopted by a two-thirds approval by letter ballot or a tallied meeting vote only after negative votes have been resolved with the voter or deemed by the Committee as nongermane or nonpersuasive. The number of affirmative, negative, and abstaining votes for each action on standards are reported to the Society. The Committee on Standards determines, on the behalf of the Society, whether the procedural requirements of the Society have been met and whether a satisfactory consensus has been reached. If the Committee on Standards takes favorable action upon the recommendation, the standard is approved, then published, and the action announced in the annual report.

ANSI no longer generates standards on occupational exposure limits but restricts itself to the sanctioning of consensus standards. The procedure is one of utilizing ANSI-accredited committees or organizations which have been sanctioned by ANSI. The documentation for a proposed exposure limit is sent to ANSI who certifies that the sponsor has followed ANSI approved procedures. ANSI then authorizes the addition of an American National Standard number to the originator's documentation. Thus, the procedures of ASTM and ANSI are aligned to the adoption of occupational exposure limits by consensus means.

Due to the large volume of chemicals routinely used in industry and the limited availability of published occupational exposure guides or limits, many industrial firms in the USA have established internal limits to protect their employees as well as the persons who purchase those chemicals (7). In addition to industrial corporations, industrial, technical, or trade associations, e.g., of manufacturers of glycol ethers, may recommend occupational exposure guides for use by producers and users. Most of the industrially derived limits relate to air monitoring; however, biological monitoring limits have also been developed.

Governmental Agencies

In the USA, the authority to promulgate local federal health standards is delegated by Congress to the Executive Branch of the government (8). The procedure is one designated as an administrative rulemaking which encompasses the processes of notice and comment. In this process, the public is given notice of a particular agency's proposed rule which would affect the conduct of activities in the workplace. The public, which includes industry, labor, academia, and government, participates in the rule-making process by presentation of written or oral comments and scientific data on the various issues addressed in the proposed rule. Subsequently, the agency publishes a final rule which is the product of the comments and data received. The final rule has legal status and is thus binding on the regulated industry. Violations may be punishable by fines or imprisonment or both.

The Occupational Safety and Health Administration, Department of Labor, has the responsibility for promulgating and enforcing health standards in the majority of work environments (9). The Mine Safety and Health Administration, Department of Labor, has the responsibility for promulgating and enforcing metal and nonmetal mining air quality standards (10). A third federal agency, the National Institute for Occupational Safety and Health (NIOSH), develops Criteria Documents recommending standards for occupational exposure to substances in the workplace, to be acted upon by OSHA. NIOSH also provides written comments and oral testimony during the OSHA rulemaking process (9).

The legal maximum allowable level of a contaminant in the worksite atmosphere, as established by the Occupational Safety and Health Administration, is referred to as the Permissible Exposure Limit (PEL). Following enactment of the Occupational Safety and Health Act of 1970, existing consensus standards were adopted as PELs. These included about 400 TLVs on the ACGIH 1968 list and 22 air standards of the American Standards Association (ANSI). Although the ACGIH revises the TLVs each year, the PELs remain as promulgated unless changes in the regulations are made. Thus the PELs are typically less restrictive than many of the current TLVs.

When data is published necessitating that a PEL be reevaluated or established to ensure adequate protection of the health of workers, NIOSH may develop a recommended exposure limit (REL) as expressed in the form of Criteria Documents, or else OSHA develops new PELs through the rulemaking process, which may include the issuance of an Emergency Temporary Standard to meet such needs.

About 12 years ago NIOSH and OSHA developed the standards completion program. The standards completion program attempted to define minimum monitoring, training, recordkeeping, medical evaluation, controls, and other requirements for protecting workers potentially exposed to many of the chemicals regulated by OSHA. Included in the standard completion program were recommendations for respiratory protection which were in part based on the concept of the Immediately Dangerous to Life and Health (IDLH) level. NIOSH defines the IDLH as the maximum concentration from which a worker can escape within 30 min without incurring any significant escape-impairing symptoms or any immediate or delayed irreversible health effects. The ANSI definition is similar except that it addresses only immediate irreversible debilitating effects on health or immediate hazard to health. It should be emphasized that this limit is only for the purpose of specifying appropriate respirator selection for a specific air concentration of a particular chemical.

NIOSH and OSHA also use health risk assessment mathematical models to aid in the setting of their respective limits, RELs and PELs. Risk assessment is the scientific process which provides an estimation of the probability that some injury will occur in an individual or a population as a result of exposure to a substance or a situation. This probability is assessed by multiplying the individual risk by the number of individuals who may incur that risk.

Current approaches used by the Federal government to establish exposure limits are predicated upon legislative, judicial, and executive actions. These include decisions of the US Supreme Court on benzene and cotton dust, the OSHA cancer policy, preparation of recommendations for entire industries or industrial processes, negotiated rulemaking, controversies surrounding the inclusion of limits governing short-term exposures, and the development of prevention strategies for prevalent work-related diseases.

As previously stated, the OSH Act states that in promulgating standards regulating toxic substances, the Secretary of Labor must set standards to ensure, to the extent feasible, that no employee will suffer material impairment of health or functional capacity, even if exposed for his or her lifetime. This section of the law has been further defined by two cases brought before the US Supreme Court. In the case of the Industrial Union Department, *AFL-CIO vs the American Petroleum Institute* (the "benzene case"), the Supreme Court held that the new benzene standard of 1 ppm was invalid because OSHA failed to establish specifically the benefits to which costs must be reasonably related. The Court also ruled that the Secretary of Labor must determine on the basis of substantial evidence that a standard is reasonable, necessary, or appropriate to remedy a significant risk of material health impairment. This decision has resulted in the implementation of quantitative risk assessments to provide a basis upon which the Secretary can make such a determination. An absolutely risk-free workplace is not required.

The second interpretation of the OSH Act was issued in the US Supreme Court case, *American Textile Manufacturers Institute vs Donovan* (the "cotton dust case"). In this ruling, the Court stated that OSHA is not required to perform a cost-benefit analysis of the impact of its standard and to balance costs and benefits, but is required to set standards that are technologically and economically feasible. Feasible was defined as "do-able" by the industry but not necessarily by individual companies.

OSHA promulgated its Carcinogen Policy as a regulation (29 CFR Part 1990). The stated purposes were to streamline the regulatory process and to provide predictable and uniform criteria for identifying and regulating substances as occupational carcinogens. This regulation included criteria and scientific policies for identifying and classifying a substance as a potential occupational carcinogen. It included a screening and priority-setting process to be followed in determining whether a proposed standard for a potential carcinogen should be issued. Guidelines were included on the substantive provisions of a draft standard. OSHA, in response to the "benzene decision," subsequently made deletions to the Cancer Policy provisions which required the automatic setting of a PEL at the lowest feasible level for a human carcinogen, a carcinogen identified in replicated animal studies, or its equivalent, and deleted provisions limiting the evidence which OSHA would consider in determining the exposure limits for carcinogens. Henceforth, exposure limits would be set for carcinogens on a substance-by-substance basis. OSHA would take into account significance of risk, feasibility, court interpretations, all relevant evidence, present occupational health policy, and its experience in regulating toxic substances. NIOSH has taken the position that engineering controls should be the primary method of controlling exposures to all chemical substances, including carcinogens, and that any attempt to balance costs and benefits is violative of the OSH Act, as was stated in *ATMI vs Donovan*. The example was given of β-napthylamine-caused cancer resulting from the failure to establish a zero-threshold at the very outset of knowledge of its carcinogenicity. NIOSH also recommended that no specific model or technique of risk assessment should be mandated because no single model will satisfy all of the requirements for performing risk assessments.

In addition to setting exposure limits for individual substances, OSHA and NIOSH have established work practice procedures with the intent to protect workers from potential exposure to all substances utilized in the industry or in an industrial process. In essence, the process is an assessment of the occupational safety and health hazards present, with recommendations of safe work practices and appropriate engineering controls.

A recent, innovative approach to establishing recommendations for new standards to federal regulatory agencies is one termed "mediated rulemaking." Mediated rulemaking is a procedure whereby a committee of government, academia, industry, and labor representatives propose new or review existing exposure limits and provide recommendations to the regulatory agency. This approach simulates procedures currently employed by certain European countries such as Sweden and Great Britain. To date, OSHA has organized mediated rule-making on 4,4'-methylenedianiline.

There is active interest from both the scientific and regulatory communities as to the role dose-rate plays in the type and severity of occupational health hazards. This topic has been pursued in the process of establishing a PEL for exposure to ethylene oxide. When a PEL has only a TLV-TWA with no excursion or short-term limits, work practices which are only a few minutes in duration and occur once or twice daily can result in exposures in ppm-minutes severalfold higher than the PEL. The scientific database is inadequate to define the relative health hazards, including oncogenic, reproductive, and mutagenic, posed by high-concentration/short-term exposures versus long-term/low-concentration exposures of equal dose. There are suggestive data and inferences that the pattern of exposure influences the type and severity of the toxicologic response as well as does the total dose.

Another approach to safeguarding the health of the worker has been the recent efforts by NIOSH to establish national strategies for the preventing of the leading work-related diseases. A major emphasis of the two NIOSH-sponsored National Symposia on the Prevention of Leading Work-Related Diseases and Injuries held 1-3 May 1985 and 28-31 October 1986 was to emphasize the implementation of disease prevention means, such as appropriate surveillance methodologies and control technologies. The implementation of these prevention strategies would ensure worker health to a far greater degree than do the contemporary methods of monitoring worker exposure.

The Mine Safety and Health Administration has the federal legal responsibility to promulgate health standards under the Federal Mine Safety and Health Act of 1977 (10). This law requires that mandatory health standards dealing with toxic materials or harmful physical agents shall assure, on the basis of the best available evidence, that no miner will suffer impairment of health or functional capacity. To fulfill this mandate, MSHA enforces the ACGIH 1973 TLVs to regulate exposures in metal and nonmetal mines, with one exception. The exception is that the 8-h TWA for asbestos dust shall not exceed two fibers /ml that are longer than five microns as determined by the membrane filter method. Coal mines are regulated differently; for underground coal mines, MSHA utilizes the 1972 TLVs, whereas for surface mining of coal, the current TLVs are applicable.

Individual state programs in the USA also exist for workers covered under the OSH Act where it is demonstrable that the state agencies have enacted the necessary legislation and possess the necessary manpower and facilities to perform their functions at least as well as the federal agencies. The numerical standards adopted by a state can be more, but not less, stringent than their federal counterparts. The manner by which states establish their standards varies between states.

Biological Monitoring and Biological Exposure Indices

In addition to the recommendations of TLVs for chemical substances and physical agents, a separate committee of the ACGIH introduced in its 1984-85 TLV booklet *Threshold Limit Values for Chemical Substances and Physical Agents in the Work Environment and Biological Exposure Indices with Intended Changes for 1984-85* a section designated "Biological Exposure Indices" (BEIs). These indices denote levels in blood, urine, or exhaled air of an industrial chemical or its resultant metabolite(s) above which adverse health effects may be expected due to inhalation, ingestion, or dermal absorption (11). BEI values are cited for one or more of these measures, together with the timing of sampling. A third point is often addressed under the Notation column in the Table of BEIs which qualifies its relative merits. Issues addressed are: variations in human susceptibilities; the specificity of the method to a particular chemical; the wide inter-individual variation of response following exposure to some chemicals; and the fact that the biologic determinant may be a specific indicator, but a poor quantitator. BEIs, like TLVs, have a published documentation delineating their bases and methodologies. In 1986, there were six chemicals with ACGIH-adopted BEIs; an additional ten chemicals have BEIs listed under the "Notice of Intent to Establish."

The classic use of biological monitoring methods in the USA has been related to exposure to inorganic lead and cholinesterase inhibitors. Monitoring of workers for blood lead and blood zinc protoporphyrin levels was incorporated in the OSHA Standard for Lead (12). Methods for biological monitoring of worker exposure may be found in certain NIOSH Criteria Documents on chemical substances. Federal agencies have sponsored symposia on the topic, and the AIHA, like the ACGIH, has a committee to recommend future BEIs.

Summary

The key question to be addressed in determining occupational exposure limits is what concentrations pose significant hazards to health and what concentrations can be accepted without undue risk to health. Development of occupational exposure limits involves review and evaluation of available technical information on a chemical substance and publication of written documentation supporting a proposed exposure limit, which then may be adopted by a sponsoring professional organization (ACGIH, AIHA, ANSI, ASTM) or promulgated into law by regulatory agencies.

Application of research findings to the development and support of workplace exposure limits in the USA is performed by several organizations, both governmental and private. Recommendations by nongovernmental organizations are not legally binding but are often voluntarily utilized by industry and may be adopted as legal standards by regulatory agencies. Industrial corporations and trade associations also develop occupational exposure limits for application to their particular facilities and their customers. This is particularly important when an industry is the sole manufacturer or user, the number of workers exposed is small and limited to a single company, and other organizations are totally committed to addressing the vast number of other chemicals in commerce. It is the function of the Occupational Safety and Health Administration (OSHA) and the Mine Safety and Health Administration (MSHA) of the US Department of Labor to promulgate and enforce legal standards. The National Institute for Occupational Safety and Health has the responsibility for developing health-related criteria and making recommendations to OSHA and MSHA for the promulgation of legal standards. Individual states also promulgate and enforce standards which are legal within their respective jurisdictions.

References

1. Stokinger HE (1981) Threshold limit values: dangerous properties of industrial materials report (May/June 1981). Van Nostrand Reinhold, New York, pp 8–13
2. Cook WA (1985) History of ACGIH TLVs, vol 12. International symposium on occupational exposure limits. American Conference of Governmental Industrial Hygienists, Cincinnati, pp 3–9
3. Carter VL (1985) Modus operandi of Committee on Threshold Limit Values for Chemical Substances, vol 12. International symposium on occupational exposure limits. American Conference of Governmental Industrial Hygienists, Cincinnati, pp 11–13
4. Stuart BD, Lioy PJ, Phalen RF (1986) Particle size-selective sampling in establishing threshold limit values. Appl Ind Hyg 3:138–144
5. Phalen RF et al (1986) Rationale and recommendations for particle size-selective sampling in the workplace. Appl Ind Hyg 1:3–14
6. American Industrial Hygiene Association (1986) Workplace environmental exposure level guide (June)
7. Paustenbach D, Langner R (1986) Corporate occupational exposure limits: the current state of affairs. Am Ind Hyg Assoc J 47(12):809–818
8. Administrative Conference of the United States (1983) A guide to federal agency rulemaking. Office of the Chairman
9. The Occupational Safety and Health Act of 1970. US Pub Law No 91-596
10. The Federal Mine Safety and Health Act of 1977: 30 USC 801-961 (1971 and Suppl 1978). US Pub Law No 91-173 as amended by US Pub Law 95-164
11. Lowry LK (1986) Biological exposure index as a complement to the TLV. J Occup Med 28(8):578–582
12. Federal Regulation OSHA 1910.1025-Lead (1979) p 790.0.22

Index